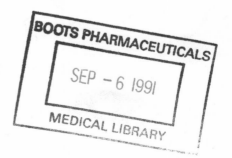

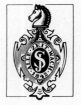

Michael S. Kramer

Clinical Epidemiology and Biostatistics

A Primer for Clinical Investigators
and Decision-Makers

With 37 Figures and 60 Tables

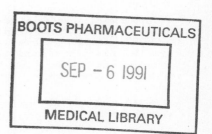
Springer-Verlag
Berlin Heidelberg New York
London Paris Tokyo
Hong Kong Barcelona
Budapest

Michael S. Kramer, M.D.

Professor of Pediatrics and of
Epidemiology and Biostatistics
McGill University Faculty of Medicine
1020 Pine Avenue West
Montreal, Quebec H3A 1A2, Canada

ISBN 3-540-18874-6 Springer-Verlag Berlin Heidelberg New York
ISBN 0-387-18874-6 Springer-Verlag New York Berlin Heidelberg

Library of Congress Cataloging-in-Publication Data. Kramer, Michael S., 1948 –
Clinical epidemiology and biostatistics / Michael S. Kramer. p. cm. Includes index.
ISBN 0-387-18874-6 (U.S.) 1. Epidemiology – Research – Methodology. 2. Epidemiology –
Statistical methods. 3. Biometry. I. Title. [DNLM: 1. Biometry – methods. 2. Epidemio-
logic Methods. 3. Research Design. WA 950 K89c] RA652.K73 1988 614.4'028 –
dc 19 DNLM/DLC

© Springer-Verlag Berlin Heidelberg 1988
Printed in Germany

Typesetting: Appl, Wemding
23/3145-54321 – Printed on acid-free paper

Preface

Does the world really need yet another textbook of epidemiology or biostatistics? Several new volumes have been published in the past few years, and the need for one more "me too" is far from obvious. The reason for adding to what is already a crowded field stems from my experience in coordinating a course in clinical epidemiology and biostatistics for first-year medical students at McGill. Unlike course offerings at most other medical schools, ours emphasized principles of analytic (cause-and-effect) inference. Unfortunately, no textbook was available for a clinical audience that focused on the acquisition of these analytic skills. Although several years have elapsed since, I still believe this to be the case.

Another problem with existing textbooks is that they tend to be textbooks of epidemiology *or* biostatistics, but not of both. Epidemiology texts are written by epidemiologists, biostatistical texts by biostatisticians. It is then usually left to the reader to make the important, but not always obvious, links between the two. One of the major goals of this book is to integrate epidemiologic and biostatistical principles by using a common language and by interweaving common examples.

Most epidemiology texts focus on the etiology of chronic diseases. Little mention is made of the application of epidemiologic techniques to studies of diagnosis, prognosis, and treatment, to evaluation of health services, and to assessment of risks and benefits. Recent books on clinical epidemiology have dealt with some of these issues, but their goals and intended audiences are clearly different, e.g., helping practicing physicians to increase their skills at clinical appraisal of the medical literature.

This book is also intended for a clinical audience, although not for those wishing only a superficial overview of epidemiologic and biostatistical concepts. It should be useful, however, to clinicians, clinicians in training, and clinical investigators who wish to develop their proficiency in the planning, execution, and interpretation of clinical and epidemiologic research, i.e., to the "doers" as well as to the "consumers" of such research.

Many of my "classical" epidemiology colleagues have objected to what may appear to be a desire to incorporate classical epidemiology within the "clinical epidemiology" rubric. My own view, developed further in Chapter 1, is that the distinctions between clinical and classical epidemiology have been overstated and are often unhelpful. While it is certainly true that "classical" epidemiology has not traditionally concerned itself with many of the nonetiologic questions of primary interest to practicing clinicians and clinical researchers, the techniques and methodologic tools required for studying health phenomena in groups of human subjects are similar, whether investigating risk factors for endometrial cancer or optimal treatment strategies in patients with unstable angina pectoris. The main reason for the "clinical" in the title of this textbook is that all of the techniques presented, as well as the examples used to illustrate those techniques, should be comprehensible and relevant to a clinical audience.

The material will be most readily understood if one begins with Chapter 1 and continues in sequence. Readers wishing to use the text only as a reference, without prior perusal, will probably find the smallest "digestible" unit to be a single chapter. Even then, many chapters refer to and build upon concepts discussed in earlier chapters.

The book is divided into three parts. Part I deals with epidemiologic research design and analytic inference, including such issues as measurement, rates, analytic bias, and the main forms of observational and experimental epidemiologic studies. Part II presents the principles and applications of biostatistics, with an emphasis on statistical inference. Part III comprises four chapters covering such "special" topics as diagnostic tests, decision analysis, survival (life-table) analysis, and causality.

Only time will tell whether this book meets an important need. I would of course enjoy hearing from clinicians and clinical investigators who have found it helpful but would also appreciate suggestions on how it can be improved.

Michael S. Kramer

Acknowledgements

Although the scope, content, and intended audience of this text differ from those of previously available texts, little of the material presented can be considered original. In addition to the many colleagues whose direct help and encouragement are acknowledged below, I owe a great debt to many authors of other texts of epidemiology or biostatistics and to numerous teachers and colleagues with whom I have come in contact over the years.

I wish to thank, first and foremost, Dr. Alvan R. Feinstein, who first "turned me on" to clinical epidemiology as a viable academic discipline. I not only cut my epidemiologic teeth with Dr. Feinstein but have continued to benefit from his support and encouragement in the years since leaving his tutelage.

I have also learned a great deal from collaborative teaching with other faculty in the McGill Department of Epidemiology and Biostatistics. Primary among these have been Drs. Tom Hutchinson and David Lane, but the list also includes Drs. John Hoey, Robert Oseasohn, and Walter Spitzer.

Several colleagues gave me extremely helpful suggestions on previous drafts of this text. They include Drs. Jean-François Boivin, F. Sessions Cole III, Erica Eason, James Hanley, David Lane, Abby Lippman, John McDowell, I. Barry Pless, and Stanley Shapiro. Drs. William Fraser, Tom Hutchinson, Paul Kramer, Samy Suissa, and Sholom Wacholder also provided helpful advice on specific items.

I cannot adequately acknowledge the peerless secretarial work of Mrs. Laurie Tesseris. Without her patience and thoroughness, this book could never have been completed, even in this era of word processors. Ms. Lenora Naimark and Ms. Tiziana Bruni provided additional secretarial assistance. Many thanks are also due to Mr. Phillip Dakin, Ms. Artemis Karabelas, and Ms. Jennifer Morrison for preparing the graphs and figures.

Lastly, and possibly most importantly, I wish to thank my wife Claire and son Eric, whose support and encouragement are so valuable to me in all my work.

To whatever extent this text succeeds in its goal, the above-named persons deserve much of the credit. Any remaining inaccuracies or lack of clarity are entirely my own.

Michael S. Kramer

Table of Contents

Part II   Biostatistics

Part III   Special Topics

Part I

Epidemiologic Research Design

Chapter I: **Introduction**

1.1 The Compatibility of the Clinical and Epidemiologic Approaches

Mr. Jones, a 55-year-old man with a recent history of myocardial infarction (heart attack), has arteriographic X-ray evidence of severe occlusion of two of his three major coronary arteries. Should his physician prescribe drug treatment or refer him to a surgeon for a bypass operation?

The traditional clinical approach to this question is based on pathophysiologic and pharmacologic reasoning. Using her[1] knowledge about coronary artery anatomy and physiology, the pathogenesis of arteriosclerotic and thrombotic changes in the arterial wall, and the mechanism of action of several potentially useful pharmacologic agents, as well as her familiarity with the individual patient (psychosocial factors, life style, personal preferences, probability of compliance with medication), the clinician arrives at a decision regarding a recommendation for medical or surgical therapy for that patient.

Epidemiologic thinking differs conceptually from clinical thinking. Epidemiology can be defined as the study of disease and other health-related phenomena in groups of persons. The word derives from the Greek *epi* (upon) and *demos* (people). The epidemiologist thus thinks in terms of groups, not individuals, and asks whether a group of patients with demographic, clinical, and psychosocial characteristics similar to Mr. Jones' will fare better, *on average,* if they receive medical or surgical therapy. He[1] will then advocate that the patient receive the treatment with the higher average rate of success.

A clinician caring for an individual patient needs to temper published data based on groups of patients with knowledge of factors about the particular case at hand. She must make decisions for *that* patient, not for some hypothetical group of patients, however similar the members of the group may appear to be to her patient. And her decisions are often all-or-none: whether to order a certain diagnostic test, whether to recommend surgery or medication, whether to continue or discontinue life-support measures. Since, in order to be effective, the clinician must believe that each of her decisions is best for her patient, she tends to think in terms of black and white, rather than shades of gray. Although she may be aware of uncertainty, she

---

[1] To avoid displays of male chauvinism or unwieldy prose (he/she, his/her), I have tried to vary the use of masculine and feminine pronouns in this text.

cannot afford to act indecisively. Consequently, she views (albeit unconsciously) the range of choices as right ones and wrong ones.

The epidemiologist is more comfortable with shades of gray. Since he is not obliged to make decisions for individual patients, he can live with uncertainty. He focuses on improving the health of populations and is less interested in the outcome of individuals within these populations; he prefers to think *probabilistically.* If 80% of patients like Mr. Jones have been shown to improve with surgery vs 60% with medical therapy, the epidemiologist would have no trouble advocating surgery for Mr. Jones. Mr. Jones' physician, however, may find it difficult to recommend a course of therapy that may not be unequivocally best for her patient.

It is important to emphasize that some fundamental clinical facts can be observed *only* in groups. No amount of pathophysiologic, mechanistic reasoning would reveal that the sex ratio at birth is not $50:50$ but $51.5:48.5$, or that males have a higher overall mortality rate than females. Predicting the sex of an individual newborn or whether a given women will outlive a given man is subject to considerable error. But the sex ratio among the next 1000 newborns or the comparative mortality of a large representative group of men and women can be predicted within a fairly narrow range.

In the past, these two different approaches, individualized and mechanistic on the one hand, group-oriented and probabilistic on the other, have had little in common. Unlike the laboratory-based sciences, epidemiology tended to remain far from the bedside. Epidemiologists concerned themselves almost exclusively with investigating the etiology of infectious and chronic diseases, and clinicians consequently found epidemiology to be of little relevance to their roles as caretakers and decision-makers. Medical, dental, or nursing school courses in epidemiology were viewed with an attitude ranging from indifference to contempt.

Recently, however, the essential compatibility and mutual benefit of the two approaches have become more evident, and this has given rise to the term "clinical epidemiology." Although all epidemiology is clinical in a broad sense, since it concerns disease and other health-related phenomena, "classical epidemiology" has usually concerned itself with disease etiology. Clinical epidemiologists also study etiology, but are equally interested in diagnosis, prognosis, therapy, prevention, evaluation of health care services, and analysis of risks and benefits.

Nonetheless, the distinction between clinical and classical epidemiology should not be overemphasized. The important point is that epidemiology and biostatistics are now recognized by clinical investigators as essential in the design and analysis of research and by practicing clinicians as useful in patient care and in interpreting and appraising the medical literature. These areas are receiving increased attention in clinical curricula, and postgraduate courses and seminars are in great demand by practitioners and researchers alike.

Happily, this marriage of the epidemiologic and individual clinical approaches is proving fruitful not only to patients, their caretakers, and researchers, but also to the disciplines themselves. Inferences based on statistical associations can lead to new avenues of laboratory investigation. For example, knowledge that exposure to a certain solvent in the work place is associated with an increased risk of liver cancer can lead to animal and in vitro experiments aiming to determine its mechanism of carcinogenesis. Conversely, knowledge of underlying mechanisms can suggest novel diagnostic or therapeutic options whose clinical utility will ultimately depend on evidence from epidemiologic studies. A new drug shown to be a potent vasodilator in dogs will need to be tested in well-designed clinical trials in hypertensive patients to assess its efficacy and safety in lowering blood pressure and preventing stroke, heart attack, blindness, or kidney failure.

1.2 Clinical Epidemiology: Main Areas of Interest

The main areas of interest within clinical epidemiology are etiology, diagnosis, prognosis, treatment, prevention, analysis of the risks and benefits of diagnostic and therapeutic maneuvers, and evaluation of health care services. To illustrate how epidemiologic principles and methods may be applied to each of these areas, we return once more to Mr. Jones, now considering him and his heart disease from this wider perspective.

1.2.1 Etiology

What are the causes of coronary artery disease (CAD)? Most of what we know about this condition derives from long-term, population-based epidemiologic studies. For example, in the well-known Framingham study [1], a two-thirds sample of the 30- to 60-year-old population of that Massachusetts town was examined at the inception of the study and periodically thereafter to identify sociodemographic and clinical *risk factors* for CAD. As a result of this and other similar studies, it is now widely acknowledged that smoking, hypertension, high blood cholesterol levels, insufficient exercise, and a high-stress (so-called type-A) personality significantly increase the risk of heart attack.

1.2.2 Diagnosis

How is CAD diagnosed? A variety of invasive and noninvasive diagnostic tests have been developed in an attempt to assess the anatomic state of the coronary arteries, the derangement in blood supply to the heart muscle, and the resulting tissue damage. These include blood tests, roentgenographic studies, electrocardiograms (at rest and during exercise), and radioisotopic tracer uptakes. Before such tests achieve wide application, they should be subjected to appropriate epidemiologic study to ascertain their ability to discriminate accurately between individuals with and without CAD or its sequelae.

1.2.3 Prognosis

What is the likelihood that Mr. Jones will still be alive in 5 years? Epidemiologic inquiry has made substantial contribution to our understanding of those clinical, demographic, and psychosocial variables in CAD patients that are significantly related to future morbidity and mortality. These *prognostic factors* are analogous to the risk factors discussed above in reference to etiology but include, in addition, various indicators of the extent and severity of the underlying disease in question. Some prognostic factors are causally related to the outcome (morbidity or mortality) of interest; others serve merely as *markers* of the underlying disease or other causal factors. Significant prognostic factors for Mr. Jones might include his age, the fact that he has significant obstruction of two of his three major coronary vessels, and the results of his postinfarction electrocardiogram exercise test. Fortunately, prognosis is a dynamic, rather than a static, process that can be influenced by treatment and prevention. In other words, therapeutic and preventive interventions can themselves be prognostic factors.

1.2.4 Treatment

This facet of clinical epidemiology has already been mentioned in reference to whether Mr. Jones should receive surgical or medical therapy. Most questions about therapeutic efficacy (surgical vs medical, drug vs placebo, drug A vs drug B, treatment vs no treatment) are best answered by means of experimental epidemiologic studies, also called *clinical trials*. In the past, many treatments that were recommended for patients with CAD, based on "clinical experience" and "cumulative wisdom" rather than well-designed clinical trials, were subsequently shown to be useless or even harmful. Intramyocardial implantation of the internal mammary artery, for example, became a popular surgical treatment in the 1950s and 1960s, following the enthusiastic, but uncontrolled, experiences of its developers [2]. Later studies with longer-term follow-up showed far less impressive results [3, 4], and the procedure was subsequently abandoned. By contrast, coronary artery bypass grafting using a portion of the saphenous vein from the leg has been the subject of several well-designed clinical trials. These trials have provided much useful information about its merits and limitations for specific groups of patients.

1.2.5 Prevention

How can CAD be prevented? Some epidemiologists distinguish here between *primary prevention* (preventing the disease from developing in the first place) and *secondary prevention* (preventing progression or complication of disease already present). Unfortunately for Mr. Jones, primary prevention is no longer an option. Perhaps, had intervention been attempted when he was a young man, he might have been prevailed upon to stop smoking, improve his diet, get more exercise, and seek treatment for his hypertension (high blood pressure). Although the evidence is not clear-cut, most epidemiologic studies suggest that such changes can be effective in lowering the risk of developing CAD. In fact, many "experts" believe that recent changes in smoking, eating, and exercise behavior and improved control of hypertension are responsible for the clearly perceptible decline in morbidity and mortality from CAD in North America. As for Mr. Jones, he may benefit from the secondary preventive efficacy of such changes, as well as (possibly) from taking aspirin or other anticlotting drugs.

1.2.6 Evaluation of Health Services

When Mr. Jones suffered his recent heart attack, he was hospitalized in a specially staffed and equipped unit called a coronary care unit (CCU). Were his chances of surviving his myocardial infarction improved by the constant attendance of specially trained nurses and the continuous intra-arterial blood pressure and electrocardiographic monitoring he received? Here we have the provision of a service (a certain mode of providing health care for coronary patients), rather than a specific treatment, but many of the epidemiologic methods (especially clinical trials) for evaluating such a service are similar to those used to study efficacy of treatment. Older epidemiologic evidence suggests that CCUs are not effective in reducing postinfarction mortality [5], but new trials are required to assess the potential benefit of more recent monitoring and therapeutic techniques.

1.2.7 Analysis of Benefits and Risks

Suppose it could in fact be shown that CCUs result in a slightly lower rate of postinfarction mortality. Suppose, however, that the constant noise, light, and tension of such units kept most patients from sleeping and resulted in some developing stress ulcers. How great a reduction in cardiac mortality would be necessary to justify this increase in noncardiac morbidity? Or, suppose it costs one million dollars in CCU expenses for each 10 years of life saved by the unit. Is it worth it? Since financial resources are limited, can a greater reduction in cardiovascular mortality be realized by spending that one million dollars on mobile emergency rescue vehicles? Or on an antismoking campaign? Weighing the potential benefits, risks, and costs of different diagnostic, therapeutic, and health care approaches comprises a set of activities including *decision analysis, cost-benefit analysis,* and *cost-effectiveness analysis.* With the growing recognition that no course of action is without adverse consequences and that choices are inevitable, these activities are receiving increased attention from clinical epidemiologists (as well as from economists and ethicists).

1.2.8 Areas of Interest vs Epidemiologic Methods

The epidemiologic section of this text could have been organized according to the areas of interest to clinical epidemiologists. Thus, I might have chosen, as several other authors have done [6, 7], to devote a chapter to etiology, another to diagnosis, a third to prognosis, and so on. A common set of principles and techniques can be applied to each of these areas, however, and the epidemiologic methods for their study often overlap.

For example, clinical trials are often applicable to the study of treatment, prevention, and health services evaluation. Rather than providing separate chapters for each of these areas of interest, I have chosen to present a general discussion of clinical trial methodology, with examples of how the methodology can be applied. Although the chapter headings will thereby follow the pattern used in more traditional (i.e., "classical") epidemiology texts, I have focused on applications and examples of interest to a clinical readership.

Before we take up the individual methodologic topics, let us briefly consider epidemiology's historical roots and its current and future role in responding to controversial questions and testing unproven hypotheses.

1.3 Historical Roots

The science of epidemiology may be said to have originated with the ancient Greeks and their change from supernatural to natural explanations of disease. Hippocrates (in his *On Airs, Waters, and Places*) [8] was perhaps the first to recognize the important relationship between disease and environment, including the effects of climate and life style. Physicians over the next 2000 years were nonetheless hampered by two factors: (a) a tendency to "lump" distinct diseases together and (b) a failure to quantify (count) cases occurring in specific locations and time periods. Major advances on both of these fronts occurred in seventeenth-century London with the works of Thomas Sydenham and John Graunt respectively.

Sydenham revived the Hippocratic practice of careful clinical observation and recording and became convinced of the individuality of different disease entities and of the need for their classification [9]. Graunt is often regarded as the founder of vital statistics. In 1662, he published his *Natural and Political Observations Mentioned in a Following Index, and Made Upon the Bills of Mortality* [10]. By analyzing the weekly Bills of Mortality and registers of christenings collected by parish clerks, he may have been the first to recognize the importance of denominators (the group or population at risk) in calculating rates and in deriving valid inferences about mortality and fertility on the populational, rather than individual, level.

The concept of rates of disease in population groups was extended in the eighteenth century with the development of experimental studies (clinical trials), in which rates were compared in groups receiving or not receiving a given intervention. In 1747, James Lind carried out a famous controlled trial showing that citrus fruits were capable of curing scurvy among British sailors (subsequently nicknamed "limeys") [11]. In 1796, Edward Jenner conducted a small-scale clinical trial demonstrating the efficacy of cowpox vaccination in preventing smallpox [12].

In the nineteenth century, modern epidemiology truly came into its own. Pierre Louis became probably the first physician to use what he called *"la méthode numérique"* (a statistical comparison of rates or other quantitative measures of disease) to derive inferences about disease etiology and treatment efficacy within his own clinical practice [13]. His controlled observational study of bloodletting [14] clearly indicated its lack of efficacy in treating disease and was instrumental in its eventual discontinuation. One of Louis's students, William Farr, organized the first vital statistics registry [15] and, by applying mathematical concepts, developed methods for measuring excess risk. He also identified potential biases in attributing causation to factors affecting different groups, as well as quantitative ways of reducing such biases.

John Snow is regarded by many as the father of modern epidemiology, although "paternity" has also been claimed for Graunt, Syndenham, Louis, and Farr. Snow's studies of cholera deaths in London from 1849 to 1854 demonstrated a striking association with a contaminated water supply [16], several decades before acceptance of the germ theory of disease and demonstration of the cholera *Vibrio*.

The current century has seen the extension of epidemiologic principles and techniques to the study of a variety of diseases, treatments, and preventive measures. In 1920, Joseph Goldberger carried out a community trial of diet in the treatment of pellagra, thus demonstrating it to be a nutritional, rather than an infectious, disease [17]. This was long before the biochemical demonstration of the vitamin involved (nicotinic acid) and the understanding of its importance in intermediary metabolism. In 1941, N. M. Gregg, an astute Australian ophthalmologist, recognized the association between certain congenital deformities and maternal rubella (German measles) infection early in pregnancy [18].

In more recent decades we have had the trials of poliomyelitis vaccines [19], the observational studies by the U.S. Public Health Service [20] and subsequent community trials by the New York State Department of Health [21] demonstrating that fluoride in drinking water protects against dental caries, the recognition by Doll and Hill of the strong association between cigarette smoking and lung cancer [22], and the Framingham and other studies of risk factors for the development of cardiovascular disease [1]. Epidemiology has not abandoned its historical role in establishing the etiology of presumed infectious disease, however, and in the past few years, epidemiologists have been instrumental in discovering the causal agent in Legionnaire's disease, the relationship between tampon use and toxic shock syndrome, and the importance of aspirin as a cofactor in causing Reye's syndrome in children with influenza or chicken pox. Much of what we know now about AIDS (acquired immunodeficiency syndrome) is based on epidemiological data obtained well before the recent discovery of the responsible human immunodeficiency virus (HIV). The efficacy of future vaccines and other preventive measures for AIDS will also require evaluation by epidemiologic studies.

1.4 Current and Future Relevance: Controversial Questions and Unproven Hypotheses

Many of the current controversies and unproven hypotheses in medicine will require epidemiologic research. Does coffee consumption increase the risk of developing pancreatic cancer? Will daily aspirin administration lower the risk of myocardial infarction or sudden cardiac death? What are the risks and benefits of home labor and delivery? Does tonsillectomy and/or adenoidectomy lessen recurrence of pharyngitis (throat infection) or otitis media (middle ear infection)? Does "tight" control of blood sugar improve long-term prognosis in patients with insulin-dependent diabetes? What are the diagnostic benefits of new imaging techniques, such as positron emission tomography (PET) and magnetic resonance imaging (MRI)?

These are but a small sampling of the questions whose answers will require epidemiological data. Training and skill in research design and statistical analysis are of course essential to the researchers who will be providing these data. But practicing clinicians will also require considerable knowledge of epidemiology if they are to interpret and apply published research to the best advantage of their patients. The goal of this volume is to help the "doers" of clinical research in improving the scientific quality of their investigation, and the "users" of research in developing their skills of appraisal and application.

References

1. Dawber TR (1980) The Framingham study: the epidemiology of atherosclerotic disease. Harvard University Press, Cambridge
2. Vineberg A, Walker J (1964) The surgical treatment of coronary artery heart disease by internal mammary implantation: report of 140 cases followed up to thirteen years. Dis Chest 45: 190–206
3. Urschel HC, Razzuk MA, Miller ER, Nathan MJ, Ginsberg RJ, Paulson DL (1970) Direct and indirect myocardial neovascularization: follow-up and appraisal. Surgery 68: 1087–1100
4. Sethi GK, Scott SM, Takaro T (1973) Myocardial revascularization by internal thoracic arterial implants: long-term follow-up. Chest 97: 97–105
5. Hill JD, Holdstock G, Hampton JR (1977) Comparison of mortality of patients with heart attacks admitted to a coronary care unit and an ordinary medical ward. Br Med J 2: 81–83
6. Fletcher RH, Fletcher SW, Wagner EH (1982) Clinical epidemiology – the essentials. Williams and Wilkins, Baltimore
7. Sackett DL, Haynes RB, Tugwell P (1985) Clinical epidemiology: a basic science for clinical medicine. Little, Brown, Boston
8. Hippocrates (1939) The genuine works of Hippocrates. Williams and Wilkins, Baltimore
9. Dewhurst K (1966) Dr. Thomas Sydenham (1624–1689). University of California Press, Berkeley
10. Wilcox WF (ed) (1937) Natural and political observations made upon the bills of mortality by John Graunt. Johns Hopkins Press reprint, Baltimore
11. Lind J (1793) A treatise of the scurvy. Sands, Murray, and Cochran, Edinburgh
12. Jenner E (1910) Vaccination against smallpox. In: Eliot SW (ed) Scientific papers. Collier, New York, pp 153–231
13. Bollet AJ (1973) Pierre Louis: the numerical method and the foundation of quantative medicine. Am J Med Sci 266: 92–101
14. Louis PC-A (1836) Researches on the effects of bloodletting in some inflammatory diseases, and on the influence of tartarized antimony and vesication in pneumonitis. Milliard, Gray, Boston
15. Farr W (1975) Vital statistics: a memorial volume of selections from the reports and writings of William Farr. New York Academy of Medicine, Metuchen, NJ
16. Snow J (1936) Snow on cholera. The Commonwealth Fund, New York
17. Goldberger J (1964) Goldberger on pellagra. Louisiana State University Press, Baton Rouge
18. Gregg NM (1941) Congenital cataract following German measles in the mother. Trans Ophthalmol Soc Austr 3: 35–46
19. Francis T, Korns RF, Voight RB, Boisen M, Hemphill FM, Napier JA, Tolchinsky E (1955) An evaluation of the 1954 poliomyelitis vaccine trials: summary report. Am J Public Health 45 [Part II Suppl]: 1–630
20. Dean HT, Arnold FA, Elvove E (1942) Domestic water and dental caries. V. Additional studies of the relation of fluoride domestic waters to dental caries experience in 4425 white children, aged 12 to 14 years, of 13 cities in 4 states. Public Health Rep 57: 1155–1179
21. Ast DB, Schlesinger ER (1956) The conclusion of a ten-year study of water fluoridation. Am J Public Health 46: 265–271
22. Doll R, Hill AB (1952) A study of the aetiology of carcinoma of the lung. Br Med J 1271–1286

Chapter 2: **Measurement**

2.1 Types of Variables and Measurement Scales

The attributes or events that are measured in a research study are called *variables,* since they vary, i.e., take on different values in different subjects. Variables are measured according to two broad types of *measurement scales:* continuous and categorical.

Continuous variables (also called *dimensional, quantitative,* or *interval* variables) are those expressed as integers, fractions, or decimals, in which equal distances exist between successive intervals. Age, systolic or diastolic blood pressure, serum sodium concentration, and the number of children in a family are all examples of continuous variables.

Categorical variables, which are also called *discrete* variables, are those in which the entity measured is placed into one of two *(dichotomous)* or more *(polychotomous)* discrete categories. Examples of dichotomous categorical variables include vital status (dead vs alive), yes vs no responses to a question, and sex (male vs female). Polychotomous categorical scales can be either *nominal* or *ordinal.* Nominal scales contain named categories that bear no ordered relationship to one another, e.g., hair color, race, or country of origin. In ordinal scales, the categories bear an ordered relationship to one another. Unlike continuous scales, however, the intervals between ordinal categories need not be equal. For example, an ordinal pain scale might include the following ranked categories of pain severity: none, mild, moderate, and severe. Some ordinal scales are "pseudocontinuous," in that the intervals between categories appear equal. In a neurologic examination, for example, deep tendon reflexes are usually measured as absent, $1+$, $2+$, $3+$, or $4+$. Although criteria exist for assigning these categories, the difference between $1+$ and $2+$ is not necessarily the same as that between, say, $2+$ and $3+$.

2.2 Sources of Variation in a Measurement

When a measurement is performed on a single subject, two sources of variation can affect the result: *biologic variation* and *measurement error.* Biologic variation reflects the dynamic nature of most biologic entities and leads to differences between individuals of different age, sex, race, or disease status. Another source of biologic variation can occur within the same individual over time *(temporal variation)*; unlike the physical measurement of inanimate objects (e.g., the length of a desk), a subject's biologic attributes can vary over time in response to a variety of physiologic functions and other factors. To the degree that such changes are regular and predictable, intraindividual temporal variation can be reduced by the investigator. For example, in measuring a variable such as plasma cortisol concentration, which is known to have a regular diurnal cycle, variability is reduced by drawing the blood sample at a specified time of day.

Every measurement is subject to some degree of measurement error. There are two different types of measurement error: (a) random (chance) error and (b) bias. When a single (nonrepeated) measurement is obtained, there is simply no way of knowing if the difference (error) between the measured value and the true biologic value is due to chance or bias. The distinction can be made only when the measurement is repeated. If the average value of a large number of repeated measurements is the same as the true biologic value, then the reason for the disparate single measurements is random error. If the average value is also erroneous, then the explanation is bias (with or without additional random error).

These relationships are illustrated in Fig. 2.1. Each measurement has been repeated eight times. Measurement A is biased but subject to little random (chance) error. B is unbiased but subject to considerable chance variation. C is both biased and highly variable. Measurement D has the smallest propensity for error; it is both unbiased and relatively invariable.

Measurement error can arise from either the method (measuring instrument[1]) or the observer (the measurer). When measurements are repeated, therefore, we can talk about the variability between methods of making the measurement or between the observers using those methods. We can also distinguish between the variability that occurs when the same method or observer is used to repeat the measurement *(intramethod* or *intraobserver variability)* and that which occurs between two or more methods or observers *(intermethod* or *interobserver variability).*

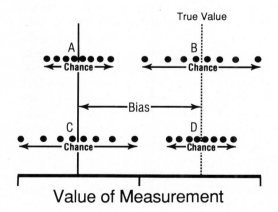

Fig. 2.1. The roles of chance and bias in measurement error. [Each measurement, A–D, has been repeated eight times. Vertical lines represent average values for measurements A and C (solid line) and measurements B and D (broken line).]

---

[1] A measurement "instrument" need not be a mechanical device. Death certificates, questionnaires, and psychologic tests are examples of instruments commonly used to measure subjects' attributes in epidemiologic studies.

When repeated measurements are obtained, biologic variation and measurement error interact to produce a phenomenon known as *regression toward the mean.* For many biologic attributes, most individuals in a group will have true values for that attribute closer to the group average, or mean, value than to either (high or low) extreme. Since each individual measurement is subject to both biologic variation and measurement error, an extremely high or low value obtained in an individual from that group is more likely to be in error than is an intermediate value. Thus, when the measurement is repeated, the tendency toward a less extreme repeat value, i.e., a "regression toward the mean," is greater than the tendency for an intermediate value to become more extreme.

2.3 Properties of Measurement

There are three essential properties of measurement: (a) validity, (b) reproducibility, and (c) detail.

The *validity* of a measurement is the extent to which it corresponds to the "true" biologic value or some accepted "gold standard." (Some statisticians prefer the term *accuracy* for this property, although the common English usage of this term may cause confusion with the detail of the measurement). Validity depends on minimizing measurement error caused by bias. A valid measurement thus requires both a valid method (instrument for measurement) and a valid observer (measurer).

Unfortunately, no gold standard exists for many of the variables of interest in clinical research. It is impossible to know with certainty how much pain or anxiety a patient is experiencing or the extent of cellular dysplasia in a cervical smear. The validity of such measures thus cannot be assessed. Instead, a variety of "proxy" indexes of validity are used.

Face validity is the extent to which the measure appears apposite or appropriate to the entity measured. *Content validity* pertains to the appositeness of the individual items or components of the measurement, e.g., the individual questions in a questionnaire (scale) designed to measure depression. *Concurrent criterion validity* is the degree to which the measurement correlates with other accepted measures (criteria) of the entity obtained at the same time, e.g., the presence of tears in patients scoring high on our depression scale. *Predictive criterion validity* is the extent to which the measurement predicts some accepted criterion of the entity that occurs in the future. If, for example, only those patients who appear severely depressed on our scale subsequently commit suicide, the depression scale measurement can be said to be a valid predictor of suicide. Finally, *construct validity* is the extent to which the underlying entity itself, i.e., the theoretical construct, is valid. The validity of depression as a construct is well accepted. Were it not, however, we would need to hypothesize relationships with other measurable variables, based on theoretical considerations, and then design ways of testing these hypotheses.

The *reproducibility* of a measurement is the degree to which the same results are obtained when the measurement is repeated. (In practical terms, however, few measurements are actually repeated, and reproducibility represents the extent to which the same result *would* have been obtained had repeated measures been taken.) It may reflect either (temporal) variation in the underlying biologic attribute or random measurement error (due to method and or observers). Many other terms exist for the property of reproducibility, and this is a major source of confusion among persons encountering these concepts for the first time. The most commonly encountered term for this measurement property is *reliability*, but the term is misleading, since it seems unwise to *rely* on a measurement that may be invalid, merely because it is reproducible. Statisticians prefer the word *precision*, which unfortunately can be confused in its normal English usage with measurement detail. Perhaps the best word is *consistency*, but this has not achieved general acceptance. The important thing here, however, is the concept: the extent to which the same answer is obtained when the measurement is repeated.

As shown in Fig. 2.1, a measurement may be highly reproducible but biased, and therefore invalid (measurement A in the figure). It may be biased systematically upward or downward, e.g., an incorrectly calibrated serum glucose autoanalyzer that reproducibly gives values 30 mg/dl above the true concentration. Or it may be consistently biased toward a given value; a broken watch, for example, will reproducibly give the time but will be valid only twice a day.

As also shown in Fig. 2.1, a measurement may be poorly reproducible but unbiased (measurement B). When such a measurement is taken with several replications, the average value of the replicates may have fairly good validity. This is common practice in epidemiologic studies for variables such as height and blood pressure, which are subject to considerable (random) intra- and interobserver error.

The final measurement property of interest is *detail*. The detail of a measurement is equivalent to the amount of information provided. For continuous variables, this usually means the number of "significant figures" or decimal places. For categorical variables, detail refers to the number of categories contained in the scale.

Ideally, a measurement should be sufficiently, but not excessively, detailed. Detail should be sufficient to distinguish individuals or groups with true differences in the entity of interest, but it should not be excessive, in the sense that measured differences are of no biological importance. Furthermore, the detail of a measurement should not exceed its validity and reproducibility. Serum glucose concentration, for example, is usually measured to the nearest mg/dl. Measurement to the nearest 100 mg/dl would be insufficient in distinguishing normal subjects from those with hypoglycemia, on the one hand, or diabetes, on the other. Even measurement to the nearest 10 mg/dl might be insufficient to document improvement or deterioration in diabetic control after changes in insulin dosage. Conversely, measurement to the nearest 0.1 mg/dl would probably be excessive, since changes of this magnitude have no known clinical significance and since existing technology for measurement does not yield this degree of validity or reproducibility.

To illustrate the same concept using categorical variables, consider the question "How would you describe your mood today?" The range of responses (scale of categories) to a question of this type is often given according to what is called a Likert format, e.g., depressed, neutral, or happy. Such a 3-point scale might be insufficient to distinguish mildly depressed from suicidal patients, however, and expansion to five categories (e.g., severely depressed, mildly depressed, neutral, slightly happy, very happy) is probably preferable. A further increase in the number of categories, on the other hand, may exceed the respondent's ability to characterize his or her mood.

2.4 "Hard" vs "Soft" Data

Many laboratory measurements are performed by modern, highly sophisticated mechanical devices. With adequate quality control by the manufacturer and the measuring laboratory, the resulting measurements are often highly reproducible and valid. The data are usually displayed on a continuous scale as a digital readout or computer printout, thus effectively reducing or eliminating the effect of the technician or other observer making the measurement. Such data are often referred to as "hard" to distinguish them from more subjective ("soft") measurements with greater potential for bias or variability on the part of the observer. Most hard measurements are continuous, although a few categorical variables (e.g., vital status, sex, and race) have also been admitted to the "club," despite their dependence on human observation.

Unfortunately, many of the variables that are most important in caring for patients are soft and subjective. In evaluating the efficacy of a new cancer chemotherapeutic agent, for example, pain, mood, and ability to work may be of far greater concern to a patient and his family than the size of his tumor and may even be more important than the duration of his survival. As Feinstein has emphasized, the tendency of clinical investigators to focus on hard rather than soft measurements can result in research that is both dehumanizing and irrelevant [1]. Furthermore, many data traditionally considered hard can be seen, at closer inspection, to have feet of softer clay. Roentgenographic and cytopathologic diagnosis, despite their reputation for hard objectivity, have repeatedly been shown to be subject to considerable intra- and interobserver disagreement, even among experts [2, 3].

Much can be done to harden soft data. Scales can be constructed in which objective criteria are used to specify the score or category appropriate for each subject. *Operational definitions* are often helpful; they tell the observer (the measurer) what operations to perform to arrive at a correct classification.

The use of objective criteria and operational definitions can result in substantial improvements in the reproducibility and validity of many soft measures. As an example, consider the problem of identification of adverse drug reactions (ADRs). Adverse events are unfortunately common in ill patients treated with drugs, and attribution of responsibility for such events in persons with several underlying diseases under treatment with numerous drugs is exceedingly complex. Even experts disagree substantially when asked to assess the probability of an ADR in a given case or series of cases [4, 5]. The use of a diagnostic algorithm, however, which provides rules for ADR identification in response to information elicited about a specific case, results in considerable improvement in both reproducibility and validity [6, 7].

2.5 Consequences of Erroneous Measurement

As we have seen, a measurement may be erroneous either because it is systematically biased or because it tends to vary (randomly) around its true value. When individuals are considered, the consequences are the same. If the measurement is wrong, it makes little or no difference whether the error is systematic or random, and besides, we usually have no way of finding out. If a woman participating in a "hypertension screening clinic" in a local shopping center has her blood pressure erroneously recorded as 160/100 instead of her usual true pressure of 130/80, it matters little whether the reason is an insufficiently wide blood pressure cuff (bias), an inexperienced person taking the reading (random measurement variation), or the fact that she is under some stress because the time has expired on her parking meter (biologic variation). Regardless of the reason for the error, she may be labeled as "hypertensive" and suffer all the worries attendant upon receiving such a diagnosis, at least until such time as she is rechecked when calm by her own physician using a proper cuff.

When groups instead of individuals are considered, however, the situation is quite different. Variability (poor reproducibility), in the absence of bias, should not change the average group value, since there is just as much a chance that any individual measurement is too high or too low with respect to its true value. In the absence of bias, therefore, the average measurement for a group (if sufficiently large) will be valid even if many of the individual measurements from which it derives are not. To use engineering parlance, the "signal" may be correct despite considerable "noise." If adequate numbers of subjects are studied (to improve the signal-to-noise ratio), a valid measure of the group average will be revealed even in the presence of considerable random measurement error. When the individual measurements are biased, however, the group signal will also be erroneous, despite inclusion of a large sample of study subjects.

Random measurement error can nonetheless have deleterious consequences when one is seeking associations or correlations between two measured variables in a group of subjects. In these situations, random errors in the individual measurements will lead to an *analytic bias* by diminishing the extent of association or correlation between the two. Say, for example, that we wish to study the correlation between weight and systolic blood pressure. Poorly reproducible (i.e., randomly erroneous) but unbiased measurements of weight and/or blood pressure might reveal valid group averages for each of these variables, but the correlation between the two would be reduced below its true value. Similarly, in a study of a possible association between smoking and myocardial infarction (MI), random errors in classifying study subjects as to their smoking status and/or diagnosis (MI or no MI) will tend to reduce (bias) the measure of association between the two. The type of analytic bias that occurs in the statistical relationship between variables as a result of errors in measuring those two variables is called *information bias* and will be discussed in greater detail in Chapter 5.

In summary, then, poorly reproducible measurements are more tolerable in epidemiologic research than in the assessment of individual patients for clinical purposes. The effects of random measurement errors can be overcome, in part, by increasing the number of subjects measured, and statistical relationships between variables that result from such random errors will generally lead to conservative inferences. Thus, even "sloppy" measurements should not, in the absence of bias, create false statistical associations where none exist. Depending on one's point of view, this built-in conservatism can be considered either beneficial (preventing the too-ready acceptance of new findings) or harmful (hindering scientific progress).

2.6 Sources of Data

In clinical research, measurement data may be gathered from a variety of sources. The choice of data source is often dictated by practical and economic, as well as scientific, considerations. It is important to distinguish between *primary* and *secondary* sources. Primary data derive from those measurements planned and carried out in the course of a research study by the study's investigators. Secondary data are those routinely collected by clinicians or public health authorities, as well as those obtained in the course of some other study.

2.6.1 Clinical Observations

Clinical observations include the elements of a medical history, physical examination, and laboratory data that are obtained in the clinical care of patients. They may be either primary or secondary, the latter usually being obtained from existing medical records.

The quality of data obtained from medical histories depends on how the questions are asked, and therefore on language, understanding, alertness, and other characteristics of both the history taker and patient. These factors can affect either the reproducibility or validity of data obtained by history. As reviewed by Koran, interobserver agreement is often poor when two or more observers obtain a medical history from the same patient [8]. Furthermore, if the observer obtaining the history has a preconceived notion or hypothesis in mind, the resulting measurement is susceptible to bias, especially when that observer is not "blind" to the characteristics of the patient whose history is being taken.

Suppose, for example, we wish to know whether our patient, Mrs. Jones, has experienced hemoptysis (coughing up blood) within the past year. Here are two (admittedly extreme) ways of asking her:

1. Mrs. Jones, it is not at all uncommon for people with a bad cough or cold to notice, on occasion, the appearance of small flecks of blood in their phlegm. Has this happened to you at any time during the past year?
2. Mrs. Jones, you haven't been so unfortunate, so obviously ill, so utterly doomed as to have coughed up blood in the past year, have you?

It would hardly be surprising to receive opposite responses to these questions. Although such extreme examples of attempting to bias a response are probably rare, subtle shadings of wording and inflection can have a significant impact on the data obtained and can create statistical associations where none exist or eliminate those that do exist. The impact of this type of systematic information bias will be discussed more fully in Chapter 5.

Even in the absence of observer bias, some items in the medical history tend to be biased by the subject. In particular, people are generally believed to overreport minor symptoms (abdominal pain, headache, insomnia) and to underreport bad habits (smoking, drinking, drug abuse).

Physical examination depends on the skill, training, experience, and mental state of the examiner, and many of the measurements obtained are thus somewhat subjective (e.g., the presence or absence of liver enlargement). As with history taking, interobserver agreement has been shown to be poor for a variety of aspects of the physical examination [8]. Here, too, the use of nonblind examiners increases the potential for biased measurement.

Laboratory data are usually more valid and reproducible than those obtained by history and physical examination, but they depend on the quality control utilized by the clinical laboratory or X-ray facility. As reviewed by Koran, interobserver agreement is not as high as one may be led to believe by the impressive technologic advances in recent years [8]. In general, the greater the potential for subjectivity ("clinical judgment") in obtaining the laboratory measurement, the poorer the reproducibility and the greater the opportunity for bias.

When clinical observations are planned and carried out by a study's investigators (i.e., the data source is primary), the reproducibility and validity of the measurements can be improved by adequately training and blinding the observers (clinicians and laboratory personnel) and by providing objective, operational criteria for performing and recording the measurements. When the data come from secondary sources, the recording of the observations cannot (by definition) be controlled by the investigators, but medical record abstractors should be provided with operational rules and criteria for extracting their observations and should be kept blind, as far as possible, to the study's principal hypotheses. Medical records may have the additional problem, of course, that data may be missing or insufficiently detailed for use in the study.

2.6.2 Questionnaires and Interviews

Since questionnaires and interviews are often highly structured and designed by investigators for a specific study, the resulting data are usually primary. These data sources share some of the same characteristics as the medical history. As with history taking, responses depend on how questions are asked. Similarly also, subjects are generally believed to overreport minor symptoms and underreport bad habits.

Self-administered questionnaires suffer from three additional problems. First, since many questionnaires designed for a specific study utilize a fixed format (i.e., the range of possible responses to each question is limited to those printed on the questionnaire), they occasionally provide insufficient or excessive detail. The pretesting of such questionnaires prior to use in an actual research study is thus essential to improve the quality of data obtained therefrom. Second, inconsistent responses cannot be resolved, unless provision is made for follow-up contact by mail, telephone, or personal visit. Third, since self-administered questionnaires are usually sent by mail, nonresponse can be a major problem. Many people simply do not return questionnaires sent to them in the mail. Even with repeated mailings, response rates above 80% are unusual. Of even greater concern, those who do return the questionnaire may differ in important ways from those who do not, thus leading to a potential for bias due to nonresponse.

The data presented in Table 2.1 are taken from a study by Burgess and Tierney

Table 2.1. Smoking habits among 1184 Rhode Island physicians [9]

Subjects	Number	% of Total	% Smoking
Respondents			
First mailing	837	70.7	21.7
Second mailing	189	16.0	26.5
Total	1026	86.7	22.6
Nonrespondents	158	13.3[a]	45.5

[a] Based on a sample of 33 of the 158 nonrespondents.

[9]. In 1968, short questionnaires concerning (among other items) cigarette smoking were mailed to 1184 licensed physicians in Rhode Island. The first mailing produced a 70.7% response; 21.7% of the respondents admitted to being current cigarette smokers. A second mailing netted an additional 189 (16.0%) respondents, 26.5% of whom reported smoking. When a sample of the 158 (13.3%) remaining nonrespondents (or their families or friends) were approached in person, it was found that 45.5% were smokers. In other words, nonrespondents were about twice as likely to smoke as respondents.

It should be emphasized, however, that nonresponse does not always lead to bias [10]; data based on low response rates can indeed be valid. The problem is that the characteristics of the nonrespondents are usually unknown, and the potential for bias is unassessable and therefore capable of undermining the findings of a study.

Personal interviews, either by telephone or direct questioning (often in the home), have several advantages over mailed, self-administered questionnaires. The response rate is often higher when the study subject can meet, or at least talk to, the person asking the question. People are far more likely to throw away or ignore a written questionnaire received by mail from an investigator or study group they have never met or talked to than to refuse to answer questions asked by telephone or in person by someone who adequately introduces him- or herself. Another advantage of the personal interview is that inconsistencies between two or more responses can be resolved by the interviewer. One disadvantage of personal interviews relative to self-administered questionnaires is their potential for systematic measurement bias. This can be minimized by thoughtful a priori structuring of the interviews and by careful training, periodic quality control, and "blinding" (to preselected characteristics of study subjects and the study hypothesis) of interviewers.

2.6.3 Reportable Diseases and Disease Registries

In order to initiate control measures for outbreaks of communicable diseases, the reporting of a number of infectious diseases is mandated by public health authorities in most industrialized countries. Physicians, hospitals, and laboratories are required to report documented cases of these diseases. The major difficulty with the quality of data obtained from this source is that, except for rare and serious diseases like bubonic plague and rabies, most of these diseases are underreported, despite the legal mandate.

Furthermore, the degree of underreporting is variable and usually unknown. For example, socially embarrassing diseases (e.g., sexually transmitted diseases) are systematically underreported. Second, the detection of many diseases (e.g., tuberculosis) depends on how actively they are looked for, that is, on the intensity of surveillance. Third, diagnosis may require special diagnostic facilities or techniques (e.g., Legionnaire's disease or AIDS). Nonetheless, reportable disease data can be useful for documenting secular trends in the local, regional, or national occurrence of the diseases reported.

In disease registries, which may be legally required or voluntary, newly diagnosed cases meeting specific criteria are identified through reports submitted by physicians and hospitals tó a central agency or repository. Baseline demographic and clinical data are recorded, and the registry is updated through periodic follow-up. As with reportable diseases, the quality of data obtained from disease registries depends on the intensity of surveillance and the availability of special techniques. Underreporting and even some overreporting are common. For example, the U.S. Food and Drug Administration maintains a registry of adverse drug reactions (ADRs) based on voluntary reports submitted by individual physicians, occasionally supplemented by follow-up information obtained by mail or telephone. Minor adverse reactions are, of course, systematically underreported, whereas rarer and more serious adverse events, which might be caused by underlying diseases or other factors, may be falsely labeled as ADRs. For some diseases, however, special registries appear to work quite well. The state of Connecticut has long had an excellent cancer registry, and the Scandinavian countries are leading the way in registries for birth defects.

2.6.4 Health Records for Defined Population Subgroups

This general category of (secondary) data source includes school and industry records of baseline and periodic physical examinations and of absenteeism, health records of the armed forces and the Veterans Administration, and data from insurance programs. Although the data from such sources is often conveniently computerized and of high quality, the major limitation concerns generalizability to persons outside of the specific group from which the data derive. Military data are highly nonrepresentative with respect to age and sex, employers and life insurance companies are likely to exclude persons with significant illness, and prepaid health insurance plans (e.g., Kaiser Permanente in the Western United States and the Health Insurance Plan of Greater New York) underrepresent the economically disadvantaged.

Nonetheless, the quality and size of these data bases have facilitated a number of important epidemiologic studies. For example, data on height and weight routinely collected by the Metropolitan Life Insurance Company have been useful in understanding the relationship between obesity and life expectancy. One of the best of these data sources has been the Mayo Clinic and the Olmstead Country Medical Group, which provide medical care for the vast majority of residents in the Rochester, Minnesota, area. Although underrepresentative of poor and minority groups, the exploitation of this data source has contributed to our understanding of the natural history of several chronic diseases.

2.6.5 Vital Statistics and Other Population-Based Data Sources

When their completeness and validity can be assured, as is the case in most industrialized countries, national or other population-based statistics can be valuable secondary data sources for epidemiologic investigation. The *census* is taken every 10 years in the United States and Canada and includes data on age, sex, race, education, and socioeconomic status. Although illegal immigrants are uncounted and certain other groups (e.g., infants, racial minorities, and vagrants) are under-counted, the census often provides the best source of denominator data for many of the epidemiologic rates that will be discussed in the next chapter.

Vital statistics consist of population-based data bearing on births, deaths, marriages, and divorces. Birth and death certificates provide fairly valid data for counting numbers of births and deaths, except in remote areas where such events occur without contact with hospitals or medical care personnel. In addition to the fact of the birth, birth certificates also include useful information concerning the parents' race and education, the mother's pregnancy history and use of prenatal care, and evidence of (obvious) congenital anomalies. Death certificates include data on the age, sex, marital status, and occupation of the deceased.

The main problem with death certificates concerns the *cause* of death, because it depends on the attribution of cause by the attending physician. One problem is that socially undesirable causes of death, such as suicide and alcohol or drug abuse, are systematically underreported. But even more importantly, death certificates require the physician to specify an *underlying* cause. Not only does this require a judgment by the physician as to which of several diseases the patient may have been suffering from was the underlying fatal one, but the cited cause is not usually changed by the results of autopsy or other data that may subsequently become available. Fortunately, although published mortality statistics are based on the single underlying cause of death, data concerning other conditions listed on the death certificate are also entered into the computerized data base and are thus available to investigators having access to that data base.

In an attempt at international standardization, most countries adhere to the classification codes established by the International Classification of Disease (ICD), which is now in its ninth revision. Secular changes in causes of deaths, however, may be confounded by changes in nosology. For example, the disease "dropsy" (swelling of the ankles) has, in this century, been replaced by more specific causes of death, such as heart, liver, or kidney failure. Important changes in diagnostic technology have also resulted in some artificial changes. The recent drop in the number of deaths from stomach cancer, for example, is probably at least partly attributable to a previous tendency to label any abdominal mass or tumor as stomach cancer. It is now known that most of these masses are caused by cancer of the colon, ovary, pancreas, or other intra-abdominal organs. Conversely, the death rate for hypertension increased about tenfold in English and Welsh men 45–54 years old between 1930 and 1950. This increase did not reflect a true increase in either the occurrence or fatality of hypertension, but rather the increasing availability and use of the sphygmomanometer and the recognition of the role of hypertension in causing fatal heart disease and stroke. Finally, geographic differences in terminology may also lead to spurious differences in mortality. The same chronic obstructive lung disease may be called *emphysema* in the United States and *bronchitis* in the United Kingdom.

Abortion (fetal death) rates are worthy of special comment. Many early pregnancies go unrecognized, and requirements vary as to stage of gestation at which registration is required. Because of these factors, as well as the obvious difficulties in determining cause of death in many cases, data concerning fetal deaths (which require a distinct certificate form) are of notoriously poor quality and completeness.

Because of the legal requirements for registration of births and deaths, population-based data concerning fertility and mortality are both more complete and of higher quality than data concerning morbidity. For countries like the United Kingdom, where the National Health Service assigns each individual to one general practitioner, physicians' records can serve as a base for collecting morbidity data. In the United States, such data have been produced by the National Center for Health Statistics (NCHS) over the past 30 years by a series of interviews and examinations (the Health Interview Surveys and Health and Nutrition Examination Surveys) of random samples of the U.S. population. These data are supplemented by sampling physicians' offices (the National Ambulatory Care Survey).

The NCHS data are limited by the fact that the surveys are cross-sectional in nature, i.e., they measure only morbidity present at the time of the interview, examination, or physician visit. Furthermore, the size of the samples studied is insufficient to study infrequent diseases. Nonetheless, they have provided a valuable source of national data concerning anthropometric measurements and nutritional status, minor illnesses and disabilities, and utilization of health care services.

Perhaps the best population-based data sources are the extensive data linkage networks in the Scandinavian countries. In Sweden, for example, each person has a unique identification number assigned at birth. Information about birth, employment, health, and death is stored in computer data banks accessible through this number. Individuals listed in birth defects registries and cancer registries can also be identified through this number, and linkage to other data bases is readily achieved. The availability of such information for virtually the entire population is an invaluable resource for epidemiologic investigation.

2.6.6 Sources of Data: Concluding Remarks

An important distinction to be made concerning the various sources of data discussed above relates to whether group data that are aggregated for presentation can be disaggregated to obtain data on the individual members of that group. When a single variable is considered in isolation, this distinction is of little importance, since, as we have seen, the group average for that variable should be valid if the individual measurements are unbiased. When the main interest is in the possible association between two variables, however, aggregate data can lead to a spurious association that would not be found on analysis of the same two variables presented by individual subjects.

For example, consider the relationship between death from colon cancer and dietary fiber intake. Analyses based on aggregated vital statistics and food consumption data by country have revealed a very tight inverse association: the higher a country's per capita fiber intake, the lower its colon cancer mortality [11]. An obvious conclusion is that eating dietary fiber protects against colon cancer. This conclusion might be false, however. It is possible that on an individual basis, no association exists between fiber intake and the development of colon cancer. In other words, *within* countries having a given per capita fiber intake, individuals consuming a high-fiber diet might be just as likely to develop colon cancer as those consuming a low-fiber diet. The spurious association derived from the country-by-country (aggregated) analysis might then be explained, for example, by the fact that high-fiber foods are consumed (for cultural or climatic reasons) in countries lacking heavy industry, and that it is the industrial air pollution in other countries that leads to higher colon cancer death rates, rather than any protective effect of fiber in the nonindustrial countries.

The false inference that can result from analysis of aggregate, rather than individual, data is called an *ecological fallacy.* Data on individuals is always to be preferred to aggregated data on groups when investigating statistical associations between variables.

Finally, I should re-emphasize here another important distinction among data sources: the distinction between primary and secondary data. Because secondary data are collected largely for general documentation and descriptive purposes, key data items may be missing or inadequately detailed to answer specific questions or test specific hypotheses. Furthermore, as we saw in Section 2.4, poorly reproducible measurements tend to reduce the magnitude of statistical associations between measured variables. For these reasons, many epidemiologic studies make use of primary data collected by the study's investigators. Secondary and primary sources can often be profitably combined, however, as when follow-up data are obtained from patients with a specific tumor who are identified from a cancer registry.

Whether individual or aggregated, primary or secondary, data concerning death, illness, recovery, and other discrete (i.e., categorical) events are usually expressed as epidemiologic rates. The definition and interpretation of these rates is the focus of the next chapter.

References

1. Feinstein AR (1972) The need for humanized science in evaluating medication. Lancet 2: 421–423
2. Yerushalmy J (1969) The statistical assessment of the variability in observer perception and description of roentgenographic pulmonary shadows. Radiol Clin North Am 7: 381–392
3. Feinstein AR, Gelfman NA, Yesner R (1970) Observer variability in the histopathologic diagnosis of lung cancer. Am Rev Respir Dis 101: 671–684
4. Karch FE, Smith CL, Kerzner B, Mazzullo JM, Weintraub M, Lasagna L (1976) Adverse drug reactions – a matter of opinion. Clin Pharmacol Ther 19: 489–492
5. Koch-Weser J, Sellers EM, Zacest R (1977) The ambiguity of adverse drug reactions. Eur J Clin Pharmacol 11: 75–78
6. Kramer MS, Leventhal JM, Hutchinson TA, Feinstein AR (1979) An algorithm for the operational assessment of adverse drug reactions. I. Background, description, and instructions for use. JAMA 272: 623–632

7. Hutchinson TA, Leventhal JM, Kramer MS, Karch FE, Lippman AG, Feinstein AR (1979) An algorithm for the operational assessment of adverse drug reactions. II. Demonstration of reproducibility and validity. JAMA 242: 633–638
8. Koran LM (1975) The reliability of clinical methods, data and judgments. N Engl J Med 293: 642–646, 695–701
9. Burgess AM, Tierney JT (1970) Bias due to nonresponse in a mail survey of Rhode Island physicians' smoking habits – 1968. N Engl J Med 282: 908
10. Siemiatycki J, Campbell S (1984) Nonresponse bias and early versus all responders in mail and telephone surveys. Am J Epidemiol 120: 291–301
11. Armstrong B, Doll R (1975) Environmental factors and cancer incidence and mortality in different countries, with special reference to dietary practices. Int J Cancer 15: 617–631

Chapter 3: **Rates**

3.1 What is a Rate?

Much of the last chapter focused on the principles, properties, and sources of individual measurements on individual subjects. As emphasized in Chapter 1, however, epidemiology is primarily concerned with groups rather than individuals. Consequently, methods are needed for summarizing or describing measurements in groups. For continuous variables, such summary measures include the mean, median, standard deviation, and other descriptors of the central tendency and spread of individual values within the group. These concepts and terms will be developed in Chapter 11.

For categorical variables, the usual summary measure is called a *rate*, or *proportion*, and is defined as the number of individuals in the category of interest divided by the total number of individuals in the group. For example, for the dichotomous variable vital status (alive vs dead), we can summarize the data for a group by reporting the death rate during a specified period of time, which is the number of deaths during the period divided by the total number of subjects in the group. Since vital status is dichotomous, we could equally well use the complement of the death rate [i.e., (1 − death rate)], or survival rate, to provide a summary measure for the group. For polychotomous variables, a full description of a group requires a rate for each category contained in the scale. To describe the degree of retinopathy in a group of patients attending a hypertension clinic, for example, we would give rates for each of the grades 0 (none) to IV (severe), according to the Keith-Wagener classification. Because categorical attributes or events assume such an important role in clinical and epidemiologic research, an understanding of rates is an important prerequisite to discussions of research design and statistical analysis.

A rate contains two essential components, a *numerator* and a *denominator*. Numerators alone convey little information and may be quite misleading. The number (or *count*) of individuals sharing some attribute or experiencing some event does not tell us whether that attribute or event is common or rare. Counts convey only anecdotes; rates are required to convey *frequency*. A report that ten patients with arthritis experienced a serious form of hepatitis (liver inflammation) while taking a certain medication might well alarm an unsophisticated public. The data become far less worrisome when this numerator is divided by the total number of arthritis patients taking the medication (e.g., 1 000 000) to yield a rate of 10/1 000 000, or 1 per 100 000. Our concern might disappear entirely if we then discover that this rate is no higher than the rate of hepatitis occurring in arthritis patients taking some other medication, or even in those taking no medication at all.

The importance of denominators can be illustrated further by analogy with batting averages. A baseball player's batting average is defined as the number of hits he obtains divided by his number of opportunities, i.e., appearances at bat, and is represented by a rate (to three decimal places) between 0 and 1. The professional baseball leagues award separate trophies for the player getting the most hits (counts) and the player achieving the highest average (rate). They are usually not the same player, however, since batters at the beginning of the lineup invariably get considerably more at bats, and thus a greater number of opportunities for hits. Their numerators are higher because their denominators are higher, but their average may be somewhat lower than those of players further down in the lineup, who have fewer at bats but a higher rate of success.

In constructing rates, the nature of the relationship between the numerator and denominator is of crucial importance. There are two main requirements:

1. The individuals counted in the numerator must be members of the group represented by the denominator. If we were interested in the rate of skin-test positivity for tuberculosis (TB) in a given community, the community census would provide the data for the denominator. Consequently, transients or recent immigrants not counted in the census should not appear in the numerator. Similarly, if the numerator is restricted to certain characteristics, the denominator should be similarly restricted. Rates restricted in this manner are called *specific rates*. Rates may be specified by age, sex, race/ethnic origin, or any other attribute of interest. The rate of TB skin-test positivity among white men 20–34 years of age is an example of a race-, sex-, and age-specific rate.
2. All "members" of the denominator group should be *eligible* to have the attribute or to experience the event counted in the numerator. In constructing uterine cancer rates, for example, women with prior hysterectomies and men should be removed from the denominator. (That this requirement is sometimes violated, however, is illustrated by the crude birth rate, in which the numerator is the number of live births, and the denominator is the *total* population rather than the number of women of child-bearing age.)

Occasionally, the sources of data for the numerator and denominator are different, and the requirements for constructing a rate are violated. Such measures are more properly called *ratios,* rather than rates, although the latter term is often loosely (and incorrectly) applied. For example, the annual maternal mortality "rate" of a population is defined as the number of deaths due to pregnancy, labor, or delivery divided by the number of live births occurring in that population during a given year. The true denominator is falsely lowered by excluding spontaneous and induced abortions, as well as unrecognized pregnancies, and is falsely (although only slightly) inflated by twin and triplet births.

I conclude this section with a semantic warning. As is unfortunately the case with many epidemiologic terms, *rate* can convey different meanings. For some epidemiologists, the notion of rate implies change over time, or slope, and they prefer to restrict the use of the word to this context [1]. Since *rate* has achieved such wide acceptance, however, both within and outside the field of epidemiology, I shall continue to use the term in the traditional and more general sense discussed above.

The concept of change over time is nonetheless of great relevance to the measurement of rates – so much so, in fact, that two different types of rates are used. One, called *prevalence,* is a static measure of rate at a single point in time. The other, *incidence,* is dynamic and measures the rate at which some attribute or event *develops* over a specific period of time. The distinction between prevalence and incidence is of fundamental importance in epidemiology and will be the focus of the following section.

3.2 Prevalence and Incidence Rates

3.2.1 Definitions

The *prevalence rate* (P) of an attribute or event in any group is the proportion of individuals in the group *having* that attribute or event at one point in time:

$$P = \frac{\text{number of individuals with attribute or event}}{\text{total number of individuals in group}}$$

It is thus a static measure, or "snapshot," of the frequency that *prevails* at a given moment.

In a *fixed group* of individuals, group membership is fixed at the beginning of the study, i.e., no new members are added during the study period. The *incidence rate* (I) is the proportion of any fixed group *developing* an attribute or event *within a specified time period.* The numerator consists of those individuals who were free of the characteristic at the beginning of the period and who developed it during the period. The denominator is the total number of individuals originally free of the characteristic who *could have* developed it during the period:

$$I = \frac{\text{number of individuals who develop attribute or event}}{\text{total number of individuals in group who could have developed attribute or event}} \quad \begin{array}{l}\text{per specified}\\ \text{time period}\end{array}$$

Incidence is thus a measure of frequency over time. It refers to change in status over a specified period, e.g., monthly incidence or annual incidence. Despite these clear differences between prevalence and incidence, clinicians and clinical investigators commonly confuse the two. In particular, "incidence" is often used as a generic term for "frequency," e.g., "The incidence [sic] of retinopathy among insulin-dependent diabetics at our medical center is 15%," or "The incidence [sic] of hepatic adenomas (benign liver tumors) in rats killed at 1 month was 4%." "Incidence" should be reserved for describing the frequency of newly occurring characteristics and should *always* be expressed as a function of time.

A problem arises in measuring the incidence of attributes or events that are transient and recurrent. For such characteristics, a choice must be made between the proportion of individuals in a group who develop one or more episodes within a period (the usual meaning of incidence) vs the number of episodes developing among group members within that period. The meaning of the two rates differs substantially: the proportion of individuals having at least one episode during the time period vs the average number of episodes per individual during the period. In measuring the yearly incidence of gastroenteritis among 50 infants attending a day-care center, for example, the incidence for episodes might be 100 for the 50 infants, or 200% per year. This figure might arise, however, as a result of five episodes each in 20 infants. The incidence of ≥ 1 episode for individuals would then be 40% per year. Unless otherwise specified, incidence rates are assumed to be based on individuals, rather than episodes.

The distinction between prevalence and incidence can be more easily appreciated if we consider the factors that can affect prevalence. In general, as incidence increases, so does prevalence. Duration of disease also has a marked effect, however: the longer the average duration (D) of an attribute or event, the higher the prevalence. Thus,

$$P \, \alpha \, I \cdot D$$

i.e., prevalence is proportional to the product of incidence and average duration. The average duration of any characteristic is dependent on two primary determinants: (a) its mortality and (b) its rate of disappearance (either spontaneously or in response to some treatment or other intervention).

A disease with a high incidence may therefore have a low prevalence if it is of short duration, e.g., the common cold or lung cancer. Conversely, a disease of low incidence can attain a high prevalence if it is incurable but nonfatal. In fact, medical treatment can (paradoxically) increase the prevalence of disease. A good example is end-stage kidney disease, where the availability of dialysis and transplantation has turned a previously rapidly fatal disease into a chronic illness with a prevalence that continues to rise.

Figure 3.1 depicts the experience of 40 subjects followed up for 1 year for the development of a (hypothetical) disease lasting 1 month. The distinction between incidence and prevalence can be clearly seen if we examine the situation at 6 months. The incidence of the disease over the first 6 months is 10/40, or 25%. The prevalence at 6 months, however, is 0%, i.e., none of the 40 subjects has the disease at that time. It is also apparent that if the average disease duration were, say, 1 year instead of 1 month, the prevalence would increase markedly. At 12 months, the prevalence would then be 20/40, or 50%, rather than 0%.

In groups or populations in which the occurrence of attributes or events is stable,

$$P \, \alpha \, I \cdot D \text{ becomes}$$
$$P = I \cdot D$$

"Stability" here means that incidence and average duration remain constant over time. Thus, if the incidence of a certain characteristic remains stable, and no change occurs in its rate of disappearance, its prevalence will also remain unchanged. In such situations, any two of these three quantities, if known, can be used to calculate the third. This is frequently the case for nonfatal, chronic illnesses such as arthritis

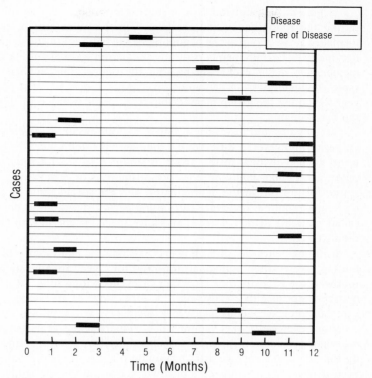

Fig. 3.1. Forty subjects followed up for 1 year for the development of a hypothetical disease with 1-month duration

and asthma. It is also true for fatal diseases (e.g., certain cancers) for which no effective treatment is available.

3.2.2 Incidence Rates for Prolonged Follow-up and Dynamic Groups

The definition of incidence presented so far applies only to fixed groups and outcomes that develop quickly, i.e., where the period of follow-up is exceedingly short. For many outcomes, including many chronic diseases of interest to epidemiologists, longer periods of follow-up are required, and study subjects may die, withdraw, or be lost to follow-up during the study period. With prolonged follow-up, it is highly unlikely that the individuals constituting the group at the end of the period will be the same as those present at the beginning. Which numerators and denominators should then be used in calculating the incidence rate?

The same questions arise in the study of *dynamic groups*. Dynamic groups differ from fixed groups in that new members can be added during the study period. If such individuals are counted in the numerator when they develop the outcome, how should the denominator be adjusted to reflect their shorter duration of follow-up?

In general, all individuals in a study group who develop the attribute or event during the follow-up period are placed in the numerator, even if they were not members of the group at the beginning of the period. For the denominator, the *average* number of group members during the period is usually used. If changes in group membership occur evenly throughout the period, the number at mid-period will serve adequately as the denominator. Thus, an incidence rate for a given calendar year would use the group membership (e.g., population) as of July 1 of that year for the denominator.

When gains and losses for a dynamic group occur *irregularly* during the follow-up period, however, a different denominator is often used. The duration of follow-up of each individual in the group is summed to yield a total number of person-durations. *Person-durations* (e.g., person-months or person-years) would then substitute for persons in the denominator, and the specification of time period is then no longer required. Incidence rates using person-durations as denominators are also called *incidence density rates* [2] and have special properties, to be discussed later in the text.

Even incidence densities, however, assume the equivalence of equal units of follow-up, i.e., that ten individuals followed for 1 year are equivalent to one individual followed for 10 years. For attributes or events with a long *latent period* (the period between exposure to a cause and the appearance of an effect), such an assumption can lead to an erroneous measure of incidence. For example, a group's adoption of a certain exercise or diet regimen may require many years before resulting in any subsequent reduction in cardiovascular mortality. If most individuals are followed up for only a year or two after beginning the diet, no beneficial effect may be seen, even if tens of thousands of individuals participate in the study. In other words, a large number of individuals followed up for a short period of time will lead to an underestimate of the true incidence. Adjustment of incidence for differential durations of follow-up is accomplished by means of life-table techniques. These will be taken up in Chapter 18.

3.2.3 Incidence Rates: Specific Examples

There are several attributes or events of particular interest to epidemiologists, and their incidence rates carry special names. The *death rate* (or *mortality rate*) is the number of individuals in a group who die within a given number of person-years of follow-up. When restricted to deaths caused by a specific disease, the incidence is referred to as the *disease-specific death* (or *mortality*) *rate*. This is to be distinguished from the disease-specific *case fatality rate*. Both rates have the same numerator, i.e., the number of individuals who die of the disease within the given period. The denominators are entirely different, however. For disease-specific mortality, the denominator consists of the total person-years of follow-up, whereas for case fatality, it is restricted to the number of individuals in the group who are affected by the disease.

When the time period at risk for development of a given attribute or event is limited, the incidence may be expressed as an *attack rate* without specifying the duration of time during which cases developed. The attack rate is of particular use in describing incidence during epidemics, when the susceptible population may be at risk only briefly following a single ("point") exposure to the responsible agent or until control measures (elimination of agent, quarantine of cases, or immunization of susceptibles) are successful in stopping the spread of the disease. For example, the incidence of staphylococcal "food poisoning" occurring after a picnic at which a contaminated food is consumed can be expressed as an attack rate, i.e., the proportion of individuals attending the picnic who developed symptoms of gastroenteritis during the ensuing hours. For outbreaks of contagious diseases, the *secondary attack rate* is often used to describe the incidence among susceptible contacts after the occurrence of a primary case.

The definitions of several kinds of annual incidence rates commonly used in reporting vital statistics are contained in Table 3.1.

3.2.4 The Uses of Incidence and Prevalence Rates

The incidence rate of an attribute or event is the frequency measure of choice when interest focuses on the *cause* of that attribute or event. Because causal factors operate prior to the development of the effects they cause, causal reasoning is enhanced by knowing that individuals are free of a characteristic (effect) before being exposed to the causal factor under suspicion. Furthermore, rapid recovery or death from the characteristic of interest will prevent its detection if only prevalence is known. In order to ensure detection of all new cases, however, calculation of incidence requires measurement of the characteristic in all individuals within a group at the beginning of follow-up and systematic assessment of its occurrence until the end of follow-up.

Table 3.1. Annual incidence rates used in vital statistics

Name	Numerator	Denominator	Expressed
Crude birth rate	Number of live births[a]	Mid-year population	per 1000
General fertility rate	Number of live births[a] to women 15–44 years	Mid-year population of women 15–44 years	per 1000
Crude mortality rate	Number of deaths	Mid-year population	per 1000
Maternal mortality rate	Number of deaths due to pregnancy, labor, and delivery	Number of live births[a]	per 100 000
Perinatal mortality rate[b]	Number of fetal deaths ≥ 20 wks gestation[a] plus infant deaths <7 days	Number of live births *plus* fetal deaths ≥ 20 wks gestation[a]	per 1000
Neonatal mortality rate	Number of deaths in infants <28 days	Number of live births[a]	per 1000
Infant mortality rate	Number of deaths in infants <1 year	Number of live births[a]	per 1000

[a] The definitions of "live birth" and "fetal death" are far from uniform. Some U.S. states, for example, require that a newborn or fetus weigh ≥ 500 g to count as either a live birth or fetal death, respectively [3].

[b] This measure is more appropriately called a *ratio*, rather than a *rate* (see p. 26).

Prevalence, on the other hand, is much easier to calculate, since it requires only one measurement of individuals in a group at a single point in time. No follow-up or repeat measurements are required. Furthermore, prevalence is quite useful for describing the extent or "burden" of an attribute in a given community, clinic, etc. Prevalence is therefore of great importance from a public health perspective, since health care services are often distributed according to need, i.e., existing health and disease status. For example, conditions like arthritis and heart disease usually consume far greater resources than do more commonly occurring but shorter-lived diseases like the common cold or viral gastroenteritis.

Finally, although not generally appropriate for making causal inferences, prevalence rates can occasionally be useful in suggesting hypotheses when incidence rates are unavailable. Comparison of the prevalence of cardiovascular disease among different types of societies, for example, might give rise to etiologic clues based on differences in diet, physical activity, or other characteristics of those societies.

One peculiar kind of rate, called the *period prevalence rate,* represents a hybrid of incidence and prevalence. It is defined as the proportion of individuals in a fixed group who *either* have a given characteristic at the beginning of a specified period or develop it during the period. It is thus the sum of the initial prevalence (also called the *point prevalence*) and the subsequent incidence. But since period prevalence has neither the etiologic advantages of incidence nor the public health utility of prevalence, it is little used in modern epidemiology.

3.3 Stratification and Adjustment of Rates

Comparisons are often made between rates in two or more groups for the purposes of generating or testing etiologic hypotheses. An important difference in death rates in two separate communities might, for example, lead to research into possible genetic, dietary, environmental, or psychosocial factors that might explain the difference. As in all comparisons, however, we must ensure that we are comparing like with like and that the presence of some extraneous factor is not biasing the comparison.

When we speak of bias in this context, we are referring to bias that occurs in comparing groups on some measured attribute, rather than bias in the individual measurements themselves. To be sure, as mentioned in Chapter 2, the latter can lead to information bias, which can indeed affect the statistical relationship between two variables. But even if the measurements themselves are perfectly valid, a comparison between groups on a given attribute can be biased if some extraneous factor that can affect that attribute *independently* of group membership is unequally distributed between the groups. This kind of bias is called *confounding bias,* and the factor responsible for creating the bias is called a *confounding factor* or *confounding variable.*

The concept of confounding is fundamental in epidemiology, and I shall have much to say about it throughout this text (especially in Chapter 5). For now, I shall limit the discussion to showing how it may bias a comparison between rates and how so-called *crude rates* may be *stratified* or *adjusted* to reduce or eliminate such bias.

Consider the example shown in Table 3.2, which compares the annual death rates in two (hypothetical) small U.S. communities, one a northeastern industrial town (Millville), the other a sun-belt retirement colony (Sunnyvale). The overall crude death rates in the two communities are shown in the last row of the table (columns 4 and 7). Contrary to what we might expect, Sunnyvale appears to be a considerably more lethal habitat than Millville, with an annual death rate twice as high (23.8 vs 11.0 per 1000 per year). A closer examination of the individual rows corresponding to different age groups or *strata,* however, reveals just the opposite. In each age stratum, the death rate in Sunnyvale is in fact lower than that in Millville. The discrepancy is caused by an age distribution that is quite different in the two communities, with Sunnyvale having a much older age structure (columns 2 and 5); 74% of the Millville population is under 45, compared with only 28% in Sunnyvale. Age is thus a confounding factor here. It is unequally distributed between the two groups and is independently related to the attribute of interest (death).

Stratification of rates is accomplished by comparing the stratum-specific, rather than overall, rates and is one method of eliminating bias due to confounding. We might, however, prefer some overall measure that combines the data from all strata without reintroducing bias. This is especially important when the stratum-specific rates reveal a mixed picture, with some rates higher in one group and other rates higher in the second. There are two frequently used methods for this overall type of adjustment: direct and indirect standardization.

For *direct standardization,* the observed stratum-specific rates in the two groups are applied to a third ("standard") group or population with known stratum structure. In Table 3.3, the age-specific death rates in Millville and Sunnyvale are applied to a standard population of 12 000 with an age distribution as shown in column 2. For each age stratum in column 1, the number of persons from the standard population in each stratum (column 2) is multiplied by the age-specific death rate for Millville (column 3) and Sunnyvale (column 5) to yield the number of deaths (columns 4 and 6, respectively) that *would be expected* if each community had the age structure of the standard population. The total number of "expected" deaths for each community (last row, columns 4 and 6) is then divided by the total population of 12 000 to yield the standardized death rates shown in the last row, columns 3 and 5. In con-

Table 3.2. Comparison of annual death rates in two (hypothetical) U.S. communities

Age stratum (1)	Millville Population (2)	Deaths (3)	Deaths/1000 (4)	Sunnyvale Population (5)	Deaths (6)	Deaths/1000 (7)
0–14	500 ⎫	2	4	400 ⎫	1	2.5
15–29	2000 ⎬ 74%	8	4	300 ⎬ 28%	1	3.3
30–44	2000 ⎭	12	6	1000 ⎭	5	5
45–59	1000 ⎫	10	10	2000 ⎫	18	9
60–74	500 ⎬ 26%	20	40	2000 ⎬ 72%	70	35
≧75	100 ⎭	15	150	400 ⎭	50	125
Total	6100	67	11.0	6100	145	23.8

Table 3.3. Direct standardization of annual death rates shown in Table 3.2

Age stratum (1)	Standard population (2)	Millville		Sunnyvale	
		Deaths/ 1000 (3)	"Expected" deaths (4)	Deaths/ 1000 (5)	"Expected" deaths (6)
0–14	500	4	2	2.5	1.25
15–29	2500	4	10	3.3	8.25
30–44	3000	6	18	5	15
45–59	3000	10	30	9	27
60–74	2500	40	100	35	87.5
≧75	500	150	75	125	62.5
Total	12000	19.6	235	16.8	201.5

formity with the stratum-specific rates, the overall standardized rates reveal a higher annual death rate in Millville (19.6 vs 16.8 per 1000).

Note that the choice of "standard" population is arbitrary. Generally speaking, the standard population should reflect the age distribution of the population to which one wishes to generalize the results. In the above example, the standardized rates tell us the deaths we could expect if the standard population of 12000 lived in Millville or Sunnyvale. A better standard might have been the entire U.S. population, as based on the most recent census. When no standard is available, the groups being compared are often combined into a single "standard." If the groups are of markedly unequal size, however, the larger group will have an undue influence on the adjusted overall rates.

Indirect standardization is used in one or more of the following circumstances:

1. When small numbers lead to potentially unstable (i.e., poorly reproducible) stratum-specific rates.
2. When the stratum structure (number of individuals in each stratum) of the standard population is unknown.
3. When the overall death rates and stratum structures are known for the compared groups but their stratum-specific rates are unknown.

Indirect standardization always requires knowledge of the stratum-specific rates for the standard population, however.

The method is illustrated for our Millville-Sunnyvale example in Table 3.4. Column 2 lists the age stratum-specific death rates for the standard population. These rates are then multiplied by the population in each stratum for Millville (column 3) and Sunnyvale (column 6) to yield the number of deaths (columns 4 and 7 respectively) that would be expected if the two communities experienced the same stratum-specific rates as the standard population. The total number of observed deaths for each community (last row, columns 5 and 8) is then divided by the total number of expected deaths in that community (last row, columns 4 and 7) to obtain a *standardized mortality ratio* (SMR) for each community. [Note that, as cited under point 2 above, the number of observed deaths in each stratum (columns 5 and 8) is

Table 3.4. Indirect standardization of annual death rates shown in Table 3.2

Age stratum	Deaths/1000 in standard population	Millville Population	"Expected" deaths	Observed deaths	Sunnyvale Population	"Expected" deaths	Observed deaths
(1)	(2)	(3)	(4)	(5)	(6)	(7)	(8)
0–14	3	500	1.5	2	400	1.2	1
15–29	4	2000	8	8	300	1.2	1
30–44	5	2000	10	12	1000	5	5
45–59	10	1000	10	10	2000	20	18
60–74	38	500	19	20	2000	76	70
≧75	140	100	14	15	400	56	50
Total	18.5[a]	6100	62.5	67	6100	159.4	145

$$\text{Standardizated mortality ratio (SMR)} = \frac{\text{Observed deaths}}{\text{Expected deaths}}$$

For Millville, $\text{SMR} = \dfrac{67}{62.5} = 1.072$

For Sunnyvale, $\text{SMR} = \dfrac{145}{159.4} = 0.910$

Indirectly standardized death rate = SMR × death rate in standard population
For Millville, standardized rate = 1.072 × 18.5 = 19.8 per 1000
For Sunnyvale, standardized rate = 0.910 × 18.5 = 16.8 per 1000

[a] Note that the overall death rate in the standard population must be known. It cannot be derived from the stratum-specific death rates without one also knowing the population in each stratum.

not required in making this calculation. Only the total is necessary.] Finally, each community's SMR is multiplied by the overall death rate in the standard population to obtain the indirectly standardized death rate. Once again, we see that the standardized rate is lower in Sunnyvale (16.8 vs 19.8 per 1000) despite its higher observed overall crude (unstandardized) rate.

In a way, the two methods of standardization are mirror images of one another. With the direct method, we calculate the number of "expected" deaths in the *standard population* based on *its* age distribution and the study group's stratum-specific death rates. With the indirect method, we calculate the number of "expected" deaths in the *study group* based on *its* age distribution and the standard population's stratum-specific death rates.

Since age affects many of the attributes and events of interest to epidemiologists, it is often a confounding factor when rates are compared. Depending on the attributes or events measured and the characteristics of the groups compared, other variables may have an equal or greater potential for confounding. For example, a comparison of death rates from lung cancer in asbestos vs coal miners should standardize by cigarette smoking status unless there is good reason to believe that the two groups of miners have similar smoking habits. The choice of variables by which to standardize thus depends on existing biologic and clinical knowledge (e.g., of the relationship between cigarette smoking and lung cancer), and on how well those variables can be measured.

3.4 Concluding Remarks

In this chapter I have discussed the intricacies of rates, summary descriptors of categorical variables measured in groups of individual subjects. The distinction between dynamic, time-dependent rates (incidence) and static rates (prevalence) measured at a single point in time has been emphasized. Finally, I have introduced the concept of confounding bias whenever rates are compared between two or more groups, as well as strategies for reducing such bias.

Now, before rates (or corresponding summary measures for continuous variables) are obtained, the groups of individual subjects whose characteristics are to be compared must be assembled and measured. The epidemiologic strategies for accomplishing these goals will form the basis of the next six chapters.

References

1. Kleinbaum DG, Kupper LL, Morgenstern H (1980) Epidemiologic research: principles and quantitative methods. Lifetime Learning Publications, Belmont, CA, pp 96–116
2. Miettinen O (1976) Estimability and estimation in case-referent studies. Am J Epidemiol 103: 226–235
3. Wilson AL, Fenton LJ, Munson DP (1986) State reporting of live births of newborns weighing less than 500 grams: impact on neonatal mortality rates. Pediatrics 78: 850–854

Chapter 4: Epidemiologic Research Design: an Overview

4.1 The Research Objective: Descriptive vs Analytic Studies

Broadly speaking, an epidemiologic study has one of two objectives: description or analysis. In a *descriptive study*, data are assembled and reported to summarize information (e.g., rate, mean, distribution) about one or more attributes in a group of subjects. No associations are sought, and no causes are inferred. Usually, the focus is on describing a *target population* having certain geographic, sociodemographic, and clinical attributes of interest. Since the entire target population is rarely available for study, however, the investigator must usually choose some method of selecting a study sample. Several aspects of sample selection will be discussed later in this chapter and in Chapter 5. For now, it suffices to say that the more representative the study sample is of the target population, the more valid will be the sample *estimate* of the population descriptor (e.g., rate or mean). Furthermore, the larger the size of the study sample, the more reproducible the sample estimate will be. Although assessing the reproducibility of a descriptor entails *statistical inference* (to be discussed further in Chapter 10), no *causal inference* is involved in descriptive studies.

In an *analytic study*, one or more groups are studied for the express purpose of drawing inferences about the association between two or more variables, particularly about a cause-and-effect association. In other words, the main objective in most analytic studies is *causal inference*. As in the case of descriptive studies, a sample must usually be selected from the relevant target population. The more representative the study sample is of the target population, the more valid will be the sample estimate of the association in the population. The larger the sample, the more reproducible the estimate.

The distinction between descriptive and analytic studies may not always be clear-cut. For example, a primarily descriptive study may compare and contrast descriptors between one or more subgroups within the study sample, thus examining the association (perhaps causal) between subgroup membership and the variable of interest. To the extent that inferences are drawn about such an association in the target population, such a study (or at least this aspect of it) should be considered analytic.

Most of our attention in this text will be focused on analytic research, because causal inference is usually required in studying etiology, treatment, prognosis, prevention, and health services evaluation. Even purely descriptive studies can be useful, however, in measuring the incidence and prevalence of important diseases in a population. Most of the vital statistics discussed in Chapters 2 and 3 are based on descriptive studies (even if routinely obtained by health authorities outside of any "research" context). In addition, descriptive studies are useful in describing the natural history or spectrum of clinical findings in a group of patients with a particular disease. They may also serve to generate hypotheses for future analytic studies.

In both descriptive and analytic research, the research objective must be clear and should be stated before the project is designed and before the data are collected. The importance of a clear objective cannot be overemphasized. If the purpose of the study is description, the target population and the variables to be described should be unambiguously identified. If the objective is analytic, the researcher should also indicate the attributes whose association is being investigated. The research objective for analytic studies can usually be phrased as a question and placed in the following format: "Does *exposure* of the *target population* to a putative causal agent or maneuver cause a certain *outcome?*" Thus, the target population, exposure, and outcome must all be clearly specified. Although I have already explained what I mean by target population, the concepts of exposure and outcome require fuller discussion.

4.2 Exposure and Outcome

The *exposure* is the putative causal factor, or effector, that the investigator believes may be (at least partly) responsible for the outcome under study. It may be a natural exposure, such as exposure to air pollution, cosmic rays, or environmental toxins. It may be an intrinsic characteristic of the subject, such as sex, race, or hemoglobin genotype. It may be a practice or exposure that the subject has selected for himself, such as smoking, jogging, or drunken driving. It might be a treatment that is prescribed by the subject's clinician. Finally, it could be a treatment that is imposed by the investigator himself, such as an investigational new drug. Thus, the exposure may be either active or passive.

In *observational studies* (also called *surveys*), the exposure is not assigned by the investigator. Because the exposure arises either naturally, by self-selection, or by prescription from a clinician, the investigator cannot be certain that groups with different exposures were equally susceptible to the outcome before they were exposed. This creates a potential for *confounding bias,* which, as we will see in the next chapter, poses major problems for causality inferences.

In an *experiment,* the exposure is assigned by the investigator. When assignment occurs in a randomized fashion, the potential for confounding bias is greatly reduced. This is the main reason why randomized experimental studies provide stronger evidence for causality than do observational studies.

The *outcome* in an analytic study is the effect that the investigator believes may be caused by exposure. It may be the occurrence of death or some other health or disease state (e.g., the development of emphysema after many years of cigarette smoking) or its prevention (e.g., a lower incidence of whooping cough among vaccine recipients). It could be the amelioration of a clinical condition, such as the resolution of acute otitis media (middle ear infection) following treatment with antibiotics. It may be the relief of pain, anxiety, or discomfort provided by a pharmaceutical agent or surgical procedure. Finally, it may be a change (for the better or worse) in quality of life associated with a certain treatment.

Exposure and outcome each can be measured on a continuous or categorical scale. The quantitative expression of the exposure-outcome association will depend on whether both are continuous, one categorical and the other continuous, or both categorical. It will further depend on whether categorical exposures or outcomes are dichotomous or polychotomous.

Regardless of the measurement scale, the study of an association between exposure and outcome depends on the presence of variation in both factors. If all study subjects have the same exposure, for example, measurement of their outcomes becomes a descriptive rather than an analytic study. A comparison of outcomes in two or more groups with different exposures would be considered analytic, since the association between exposure (group membership) and outcome can be assessed.

Finally, multiple exposures and outcomes can be investigated within the context of a single research study. For example, an investigator who wishes to study the therapeutic efficacy of a new cancer chemotherapeutic agent may be interested in studying the effect of that agent on survival, tumor size, relief of pain, and quality of life. All of these would be important outcome measures. Similarly, in studying possible causes (sometimes called *risk factors*) of a community outbreak of diarrhea, numerous food and water exposures might be investigated. Although efficient in practice and clinically sensible, such multiple testing for exposure-outcome associations creates certain problems for statistical inference, as we shall see in Chapter 12.

4.3 The Three Axes of Epidemiologic Research Design

Once the research objective for an analytic study has been adequately specified in terms of the target population, exposures, and outcomes, the next step is planning the *research design.* Epidemiologic research design can be considered from three distinct aspects: (a) directionality, (b) sample selection, and (c) timing.

Directionality refers to the order in which exposure and outcome are investigated: forward, from exposure to outcome; backward, from outcome to exposure; or simultaneously, exposure and outcome being determined at the same point in time, often without knowledge of which actually occurred first. *Sample selection* pertains to the criteria used to choose study subjects; it can be based on exposure, outcome, or other criteria. *Timing* concerns the relation between the time of the study proper and the calendar times of exposure and outcome: historical (exposure and outcome both occurred prior to the study); concurrent (exposure and outcome are contemporaneous with the investigation); or mixed timing. Although these three aspects of research design have often been confused, with considerable overlap between terms, what follows is an attempt to organize them into a unified nosology by using a distinct classification "axis" for each [1].

4.3.1 Axis I: Directionality

A *cohort study* is a study in which subjects are followed forward from exposure to outcome. By definition, study subjects are free of the outcome at the time exposure begins. The inferential reasoning in cohort studies is from cause to effect.

In *case-control studies,* the directionality is the reverse of that of cohort studies. Study subjects are investigated backwards from outcome to exposure. In case-control studies, we usually start with measurement of the outcome (often a classification of subjects into those with and those without the outcome), and we then ask or find out about prior exposure. The reasoning is from effect to cause.

In *cross-sectional studies,* exposure and outcome are determined at the same point ("cross section") in time, i.e., simultaneously. Since exposure and outcome have usually been present for some time prior to the study, it is not always obvious whether the exposure preceded the outcome. An outcome that occurs simultaneously with or precedes an exposure obviously cannot have been caused by that exposure. This well-recognized cart-vs-horse problem *(reverse causality bias)* often makes causality inference problematic in cross-sectional studies.

The term "simultaneous" is an approximation; the investigation focuses on exposure present around the same time as the outcome. A study subject questioned about current cigarette smoking habits is unlikely, of course, to be smoking during the actual interview. The important point is that in cross-sectional studies, the exposure measured corresponds roughly to the time at which the outcome is determined, rather than to a prior point or period of time consistent with the known or suggested biologic mechanism of causation (the so-called *latent period*).

4.3.2 Axis II: Sample Selection

Researchers can rarely study the entire target population, and therefore they usually must choose some method of sample selection. Since the main interest in epidemiologic research is the association (and presumed causation) between exposure and outcome, most studies will select their sample by either exposure or outcome. If the exposure is rare, a selection procedure that ensures a sufficient number of exposed subjects is necessary to provide a statistically meaningful result. The study may compare samples of exposed and unexposed subjects, subjects with different levels of exposure, or subjects exposed to two or more different agents or treatments. This is the kind of sample selection often employed in cohort studies. When the outcome is rare, selection by outcome may be necessary. This is the kind of sample selection usually employed in case-control studies; a sample of subjects with the outcome (cases) is compared with a sample without the outcome (controls) for their prior exposure.

Thus, sample selection is not entirely independent of directionality. Most cohort studies sample by exposure, and most case-control studies sample by outcome, while cross-sectional studies can use either method. Any of the three directionality designs, however, can use some form of subject selection from the target population other than exposure or outcome. For example, an investigator can select any group ("convenience" sample) of study subjects, measure their exposure, and then follow them forward in time (i.e., cohort directionality) to the development of the outcome. Similarly, in a case-control study, subjects can be selected without regard to exposure or outcome, classified by outcome, and then questioned about prior exposure to an agent or treatment of interest. These would not be statistically efficient strategies, however, when exposure (in cohort studies) or outcome (in case-control studies) is rare. Although cross-sectional studies often use this type of sample selection, their statistical efficiency can often be improved by selecting a sample either by exposure or outcome, depending on which is rarer in the target population.

Regardless of which criteria are used to select study subjects, those subjects should be representative of their counterparts in the target population. In other words, when a sample is selected by exposure, sample subjects should be representative of those members of the target population having the studied levels of exposure. When selected by outcome, sample cases and controls should be representative of cases and controls in the target population. Finally, when "other" criteria are used, sample subjects should be representative of the overall target population. If study subjects are truly representative of their counterparts in the target population, then the results of the study can be safely extended to that population. If the sample is not known to be representative, the main concerns are the potential for sample distortion bias (discussed in Chapter 5) and uncertainty as to whom the study results may be applied.

One way of ensuring representativeness is by *random sampling*. In *simple random sampling,* each member of the target population has an equal probability of being selected for the study, and that probability depends only on chance, i.e., a random event, and not on either the investigator or the subject. The usual way this is achieved is by obtaining a list of persons in the target population and then using a table (or computer-generated list) of random numbers to assign a number to each person.

An example of a random number table is contained in Appendix Table A.1. The table can be entered at any point, e.g., at the beginning or by pointing while "blindfolded." The investigator then continues through the table, either down the columns or across the rows, assigning successive numbers to the next person on the list. The "rules" for sample selection should be established beforehand and are based on the size of the desired sample. If a 50% simple random sample (of the target population) is needed, odd- or even-numbered persons could be selected. For a 25% sample, those persons whose number is evenly divisible by 4 could be chosen. A similar procedure can be used for any fixed fraction (e.g., 1/10, 1/30, 1/100). If a specific number of sample subjects is desired, e.g., 137, then the subjects with the 137 highest (or lowest) numbers can be chosen. The main requirement is that the method of selection is decided *before* entering the table, so that neither the subject nor the investigator can exert any influence on the choice.

In *stratified random sampling,* individuals from certain clinical or sociodemographic subgroups (strata) are selected more frequently. This strategy is often used to ensure that the study sample is representative of the target population with respect to subgroup (stratum) membership, e.g., race, sex, marital status. It is also essential in examining results separately in those subgroups that, owing to their small size, may require oversampling to provide more stable (reproducible) estimates.

Finally, *clustered random sampling* involves the random selection of natural groups (clusters) of subjects, such as households or villages. This method is often used for practical reasons: to reach a greater number of subjects with a limited amount of research personnel or other resources.

4.3.3 Axis III: Timing

When both exposure and outcome occur (or begin) prior to the selection of study subjects, the timing is *historical.* Alternatively, both exposure and outcome may occur as the investigator studies them (concurrently). Or, as is the case in many studies, the exposure may have occurred in the past, but the outcome is concurrent. This is an example of a *mixed timing* research design. Designs combining subjects with historical exposure and outcome and others with concurrent exposure and outcome are also considered to have mixed timing. These distinctions are important only to the extent that measurement of exposure is enhanced (i.e., more valid and reproducible) when planned and implemented by the investigator. Historical studies may be more prone to misclassification of exposure and/or outcome than concurrent cohort studies and hence may be less sensitive for detecting a true exposure-outcome association.

As with sample selection, timing is somewhat dependent on the directionality of the study design. Its major relevance is for cohort studies, which can easily accommodate any of the three timing strategies. Most cross-sectional studies are concurrent, while most case-control studies use a mixed timing design.

4.3.4 Summary of Three Axes

Each axis thus has three different points:

For directionality: cohort, case-control, or cross-sectional
For sample selection: by exposure, outcome, or other criteria
For timing: historical, concurrent, or mixed

Seven designs are defined by directionality and sample selection (see Table 4.1). Cohort studies can select study samples by exposure or other criteria; case-control

Table 4.1. Classification of epidemiologic research designs defined by directionality and sample selection[a]

	Directionality		
	Cohort	Case-control	Cross-sectional
Sample selection			
Exposure	A	–	E
Outcome	–	C	F
Other	B	D	G

[a] Capital letters refer to examples in the text.

studies, by outcome or other criteria; and cross-sectional studies, by any of the three.

Each of the directionalities can incorporate either incident or prevalent outcomes. *Incident outcomes* develop de novo during subject enrollment or follow-up, whereas *prevalent outcomes* are those present at a single point in time. Most cohort studies use incident outcomes, although one could imagine a design in which the (prevalent) outcome was determined at a single point in time during follow-up after exposure. For example, current blood pressure might be measured in a group of adults followed since birth, with exposure defined as salt intake during infancy or childhood. Cross-sectional studies generally utilize prevalent outcomes, but incident outcomes are also feasible. Patients presenting with myocardial infarction, for example, might be interviewed concerning their current smoking habits. Case-control studies are common using either incident or prevalent cases of the outcome.

When prevalent outcomes are used and sample selection is by criteria other than exposure or outcome, the distinction between cohort and case-control studies disappears. Directionality can be either forward or backward, and the results can be analyzed using either the cohort or case-control approach. A study of the relationship between current blood pressure and prior salt intake in a community random sample could therefore be classified as either a cohort or case-control design.

Finally, the distinction between case-control and cross-sectional studies can also become blurred under certain circumstances. When sample selection is based on outcome and the exposure variable is a permanent attribute (e.g., sex, race, or blood group) that can be assumed to have been present prior to the outcome, simultaneous and prior exposure are equivalent. Similarly, whenever simultaneous exposure is a valid proxy for exposure occurring at a time in the past consistent with the known or suspected biologic mechanism of causation, the two designs become interchangeable. Thus, it may sometimes be more useful to think about epidemiologic research designs not as discrete entitites, but as lying on a continuous spectrum without sharp boundaries.

4.3.5 Examples

The following examples constitute seven different ways of examining the same basic research question:

Does occupational exposure to asbestos increase the risk of subsequent lung cancer?

Each example listed in Table 4.1 (as indicated by its letter A to G) illustrates one of the seven basic designs defined by directionality and sample selection. Each of these seven basic combinations can incorporate historical, concurrent, or mixed timing, thus yielding a total of 21 different research designs. These are illustrated in Fig. 4.1, which represents a $3 \times 3 \times 3$ cube with two "tunnels" indicating the six impossible combinations (sample selection cannot be by outcome in cohort studies or by exposure in case-control studies). The figure also indicates the seven basic designs illustrated in the examples.

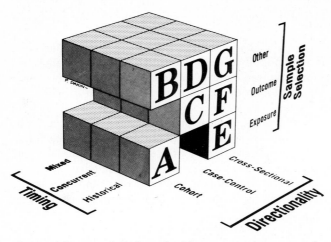

Fig. 4.1. The research design cube. The two tunnels represent the six impossible combinations of directionality and timing. Capital letters refer to the seven basic designs listed in Table 4.1 and illustrated in the text

A. *Cohort study with sample selection by exposure.* In this type of study, a group of workers who were exposed to asbestos over 30–40 years might be followed up for development of lung cancer and compared with a group of workers who were not exposed to asbestos.

B. *Cohort study with "other" sample selection.* This study would be similar to A, except that instead of sampling exposed and nonexposed workers, we might select all workers in a given plant, determine their cumulative exposure, and then follow them all up for subsequent development of lung cancer.

C. *Case-control study with sample selection by outcome.* Workers who have developed lung cancer are compared with a group of those who have not for a history of prior exposure to asbestos.

D. *Case-control with "other" sample selection.* This is similar to C, except that instead of choosing groups of cases and controls, all workers in a given plant are selected for study. Lung cancer status is determined, and workers with and without disease are compared for their history of prior asbestos exposure. This design would be inefficient relative to C, since very few workers would be expected to have lung cancer at any given point in time.

E. *Cross-sectional study with sample selection by exposure.* Workers with and without exposure to asbestos are compared for the simultaneous presence or absence of lung cancer. This design would share the same inefficiency as D but would have the additional cart-vs-horse causality inference problem of not knowing whether the exposure occurred at a biologically relevant time in the past (cf. "latent period").

F. *Cross-sectional study with sample selection by outcome.* The records of workers with and without lung cancer at a specific point in time are compared for simultaneous exposure to asbestos. This design would be more efficient than E because of the rarity of lung cancer but would share its inferential shortcomings.

G. *Cross-sectional study with "other" sample selection.* All workers in a given plant are classified simultaneously by asbestos exposure and lung cancer status. This design would share the same inefficiency as D and E and the same causality inference problem as E and F.

4.3.6 "Prospective" and "Retrospective" Studies

"Prospective" and "retrospective" are two of the most familiar, and most confusing, terms used in describing epidemiologic research designs. These terms have been applied to all three of the methodologic aspects (axes) discussed above. For example, "prospective" has been interpreted by various authors as indicating forward directionality, sample selection by exposure, or concurrent timing. Conversely, "retrospective" has been used to indicate backward directionality, sample selection by outcome, or historical timing. Some authors have even gone so far as to use a combined nomenclature, leading to such semantic difficulties as "historical prospective" studies. Furthermore, these two terms have also been used to indicate an important aspect of the statistical analysis, namely, whether the hypotheses tested were enunciated prior to data analysis ("prospective") or were "generated" by the data analyzed, i.e., arose post hoc ("retrospective"). Thus, as shown in Table 4.2, there appear to be at least four current usages of these two terms. To prevent what would otherwise be inevitable confusion, I will avoid the terms entirely.

4.4 Concluding Remarks

Because both the logic of causal inference and the statistical expressions of exposure-outcome associations depend largely on directionality, Axis I will serve as the major axis of classification, and hence as the basis for the chapter headings in the remainder of Part I of this text. I have devoted one chapter each to observational cohort studies and experimental cohort studies (also called *clinical trials*). These will be followed by chapters on case-control and cross-sectional studies.

Table 4.2. Usages of the terms "prospective" and "retrospective"

Methodologic aspect	"Prospective"	"Retrospective"
Directionality	forward	backward
Sample selection	by exposure	by outcome
Timing	concurrent	historical
Hypothesis testing	a priori	post hoc

Before discussing these designs in further detail, we need to consider a methodologic issue relevant to all epidemiologic research, regardless of design: *analytic bias*. The types, sources, and control of analytic bias are the focus of the following chapter.

Reference

1. Kramer MS, Boivin J-F (1987) Toward an "unconfounded" classification of epidemiologic research design. J Chronic Dis 40: 683–688

Chapter 5: **Analytic Bias**

5.1 Validity and Reproducibility of Exposure-Outcome Associations

In this chapter we are concerned with bias that arises in making inferences about the causal relationship between exposure and outcome in a particular target population, based on data in a study sample from that target population. As discussed in Chapter 4, both exposure and outcome can be measured on either a continuous or a categorical scale, and the measure of their association usually takes one of two forms: (a) a difference in outcome means or rates in two or more exposure groups or (b) a statistical index of the exposure-outcome interrelationship. The purpose of an analytic epidemiologic study is to provide a valid estimate of this measure, and bias is the extent to which the sample estimate *systematically* differs from the true value of the association in the target population. A biased (invalid) inference can also occur if the temporal sequence between exposure and outcome is reversed in the target population, i.e., if the study outcome actually precedes and causes the hypothesized exposure.

It is important to emphasize the distinction here between bias in estimating an association, which is called *analytic bias,* and bias in the performance of individual measurements. The latter was discussed extensively in Chapter 2. Although biased measurements are one source of analytic bias, perfectly valid measurements are no guarantee against a biased estimate of association.

In addition to speaking about the validity of an association, we can also refer to its reproducibility. Because of random variation in the individual measurements and the size of the study sample, the magnitude of the estimate of an association might not be highly reproducible. Repetitive sampling of study subjects from the same target population would result in a range of estimates for different samples. This concept is known as *sampling variation* and will be discussed in greater detail in Chapters 10 and 12. For now, it suffices to say that the smaller the sample, the less reproducible will be the sample estimate. In the absence of analytic bias, however, the *average* estimate should equal the true value of the association in the respective target population. Since we usually can study only single samples from the target populations of interest, we calculate a range in which we are reasonably confident that the true value must lie. The methods for making such calculations comprise an important aspect of *statistical inference* and will be taken up in Part II of this text. The important point here is that, as with individual measurements, exposure-outcome associations can be highly reproducible without necessarily being valid.

5.2 Internal and External Validity

The effect of analytic bias is to invalidate an inference about the causal effect of exposure on outcome in the target population. *Internal validity* is the extent to which the *analytic inference* derived from the study sample is correct for the target population. In other words, analytic bias impairs a study's internal validity. Internal validity also depends on proper statistical inference about the target population based on data obtained in the study sample.

The *external population* is a large group of persons with less restrictive attributes than those of the target population but to whom the investigators may wish to generalize the study's results. The *external validity*, or *generalizability*, of a study is the extent to which an exposure-outcome association found in the study sample is also true in the external population. Obviously, external validity is dependent on internal validity. Results that are not valid for the target population will not be valid for the external population. Thus, striving for internal validity by avoidance of analytic bias becomes the methodologic sine qua non for any analytic epidemiologic study. If internal validity is assured, an investigator can maximize external validity by selecting study subjects from a target population as similar as possible to the external population to which he (or others) may wish to generalize the study's results.

The relationships between the study sample, target population, and external population, and their relation to internal and external validity are shown in Fig. 5.1.

A good illustration of these concepts is the Veterans Administration clinical trial of the treatment of hypertension (high blood pressure [1]). The study sample consisted of 143 men who were 30–73 years of age and veterans of the U.S. armed forces, had average diastolic blood pressures ranging from 115 to 129 mm Hg, were initially free of complications of hypertension, and were compliant with treatment. The results showed a reduction in complications (death, stroke, and eye, heart, or kidney damage) in those who received the active treatment (a combination of hydrochlorothiazide and reserpine). The reduction was statistically significant, i.e., chance (random variation) could be reasonably excluded as an explanation. The study was carefully designed and analyzed and seems free of analytic bias, so its

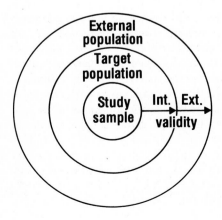

Fig. 5.1. Internal and external validity

Table 5.1. The four sources of analytic bias

---

1. *Sample distortion bias:* estimate of exposure-outcome association is biased because the study sample is unrepresentative of the target population with respect to the joint distribution of exposure and outcome.
2. *Information bias:* estimate of exposure-outcome association is biased as a result of error in measurement of exposure or outcome.
3. *Confounding bias:* estimate of exposure-outcome association is biased by one or more variables associated both with exposure and, independently of exposure, with outcome.
4. *Reverse causality bias:* estimate of exposure-outcome association is unbiased in magnitude but biased in the inferred direction of causality, because the study outcome actually preceded and caused the exposure.

---

internal validity is generally accepted. The main controversy concerns its external validity. Are the results also applicable to nonveterans? To women? To younger or older patients? To patients with lower or higher diastolic blood pressures? To those who already have complications? To those who are less compliant with treatment? These questions are difficult or impossible to answer from the study, and subsequent studies of antihypertensive therapy have been required to provide such answers.

External validity, although useful conceptually, is often difficult to evaluate, since the degree to which results valid in one population can be generalized to another depends on clinical judgment and other factors beyond the realm of research design or statistical analysis. Therefore, the remainder of this chapter will concern internal validity and, in particular, sources of analytic bias and strategies to reduce it. Proper statistical inference, the second requirement for internal validity, will be the focus of Chapters 12–15.

The sources of analytic bias can be classified into four broad categories: (a) *sample distortion bias,* (b) *information bias,* (c) *confounding bias,* and (d) *reverse causality* ("cart-vs-horse") *bias.* They are summarized in Table 5.1 and will be discussed in turn.

5.3 Sample Distortion Bias

Neither an investigator nor the public he intends to benefit is particularly interested in results that apply only to the subjects participating in a given study. Unless the study subjects are representative of some target population of interest, the results will have little meaning. Since, for reasons of feasibility, the entire target population can rarely be studied, some sample selection procedure, whether explicit or implicit, must usually be employed. When the study sample is distorted either at the time that subjects are selected or (in cohort studies) during follow-up, sample distortion bias may occur. *Sample distortion bias*[1] is a systematic error in the estimation of the

---

[1] Many authors use the term *selection bias* to refer to what I have called sample distortion bias [2]. But "selection bias" has also been used by some epidemiologists to indicate the confounding effect that can occur when study subjects (or their families, physicians, or other proxies) *select* their own exposure. To avoid confusion, I will use the term "exposure selection bias" to refer to this type of confounding (see Section 5.5).

degree of exposure-outcome association in the target population caused by a study sample that is unrepresentative (with respect to the joint distribution of exposure and outcome) of that target population.

As outlined in Chapter 4, sample selection can occur by exposure, outcome, or other criteria. If by exposure, the investigators want the sample subjects to be representative of those persons in the target population exposed or not exposed (or exposed to different degrees) to the agent or treatment under study. If selected by outcome, the sample subjects should be representative of all those persons in the target population with the outcome under study. If sample selection is by other criteria, the investigator must ensure that he knows the characteristics of the target population of which the sample is representative.

In practice, it is often difficult to list, or even identify, all the members of the target population. In most instances, the investigator does not have access to the entire target population, even if he knows who or where they are. He usually chooses some accessible group or groups, characterizes them as best he can by relevant sociodemographic and clinical attributes, and then mentally attempts to construct the theoretical target population that he believes is represented by his sample.

This process, however, is fraught with difficulty. As shown in Fig. 5.2, distortion can occur at several steps in the selection and assembly of the study sample. Persons in the investigator's geographic region may not be representative of those in the entire target population of interest. If the study sample is based on patients who are referred in from the community, further distortion may occur. Moreover, the inves-

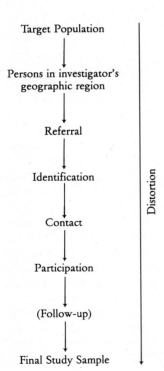

Fig. 5.2. Sources of possible distortion in the selection and (for cohort studies) follow-up of a study sample

tigator may be unable to identify all patients referred to his center, he may fail to contact some of those he can identify, and a sizeable number of those he does contact may not agree to participate.

It is important to point out, however, that nonrepresentativeness does not *necessarily* lead to bias. In particular, the association between exposure and outcome will be biased only when the sample distortion is *differential* with respect to exposure and outcome. If sample selection is by outcome, for example, bias will be introduced only if, for a given outcome status, the exposures in subjects who are studied are different from those who are not. Suppose that we wish to use a case-control design to investigate the association between cigarette smoking and lung cancer. Even if our cases (lung cancer patients) and controls are not representative of all cases and controls in the target population, no bias will occur in the estimate of the smoking-lung cancer association unless the cases (or controls) in the sample are either more or less likely to have a history of cigarette smoking than those in the target population.

In cohort studies, sample distortion can occur owing to geographic maldistribution; referral patterns; selective identification or contact of potential subjects; selective participation (response); or death, withdrawal from the study, or other loss to follow-up (see Fig. 5.2). If subjects who die, withdraw, move away, or refuse to respond before the outcome is determined are different with respect to their exposure-outcome relationship than those remaining in the study, bias will be introduced. For example, in a cohort study of the relationship between radiation exposure and subsequent leukemia, if many subjects with heavy exposure move away from the study site and are particularly likely to develop leukemia, the true magnitude of the association will be underestimated.

Case-control and cross-sectional studies share the same sources of sample distortion bias as cohort studies. The absence of follow-up in case-control and cross-sectional designs, however, means that death, withdrawal, moving away, and other losses are "hidden," in the sense that they have already occurred by the time the study samples are selected. Since the outcome status is already determined at the time the study is begun, any distortion, and, hence, bias arising therefrom, has already occurred.

A specific type of sample distortion bias can occur in case-control or cross-sectional studies carried out in a referral setting. Consider, for example, the association between two factors (usually two diseases, one of which can be thought of as the "exposure" and the other, the "outcome," i.e., one disease that is hypothesized to cause, or predispose to, the other), each of which is subject to referral. The coincidence of (positive association between) the two factors will then be falsely elevated. Persons with both factors have a higher probability of being referred into the study center than those with either factor alone, since they have two "chances" of referral instead of just one. For example, if 50% of patients with disease A and 50% of patients with disease B are referred, those with A or B alone will each have a 50% chance of referral, whereas those with both will have a 75% chance (50% referred for disease A and 50% of the remainder for disease B). Thus, among referred patients selected into a study sample, the proportion with both diseases will be higher than the proportion in the community. This problem was originally described by Berkson in case-control studies carried out in a hospital setting, and the resulting bias is often referred to as *Berkson's bias* [3, 4].

What can be done about sample distortion bias? Once the study is completed and the data are obtained, the problem may be beyond repair. The exposure and outcome status are unknown, of course, for members of the target population who were not selected or were lost to follow-up. Otherwise they would have been included. Unless at least the relative probabilities of initial inclusion and (for cohort studies) subsequent loss are known for all combinations of exposure and outcome, no adjustment can be made. Since specific data from previous studies concerning inclusion and loss as a function of exposure and outcome are not generally available, the best the investigator can do is to estimate the magnitude of the *potential* bias and mitigate his inferences accordingly.

Sometimes, even the maximum possible bias would not affect a study's overall result. In the previously cited Veterans Administration trial of antihypertensive therapy [1], the investigators ruled out possible sample distortion bias due to study dropouts by assuming a "worst case" scenario (complications in all dropouts from the active treatment group but in none of the dropouts from the control group). Even if this unlikely possibility had occurred, the results would still have favored the active treatment group.

As elsewhere in medicine, however, prevention is preferable to cure. The best way to avoid bias due to sample distortion is to strive for random (or otherwise representative) sampling when study groups are assembled and, in cohort studies, to minimize losses due to dropouts, nonresponse, or incomplete follow-up.

5.4 Information Bias

Information bias, which was mentioned in Chapter 2, is the bias that occurs in assessing the association between exposure and outcome as a result of error in measurement of exposure or outcome status. If the errors are random (i.e., the measurements have poor reproducibility), the bias will always be toward reducing the extent of association. In other words, highly variable but unbiased measurements will lead to an underestimate of the magnitude of the exposure-outcome association. In engineering parlance, the "signal-to-noise ratio" will be reduced.

Systematically biased individual measurements will have different effects, depending upon whether the bias is *nondifferential* (the same bias occurs with different exposure-outcome combinations) or *differential* (the bias changes according to exposure and outcome status or occurs only with certain exposure-outcome combinations). Nondifferentially biased individual measurements lead to a falsely low estimate of the exposure-outcome association. Differentially biased measurements, however, can lead to either a falsely low or a falsely high estimate, depending on the pattern of bias within exposure-outcome combinations.

Thus, "sloppy" or nondifferentially biased measurements usually lead to conservative estimates of the exposure-outcome association. As discussed in Chapter 2, this can be considered either beneficial or harmful, depending on one's point of view. Differentially biased measurements, however, can create statistically significant associations that do not, in fact, exist. Differentially biased measurements are particularly likely to occur when study subjects and/or observers are aware of (i.e., are not "blind" to) the research hypothesis and the subjects' exposure or outcome status.

Differentially biased measurement can also occur whenever outcome detection procedures vary with exposure. This bias (which is also called *detection bias*) may result from more frequent or thorough surveillance (in cohort studies) or from the more frequent use of diagnostic tests and is particularly likely to occur when the outcome can occur "silently," i.e., when detailed examination or special tests may be required to detect it. In a cohort study comparing rates of subsequent breast cancer in users and nonusers of oral contraceptives, for example, more frequent physical examinations or roentgenography (mammograms) might occur in users, who require regular contact with their gynecologists in order to renew their oral contraceptive prescriptions. Since many early breast cancers can be detected only by careful examination or roentgenography, this source of information bias could create a false association between contraceptive use and breast cancer.

As with sample distortion bias, little can be done about information bias once the study data are collected. Unless the direction and magnitude of the measurement errors are known for different exposure-outcome combinations (e.g., differences in surveillance and detection), the best the investigator can do is estimate the effect of the potential bias and moderate his inferences accordingly. Partial control for detection bias can sometimes be achieved, however, by stratification or multivariate statistical control for the frequency or intensity of surveillance or diagnostic testing.

On the other hand, much can be done in the design and execution stages to minimize information bias. Procedures for surveillance (in cohort studies) and detection of the outcome should be standardized, established before the study begins, and maintained until completion. Measurements of exposure and outcome should be carried out by trained observers using pretested methods, so that the reproducibility and validity of the measurements are maximized. Study subjects and observers should, whenever scientifically feasible and ethically defensible, be kept "blind" to the research hypothesis (the hypothesized exposure-outcome association). Observers should also be blind to the subjects' exposure (for cohort studies) or outcome (for case-control studies) status. In summary, information bias can be minimized by standardizing detection procedures, maintaining a high quality of individual measurements, and adequately blinding subjects and observers.

5.5 Confounding Bias

5.5.1 Definition

Confounding bias is present whenever the sample estimate of association between exposure and outcome is distorted by one or more extraneous variables. An extraneous variable will confound the exposure-outcome association whenever the variable (a) is associated with exposure; (b) is associated with outcome, independently of exposure; (c) does not lie on the hypothesized causal path from exposure to outcome. A variable that satisfies all three of these criteria is called a *confounding variable* or *confounding factor*.

A variable related only to exposure will not confound the exposure-outcome association. For example, in studying the possible association between maternal alcohol (ethanol) consumption and low birth weight, investigators know that members of certain religious groups are less likely to drink alcohol than others. Unless religion is a risk factor for low birth weight *independently* of its association with drinking, however, no bias will be introduced.

Similarly, a variable related only to outcome, and not to exposure, will not confound the exposure-outcome association. It is known, for example, that short mothers tend to have small babies. Unless short mothers differ in their drinking habits from taller mothers, however, the association between alcohol consumption and low birth weight will remain unbiased.

Cigarette smoking, on the other hand, might indeed confound an association between maternal drinking and birth weight. Not only is smoking known to be an independent risk factor for low birth weight, but it is also associated with drinking, since drinkers are more likely to smoke than nondrinkers. Thus, criteria (a) and (b) are both satisfied. Since the causal path by which maternal alcohol consumption reduces fetal growth does not involve cigarette smoking, criterion (c) is also met.

Control for a variable that lies on the causal path between exposure and outcome will lead to a biased underestimate of exposure-outcome association. In a study of the association between maternal smoking and infant mortality, birth weight is not a confounder, even though it is positively associated with both maternal smoking and infant death. Because smoking may cause infant death *through* its effect on reducing intrauterine growth (and increasing the risk of premature birth), control for birth weight would falsely reduce and perhaps even eliminate the effect on infant mortality.

When a variable satisfies all three criteria for confounding, it should be controlled for. When a variable not lying on the causal path from exposure to outcome is associated with either exposure or outcome, but not both, the estimate of exposure-outcome association will be unbiased whether or not the variable is controlled for. In studies where the variable under consideration is continuous and is associated with a continuous outcome, controlling for that variable may enhance the reproducibility of the estimate of exposure-outcome association. In other types of studies, however, such control may yield no benefit or even reduce the reproducibility of the estimate.

5.5.2 Sources of Confounding

Confounding can arise in several ways:

1. The underlying *susceptibility* or risk for developing the outcome is higher at baseline, i.e., prior to exposure, in one exposure group than in another *(susceptibility bias)*. A study designed to assess the effect of fishing (as an occupation) on the risk of skin cancer, for example, should ensure that the proportion of subjects with fair complexions is similar among the fishermen and in the control group. Because fair-skinned persons are far more susceptible to skin cancer, their unequal distribution (fishermen vs nonfisherman controls) would confound any association between fishing and skin cancer.

2. Study subjects or their families, physicians, or other proxies *select* their own exposure, and the motive or reason for selection is associated with outcome *(exposure selection bias)*. Exposure selection bias is, in fact, a special case of susceptibility bias. For example, an observational cohort study comparing maternal attachment behavior in breast-feeding and bottle-feeding mothers is likely to be confounded if mothers who select breast-feeding differ in important psychological ways that influence their behavior toward their infants.

Observational studies of treatment effects are highly prone to this type of bias, because the clinical *indications* for certain treatments may be strongly related to the outcome, independent of treatment. Miettinen refers to this as *confounding by indication* [5]. As an example, many new and experimental, but toxic, cancer chemotherapeutic agents are given only to patients with advanced disease who have been resistant to all conventional treatments. An observational study would likely reveal that patients treated with such a drug were more likely to die. The result is confounded, however, by the selection of patients who were likely to die anyway as treatment subjects.

3. The exposure is accompanied by other agents or maneuvers that can affect ("contaminate") the outcome *(accompaniment bias or contamination bias)*. This source of confounding is particularly likely to occur in studies of treatment. Patients receiving a promising new treatment may receive more attention, better nursing care, and better general supportive therapy than those receiving the "standard" treatment, and these accompaniments may be responsible for a more favorable outcome in the former group.

5.5.3 Control for Confounding Bias

Confounding can be controlled in either the research design or data analysis phase. In the design, the best way of eliminating susceptibility and exposure selection biases, where feasible, is to use an experimental design (i.e., clinical trial) and to *randomly assign* exposure to study subjects. Although, as will be discussed further in Chapter 7, randomization does not guarantee that these sources of confounding will not occur, it renders the possibility far less likely.

When a randomized clinical trial is infeasible, susceptibility and (to some extent) exposure selection bias can be reduced by *restriction* of the study sample according to certain characteristics (e.g., exclusion of men or nonsmokers) or by *matching* members of the compared groups according to the potentially confounding variables. Matching can be accomplished either within study groups (i.e., equalize the average value or distribution of the confounders within each group) or with individuals (each subject in one group is matched to one or more subjects in the comparison group). Both approaches result in bias reduction. The choice between the two will depend on the type of confounding variable, i.e., continuous vs categorical, and if categorical, on the number of categories.

Even if no control for susceptibility or exposure selection biases is incorporated in the study design, the investigator should attempt to measure factors that could potentially confound the exposure-outcome association. These factors can then be controlled for later in the analysis. Furthermore, to control for contamination bias in concurrent cohort studies, study subjects and their care-givers should be blind, where feasible, to both the study hypothesis and the subjects' exposure status.

Control for confounding in the data analysis stage can be accomplished in several, nonmutually exclusive ways:

1. *Restriction* in the analysis is, of course, automatic if restriction was incorporated in the design. If not part of the design, a restricted analysis (e.g., analyzing only the results in women or nonsmokers, rather than in all study subjects) will "waste" data in subjects not meeting the restriction criteria. This not only reduces the sample size and, therefore, the reproducibility of the resulting estimate of the exposure-outcome association, but also distorts the original study sample so that it no longer represents the original target population.

2. *Matching* should be used in the analysis if it was used in the design; otherwise, the resulting estimate of the exposure-disease association will be less reproducible. Matching in the analysis in a study without a matched design carries the same "waste" and sample size penalties as mentioned for restriction.

3. *Stratification* and *standardization* accomplish the same goal as restriction but do not waste data, because all study subjects can be included in one or another stratum. These methods were illustrated in Chapter 3 in comparing death rates in Millville and Sunnyvale. Community of residence is the "exposure" variable here, and death is the outcome. The overall death rates favor Millville but are confounded by age (the population of Sunnyvale being much older). The age stratum-specific and overall adjusted rates control for confounding bias and demonstrate that Sunnyvale, in fact, has a lower death rate for similarly aged persons. Stratification and standardization will be illustrated futher in Chapters 6 and 8.

One of the disadvantages of these methods is that simultaneous control of several confounders requires a separate stratum for the combination of each confounder with every other. This not only becomes computationally unwieldy, but also results in small (and thus poorly reproducible) numbers in each stratum.

4. *Multivariate statistical techniques* can be used to control simultaneously for several confounding variables. Modern computer technology and readily available statistical software packages enable calculations of an unbiased estimate of exposure-outcome association after adjustment for the association of each confounder with exposure, outcome, and other confounders. Although multivariate statistical techniques are largely beyond the scope of this text, they will be discussed briefly in Chapters 13–15.

5.6 Reverse Causality ("Cart-vs-Horse") Bias

An internally valid inference about causality depends on temporal sequence; obviously, exposure can cause outcome only if it precedes it. Particularly in cross-sectional studies (see Chapter 4), deciding which is the "cart" and which is the "horse" is not always straightforward. Certain exposure factors are known to be present from birth, such as sex, blood type (ABO system), and racial origin. But for other factors, it may be difficult to be sure whether exposure preceded outcome or vice versa.

Cohort studies can protect themselves against this problem by ensuring that study subjects are free of the outcome at the time exposure begins. Case-control studies can use incident outcomes and specifically inquire about *prior* exposure, although exposure histories depend on valid records or subject recall. An experimental approach (clinical trial) provides the best evidence that exposure precedes outcome, since subjects are assigned their exposures by the investigator.

5.7 Concluding Remarks

Recognition of the sources of potential analytic bias and the appropriate methods for their avoidance and reduction are of fundamental importance in epidemiologic research. The study of human beings is far more complex than experimental studies of animals, cells, or biochemical extracts. Human behavior can influence the formation of groups, sampling, measurement, and the outcome itself.

Total absence of analytic bias, however, is an illusory goal. Validity is not a dichotomous concept, and most studies are both valid and invalid to varying degrees. The presence of a small potential source of bias does not necessarily invalidate a study's findings. Black and white answers are rare; most scientific advances depend on shades of gray. It requires considerable experience to interpret shades of gray, i.e., to appreciate which biases, real or potential, are serious. Since the perfect epidemiologic study has yet to be carried out, unfettered criticism can result in a rather depressing scientific nihilism. It is useful to reflect, however, that landmark epidemiologic studies that have changed the history of medicine would all, if placed under the epidemiologic "microscope," reveal imperfections.

Epidemiologic knowledge advances in spite of analytic bias. It advances more surely, however, when careful attention is given to proper design and analysis. In the discussion of the specific research designs and statistical techniques that follow, I shall continue to emphasize the importance of controlling bias and the techniques for doing so.

References

1. Veterans Administration Cooperative Study Group on Antihypertensive Agents (1967) Effects of treatment on morbidity in hypertension: results in patients with diastolic blood pressures averaging 115 through 129 mmHg. JAMA 202: 186–192
2. Kleinbaum DG, Morgenstern H, Kupper LL (1981) Selection bias in epidemiologic studies. Am J Epidemiol 113: 452–463
3. Berkson J (1946) Limitations of the application of fourfold table analysis to hospital data. Biometr Bull 2: 47–53
4. Walter SD (1980) Berkson's bias and its control in epidemiologic studies. J Chronic Dis 33: 721–725
5. Miettinen OS (1983) The need for randomization in the study of intended effects. Stat Med 2: 267–271

Chapter 6: Observational Cohort Studies

6.1 Research Design Components

6.1.1 Introduction

An analytic cohort study is a study in which subjects are followed in a forward direction from exposure to outcome:

exposure $\longrightarrow$ outcome

Analytic cohort studies can be either experimental (exposure assigned by the investigator) or observational (exposure arises naturally, is selected by the subject, or is prescribed by the subject's clinician). Experimental cohort studies, which are usually called *clinical trials*, have achieved such widespread importance[1] that we will delay our discussion of them until Chapter 7. This chapter will be limited to a consideration of observational cohort studies.

6.1.2 Sample Selection (Assembling the Cohort)

As discussed in Chapter 4, two methods are available for sample selection in cohort studies: by exposure status or by "other" criteria. If by exposure, the study sample should be representative of exposure groups in the target population. If by "other" criteria, the sample should be representative of the entire target population. A nonrepresentative sample makes it difficult to judge the population of individuals to whom the study's results apply. Of the two choices, sample selection by exposure is usually preferable when exposure is rare in the target population, in order to have enough exposed subjects in the sample to provide statistically meaningful results. For example, studying the carcinogenic effects of exposure to an unusual environmental toxin can best be achieved by finding as many exposed subjects as feasible, rather than by choosing a "convenience" or random sample of the entire target population.

Sample selection by exposure implies the use of a discrete number of exposure categories, i.e., a dichotomous or ordinal measure of exposure. When the exposure

---

[1] In fact, when the term "cohort study" is otherwise unspecified, it usually refers to an observational, rather than an experimental, design. In accordance with this practice, we shall, in the remainder of this text, use "cohort study" for the observational design, and "clinical trial" for the experimental one.

under study is measured on a continuous scale, it is necessary to categorize the exposure data. For example, cigarette smoking can be measured as a continuous variable: the number of cigarettes smoked per day. It can be easily dichotomized or "ordinalized," however. We might compare outcomes in smokers vs nonsmokers or in light (≤ 5 cigarettes/day) vs heavy (≥ 6 cigarettes/day) smokers. Or we might use a four-category ordinal scale: nonsmokers, and those smoking 1–5, and 6–10, and ≥ 11 cigarettes/day.

The nonexposed (or least exposed) group in a cohort study is often called the *control group* or *control cohort*. When a new treatment is compared with some existing "standard" treatment, subjects receiving the standard treatment are also referred to as the control group. The degree of exposure-outcome association then becomes the difference in outcome occurring in the control and other exposure group(s).

6.1.3 The Baseline State

The *baseline state* of a cohort consists of the characteristics of its members before exposure. It includes geographic, sociodemographic (age, sex, race, marital status, socioeconomic status), and clinical attributes. Knowledge of the true baseline state is possible only when the cohort is assembled before exposure begins. In practice, however, cohorts are often assembled when exposure has already occurred, or at least begun. The investigator must then endeavor to define the baseline state that existed before onset of exposure to ensure that the study subjects' attributes are not in themselves caused by exposure. This poses no problem, of course, for "permanent" attributes like race and sex, but may be quite difficult for various health and disease states (other than the outcome under study) that might be affected by exposure.

The main importance of an adequate description of the baseline state is the control for confounding bias, particularly the bias (susceptibility bias) that can occur in estimating the exposure-outcome association when the underlying susceptibility for developing the outcome is associated with exposure, e.g., is different in exposed vs nonexposed subjects. As explained in Chapter 5, this source of confounding can be controlled in either the design or analysis. Failure to describe the baseline state adequately and to take the necessary design or analytic precautions can lead to analytic bias and an internally invalid inference regarding the exposure-outcome association.

6.1.4 Exposure

As explained in Chapter 4, the term "exposure" is to be interpreted in its broadest sense. It may represent a genetic, geographic, sociodemographic, or clinical attribute that the investigator believes to be associated with the outcome under study; a natural exposure to some environmental agent or event; a practice that the subject has chosen for himself; or an intervention prescribed by the subject's clinician.

Exposure may be measured on either a categorical or a continuous measurement scale. Although many cohort studies use a dichotomous measure of exposure (exposed vs nonexposed, high vs low exposure, treatment A vs treatment B), causality inferences can often be strengthened by finding a graded response (a *dose-response effect*) according to exposure. This can be achieved by using three or more ordinal categories of exposure and demonstrating a monotonically increasing or decreasing outcome response with higher categories of exposure. It can also be achieved with continuous exposure measures by demonstrating an important positive or negative association with outcome.

The exposure may be brief and occur only once (so-called *point exposure*), e.g., the atomic bomb explosions in Hiroshima and Nagasaki. It may consist of repeated episodes of brief exposure *(recurrent exposure)*, such as habitual drunken driving. Or it may be continuous *(chronic exposure)*, such as an infant's exposure to toxic lead paint in the home or the daily administration of estrogen to a postmenopausal woman.

The *potency* of the exposure must be clinically appropriate for the exposure-outcome association under investigation [1]. Studying the effect of an exposure that is too weak may result in a negative result (i.e., no exposure-outcome association) that may not represent the true biological consequences of degrees of exposure that commonly occur in the "real world." Conversely, the dramatic effect of an exposure that is too potent may have little clinical relevance to real-world consequences of commonly occurring exposure.

Potency includes both the quantity and quality of the exposure. *Quantity* refers to how much of the agent, maneuver, or treatment is received, i.e., the dosage and duration of exposure. Drugs that are administered in doses that are too low or too high may yield results of little relevance for clinical practice, as are those administered for too brief or too long a period of time. The *quality* of the exposure refers to how well, i.e., with what degree of skill, it is administered. An inexpert surgeon, psychotherapist, or physiotherapist may produce bad results even if the procedure performed is potentially efficacious.

The *timing* of exposure is also important. Intrauterine rubella infection leads to severe congenital malformations when it occurs early in the first trimester of pregnancy but has few if any fetal consequences when it occurs later in gestation.

When study subjects (or their clinicians) select their exposure, the opportunity arises for confounding due to exposure selection bias. This is particularly likely to occur when the exposure is a clinical treatment, and the reason for selecting the treatment is itself associated with the study outcome. Such confounding by indication, which was discussed in Chapter 5, is one of the reasons why clinical trials are usually preferable to observational cohort studies in investigating clinical treatments.

Another source of confounding associated with exposure is contamination bias. If other agents or maneuvers with independent effects on the study outcome are also associated with exposure, the effects of the study exposure will be contaminated by those of the accompanying exposures. This is particularly likely to occur in studies of treatment. For example, patients with coronary heart disease who receive a "promising" new drug may do better than those not receiving the drug, not because the drug is efficacious, but because they are subjected to intensive monitoring that allows early detection and treatment of cardiac arrhythmias (rhythm disturbances).

6.1.5 Follow-Up

The follow-up of subjects before, during, and after exposure is an important research design feature in cohort studies and can have a marked effect on the results. Follow-up begins at a point in time often referred to as *zero time* [2]. Although zero time may not be specified by name, the choice of time of entry and beginning follow-up of study subjects is often a crucial decision in the design of a cohort study. All other time measurements depend on it.

The usual choice for zero time is the time at which exposure begins. Other choices, such as the time at which subjects agree to participate or the time they become "eligible" for exposure, may be better in some situations, however. This is particularly so in studies of treatments that may require a long waiting period. A comparison of dialysis and kidney transplantation in prolonging survival of patients with end-stage kidney failure thus needs to take into account that dialysis can begin almost immediately, whereas transplant patients may have to wait months or even years for a suitable donor to appear.

Another important aspect of follow-up is that its duration should be adequate. Adequacy of the duration of follow-up is determined by the biological (clinical) relationship between exposure and outcome. It may be known from animal experiments or previous clinical studies, for example, that the potential effect of a given exposure develops only after a certain period of time (the *latent period*). For infectious diseases, the time between exposure to the infectious agent and the development of clinical symptoms and signs of infection is called the *incubation period*. This usually represents the time required for the agent to multiply and for the host to mount its response. The latent period for other types of exposures (e.g., carcinogenic, dietary, or "life-style" factors) may be years. Consequently, a cohort study of the alleged benefits of a diet low in animal fat should ensure follow-up for several decades if a difference in cardiovascular mortality is to be discerned.

It is also important that the *potential* duration of follow-up not vary according to exposure status. (The *actual* duration of follow-up may be shorter in the exposed group, however, if exposure causes death. In that case, death should be included among the study outcomes.)

Losses to follow-up (subjects who die from causes other than the study outcome, withdraw from study participation, or cannot be located by the investigators) create two kinds of problems. First, losses of large numbers of study subjects may result in a diminished sample size that prevents the exposure-outcome association from achieving statistical significance (discussed further in Chapter 12). If the outcome is categorical, too few outcome events may occur among remaining subjects to provide statistically meaningful results. The second problem is that losses may occur differentially by exposure and outcome (sample distortion bias), and the resulting measure of exposure-outcome association, even if statistically significant, may be invalid. Thus, cohort studies should attempt to maximize follow-up of study subjects and to characterize those who are lost in an attempt to estimate (if unable to quantitate) the potential bias that might have occurred.

The final important issue in follow-up is related to clinical surveillance and detection of the outcome. If the intensity (quality and quantity) of surveillance during follow-up varies according to exposure, then the observed exposure-outcome association will be biased (detection bias). This is particularly relevant for outcomes that are "silent" and require physical examination or special diagnostic tests. Avoidance of detection bias can best be achieved by ensuring that the frequency and extent of surveillance are standardized in the design protocol and are followed and maintained irrespective of exposure status.

6.1.6 Outcome

The outcome is the effect that the investigator suspects may be caused by exposure. As discussed in Chapter 4, it is usually the change (occurrence, disappearance, improvement, or relief) in some health or disease state. In many cohort studies, several outcomes are investigated simultaneously. In particular, it is often clinically important to measure "soft" as well as "hard" outcomes, especially in studying the effects of treatment. As indicated in Chapter 2, there has been a tendency in much clinical research to emphasize easily quantifiable outcomes, even if they do not best reflect the results of treatment. In a study of the effects of a new cancer chemotherapeutic agent, for example, pain and quality of life may be even more important to patients than duration of survival or the size of the tumor.

Measurement of the outcome in cohort studies provides the greatest opportunity for information bias. Although random measurement errors (for either exposure or outcome) will generally reduce the extent of exposure-outcome association, systematic errors in measuring outcome that vary according to exposure can create an exposure-outcome association in the study sample when none in fact exists in the target population (see Chapters 2 and 5). This is particularly likely to arise when observers of a "soft" (subjective) outcome are aware of both the association under investigation and the subjects' exposure status. Adequate blinding of observers is thus necessary to avoid this source of information bias. As indicated above, avoiding the assessment of "soft" outcomes is not a satisfactory solution.

The quantitative expression of the exposure-outcome association is the subject of the following section. Since the expression and analysis of the results of a cohort study depend on the measurement scales in which exposure and outcome are expressed, the discussion will be organized accordingly.

6.2 Analysis of Results

6.2.1 Exposure: Categorical
Outcome: Continuous

The main result of interest in these studies is the mean $(\bar{x})$ of the outcome variable in each of the exposure groups ($\bar{x}_1$ for exposure group 1, $\bar{x}_2$ for exposure group 2). The larger the difference in mean outcomes ($\bar{x}_2 - \bar{x}_1$) between exposure groups, the greater the exposure-outcome association.

Let us take as an example a hypothetical cohort study of the effect of exposure to asbestos on cardiopulmonary fitness as reflected by the time taken to run a 100-m race. The study subjects are 100 exposed male asbestos miners and 100 nonexposed healthy men of similar age. The exposed and nonexposed cohorts had the same mean times for running the 100-m race before exposure occurred in the miners, and both groups have been observed for 10 years without loss to follow-up. After 10 years, the mean time taken to run the 100 m in the exposed group is 14.4 sec, compared with 12.2 sec in the nonexposed (control) group. The difference of 2.2 sec is the *magnitude* of the effect of exposure on outcome and expresses the degree of association of the outcome with the exposure. Another way of expressing the results is a percent change from the control mean:

$$\text{percent change} = \frac{\bar{x}_2 - \bar{x}_1}{\bar{x}_1} (100) = \frac{14.4 - 12.2}{12.2} (100) = 18.0\%,$$

i.e., this type and extent of exposure to asbestos made the men 18.0% slower in the 100-m race.

If we had had three exposure groups (nonexposed, lightly exposed, and heavily exposed), we would have three means ($\bar{x}_1$, $\bar{x}_2$, $\bar{x}_3$) to compare instead of just two. Each exposure group could then be compared with the control (nonexposed) group to see if the mean were different. A monotonically graded dose-response effect (e.g., 12.2 sec in the nonexposed, 13.5 sec in the lightly exposed, and 15.6 sec in the heavily exposed) would strengthen the inference of causality between exposure and outcome (discussed further in Chapter 19).

6.2.2 Exposure: Continuous
Outcome: Continuous

To illustrate this situation, we will use the same example for outcome as in Section 6.2.1 (time to run 100 m), but the exposure of interest will now be cigarette smoking, expressed on a continuous scale as the number of cigarettes smoked per day. Although the investigator could choose to categorize the continuous exposure measure (e.g., 0, 1–5, 6–10, ≥11 cigarettes/day) and then express and analyze the results as was shown in Section 6.2.1, a more direct approach involves the use of linear regression and correlation. This approach assesses the extent to which a unit change (increase or decrease) in exposure (number of cigarettes smoked) is accompanied by a corresponding change (in the same or opposite direction) in outcome (time to run 100 m). Linear regression and correlation will be discussed in detail in Chapter 15.

6.2.3 Exposure: Continuous
Outcome: Categorical

Such a situation might occur, for example, if we wished to study the relationship between cigarette smoking, expressed as number of cigarettes per day, and myocardial infarction (heart attack) expressed dichotomously as present or absent. This type of study is the inverse of the study described in Section 6.2.1, in which the mean outcomes were compared between two exposure groups. One approach to the analysis of results of this type of study would be to compare the mean exposures in the two outcome groups, those with and without myocardial infarction. Such an analysis, however, ignores the forward directionality inherent in a cohort study. It bears a closer resemblance to an analysis that may be used in case-control (backwardly directed) studies. Comparing exposures among subjects experiencing different outcomes is a rather indirect way of telling us what we really want to know, i.e., a comparison of outcomes among subjects experiencing different exposures. Thus, it would be preferable to take advantage of the forward directionality of a cohort study by categorizing exposure and then analyzing the results in the fashion demonstrated in the following section.

6.2.4 Exposure: Categorical
Outcome: Categorical

Many cohort studies utilize this format, the simplest example of which is a dichotomous exposure and a dichotomous outcome. The general case is illustrated in Table 6.1, and a hypothetical example is shown in Table 6.2. The latter compares the rate of myocardial infarction (heart attack) in 200 smoking and 200 nonsmoking

Table 6.1. Two-by-two table for analyzing results of a cohort study with dichotomous exposure and outcome

	O	$\overline{O}$	
E	a	b	$a+b$
$\overline{E}$	c	d	$c+d$
	$a+c$	$b+d$	$N=a+b+c+d$

E, Exposed; $\overline{E}$, nonexposed; O, outcome; $\overline{O}$, absence of outcome

Risk of outcome in exposed $= \dfrac{a}{a+b}$

Risk of outcome in nonexposed $= \dfrac{c}{c+d}$

Relative risk (RR) $= \dfrac{\dfrac{a}{a+b}}{\dfrac{c}{c+d}}$ (Eq. 6.1)

Attributable risk (AR) $= \dfrac{a}{a+b} - \dfrac{c}{c+d}$ (Eq. 6.2)

men followed up for 20 years (without losses). Tables such as 6.1 and 6.2, which characterize groups simultaneously by two dichotomous variables, are known as 2×2 (two-by-two), or *fourfold*, *tables*. The totals to the right are called the *row totals*, those on the bottom are the *column totals*, and the total on the bottom right is the *grand total* (i.e., the total study sample).

The rate of MI among the smokers is 32/200, or 16%, compared with 15/200, or 7.5%, among the nonsmoking controls. Note that these rates are, in essence, incidence rates, since they express the occurrence of new events over a specified period of time. Thus, the incidence of MI among smokers is 16% per 20 years, or 0.8% per year. If the two cohorts (exposed and nonexposed) are *fixed* (i.e., no members are added during the period of follow-up), then the incidence of the outcome is equivalent to an individual member's *risk*, or *probability*, of developing the outcome during the study period. When the cohorts are *dynamic* (i.e., members are added during follow-up), the term *incidence density* (see Chapter 3) is probably preferable, although "risk" is often used loosely for dynamic cohorts as well.

There are various ways in which the two risks or incidence rates can be compared. The two most common are their ratio and their difference. These are called the *relative risk* (also called the *risk ratio*) and the *attributable risk* respectively,

Table 6.2. Cohort study of 200 smokers and 200 nonsmokers (controls) for occurrence of myocardial infarction (MI)

	MI	No MI	
Smokers	32	168	200
Nonsmokers	15	185	200
	47	353	400

Risk of MI in smokers $= \dfrac{32}{200} = 16\%$

Risk of MI in nonsmokers $= \dfrac{15}{200} = 7.5\%$

Relative risk (RR) $= \dfrac{\dfrac{32}{200}}{\dfrac{15}{200}} = 2.13$

Attributable risk (AR) $= \dfrac{32}{200} - \dfrac{15}{200} = \dfrac{17}{200} = 8.5\%$

$$\text{where relative risk (RR)} = \frac{\text{risk in exposed}}{\text{risk in nonexposed}} = \frac{\dfrac{a}{a+b}}{\dfrac{c}{c+d}} \qquad (6.1)$$

and attributable risk (AR) = risk in exposed − risk in nonexposed

$$= \frac{a}{a+b} - \frac{c}{c+d} \qquad (6.2)$$

The relative risk can take on any value ≥ 0. RR = 1 indicates no exposure-outcome association (thus, 1 is often called the *null value*). Values between 0 and 1 indicate a negative association, i.e., exposure protects against the outcome. Values above 1 indicate a positive association, i.e., exposure increases the risk of the outcome.

For our smoking-MI example, the relative risk is

$$\frac{\dfrac{32}{200}}{\dfrac{15}{200}}, \text{ or } 2.13$$

The attributable risk is $\dfrac{32}{200} - \dfrac{15}{200} = \dfrac{17}{200}$, or 8.5%

Both the relative risk and the attributable risk provide useful information, but their interpretations are quite different. In general, the relative risk provides the best estimate of the strength or magnitude of the exposure-outcome association and is therefore useful for making causal inferences. The attributable risk is more useful for public health purposes, since it indicates the frequency with which the outcome can be attributed to exposure in the sample studied and, by extension, to the target population of interest.

The contrast between RR and AR is illustrated in Table 6.3, which compares the two measures obtained from two cohorts, nonsmokers and heavy (>25 cigarettes/day) smokers among British male physicians from 1951 to 1961 [3]. When relative risks are compared, the relationship between cigarette smoking and lung cancer (RR = 32.43) appears stronger than that between smoking and cardiovascular

Table 6.3. Comparison of deaths from selected causes associated with heavy cigarette smoking by British male physicians

Cause of death	Death rate[a] in nonsmokers	Death rate[a] in heavy smokers	Relative risk	Attributable risk[a]
Lung cancer	0.07	2.27	32.43	2.20
Cardiovascular disease	7.32	9.93	1.36	2.61

[a] Annual death rate per 1000.

disease (RR = 1.36). A comparison of attributable risks, however, gives quite a different impression (AR = 2.20 per 1000 per year for lung cancer vs 2.61 per 1000 per year for cardiovascular disease).

Given a constant relative risk, attributable risk rises with the incidence of the outcome in the nonexposed group. The results for lung cancer and cardiovascular disease shown in Table 6.3 are thus explained by the higher "natural" (i.e., in the nonexposed) annual incidence of cardiovascular death (7.32 per 1000) compared with lung cancer death (0.07 per 1000).

An additional measure is sometimes used to indicate the impact of exposure on outcome in the target population from which the study sample derives. It is called the *etiologic fraction* (EF)[1] and measures the *proportion* of all cases of outcome in the target population that are attributable to exposure. Alternatively, the EF can be interpreted as the proportion of cases of the outcome that would disappear if exposure were eliminated in the target population. It is defined as follows:

$$EF = \frac{r_T - r_{\bar{E}}}{r_T} \tag{6.3}$$

where r_T is the risk of the outcome in the total target population and $r_{\bar{E}}$ is the corresponding risk in those who are unexposed. An algebraically equivalent form that is easier to calculate is:

$$EF = \frac{P_E(RR - 1)}{P_E(RR - 1) + 1} \tag{6.4}$$

where RR is the relative risk and P_E is the prevalence of exposure in the target population [4]. If the relative risk is assumed to remain constant from one population to another, the etiologic fraction is useful in comparing the proportion of outcome attributable to exposure in settings with different prevalences of exposure. For example, if maternal smoking doubles the risk of giving birth to an intrauterine growth-retarded (IUGR) infant, one-third of the IUGR rate can be attributed to maternal smoking in a population in which half the women smoke during pregnancy (EF $= \frac{0.5(2-1)}{0.5(2-1)+1} = \frac{0.5}{1.5} = 0.33$) vs one-eleventh in a population in which only 10% smoke.

As mentioned earlier, RR, AR, and EF all refer to fixed cohorts without losses or additions during the period of follow-up. In practice, however, most cohorts are dynamic. Some attrition (death from causes unrelated to the study outcome, withdrawal from study participation, loss to follow-up) is inevitable. Furthermore, subjects may be enrolled in a study over time, rather than simultaneously. Thus, the *period at risk* may differ for many members of the cohorts.

As discussed in Chapter 3, when the changes in cohort membership occur evenly during the period of follow-up, the *average* number of group members can be used in the denominator to calculate the incidence rate, and this will serve as an approxi-

---

1 *Population attributable risk* and *attributable risk fraction* (or *percent*) are frequently encountered synonyms.

mation of the risk. When group gains and losses occur irregularly during the follow-up period, however, it is preferable to use person-durations in the denominator. The resulting rate is called an incidence density (ID) [5]. Although many investigators use IDs to calculate relative and attributable risks, the corresponding indexes are probably better referred to as the *incidence density ratio* (IDR) and *incidence density difference* (IDD) respectively.

Another approach to the problem of unequal duration of follow-up is necessary, however, whenever equivalence of person-durations cannot be assumed. The existence of a prolonged *latent period* between exposure and outcome (particularly common with carcinogens and cancer) means that 100 subjects followed up for 1 year may not yield the same number of outcome events as ten subjects followed up for 10 years, even though both cohorts contribute 100 person-years to the denominator. In such cases, risk calculations need to be adjusted for differential duration of follow-up. The technique involved is called life-table (or survival) analysis, and this will be taken up in Chapter 18.

Finally, to illustrate how a polychotomous ordinal measurement of exposure can demonstrate a dose-response effect of exposure on outcome, let us re-examine the smoking-MI question. Instead of dichotomizing study subjects as either smokers or nonsmokers, we shall now classify them according to a three-category ordinal scale as nonsmokers, light smokers (1–5 cigarettes/day), or heavy smokers (≥ 6 cigarettes/day). The (hypothetical) results for the 400 study subjects are shown in Table 6.4. We have assumed that the 200 subjects classified as smokers in Table 6.2 distribute themselves equally between "light" and "heavy." The relative risk (RR) and attributable risk (AR) in the two smoking groups are calculated using the risk in the nonsmoking group as a "base," and the graded response is evident (RR = 1.60 among light smokers and 2.67 among heavy smokers).

When exposure is measured on a continuous scale (e.g., number of cigarettes smoked per day), classification into three or more ordinal categories, as demonstrated in Table 6.4, enables risks to be assessed as a function of exposure. Furthermore, such a classification still permits the demontration of a dose-response effect of exposure. This is the procedure often used for continuous exposures and categorical outcomes (see Section 6.2.3)

Regardless of how the sample estimate of exposure-outcome association is expressed, we must also concern ourselves with its internal validity. Internal validity requires adequate control for analytic bias and sufficient reproducibility of the sample estimate of the exposure effect, which depends on the extent of variability within the exposure groups and on the size of the sample. Assessment of the role of chance (sampling variation) in producing an observed exposure-outcome association will be discussed in detail in Chapters 12–15. The assessment and control of analytic bias is the focus of the following section.

Table 6.4. Cohort study of myocardial infarction and cigarette smoking using three-category ordinal scale of exposure

	MI	No MI	
Heavy smokers	20	80	100
Light smokers	12	88	100
Nonsmokers	15	185	200
	47	353	400

$$\text{Risk of MI in nonsmokers} = \frac{15}{200} = 7.5\%$$

$$\text{Risk of MI in light smokers} = \frac{12}{100} = 12\%$$

$$RR = \frac{\frac{12}{100}}{\frac{15}{200}} = 1.60$$

$$AR = \frac{12}{100} - \frac{15}{200} = \frac{9}{200} = 4.5\%$$

$$\text{Risk of MI in heavy smokers} = \frac{20}{100} = 20\%$$

$$RR = \frac{\frac{20}{100}}{\frac{15}{200}} = 2.67$$

$$AR = \frac{20}{100} - \frac{15}{200} = \frac{25}{200} = 12.5\%$$

6.3 Bias Assessment and Control

As in other types of analytic studies, minimizing analytic bias is essential in assuring the internal validity of observational cohort studies. Three of the four general types of analytic bias are important considerations in cohort studies: information bias, sample distortion bias, and confounding bias. (The fourth type, reverse causality bias, is less of a concern, because the forward directionality of cohort studies indicates that exposure precedes outcome, particularly if the study subjects are known to be free of the outcome in their baseline state.)

As to information bias, random measurement errors will bias the exposure-outcome association (i.e., RR) toward unity (the null value), as will systematically biased measurements that are biased in the same direction, irrespective of exposure and outcome. Nonblind observation of the outcome, however, can bias the RR away from 1 when observers are aware of both the association under study and the exposure status of the study subjects. When surveillance (detection) differs by exposure status, systematic information bias can also occur. Consequently, the best protection against information bias in cohort studies is in their design. Measurements should be of proven reproducibility and validity and should be performed by observers who are blind to the subjects' exposure status. Detection bias can be minimized by standardizing both the frequency and content (e.g., examinations, special diagnostic tests) of all follow-up procedures, to ensure that they occur independently of exposure.

Sample distortion bias can occur in assembling the cohort as a result of non-representative sample selection from the target population. It may also occur during follow-up if losses occur preferentially in some exposure-outcome combinations or if the duration of follow-up varies according to exposure and is independently related to the outcome. It can be guarded against by using a sample selection procedure that ensures representativeness of the target population, by standardizing follow-up procedures, and by minimizing losses.

Confounding bias may result from exposure selection, unequal (by exposure) susceptibility at baseline, or exposure contamination.

Exposure selection bias can be controlled for only to the extent that the reasons for subjects' (or their clinicians') choice of exposure can be reproducibly and validly measured. In that (unusual) case, confounding from this source can be dealt with, in either the design or analysis stage, as any other sort of susceptibility bias (see below). The reasons for choosing a certain exposure are often unknown, however. Even if appreciated in a general way, the reasons often involve subtle psychological or motivational factors that are difficult to measure. This is perhaps the major reason why experimental studies, particularly randomized clinical trials, are often preferable to observational cohort studies, since even unmeasurable factors are unlikely to be associated with exposure if exposure is assigned on a random basis.

Measurable differences in susceptibility that vary according to exposure can be controlled at either the design or the analysis stage. When sample selection is by exposure, the resulting exposure groups can be matched, during the design, according to the suspected confounding susceptibility factors. When matching is included in the design, the analysis should (as discussed in Chapter 5) take account of the matching. When exposure is dichotomous, the outcome is continuous, and the matching is by pairs, paired tests of group means can be performed, as will be shown in Chapter 13.

When both exposure and outcome are dichotomous and the matching is by pairs, the results can be expressed in a matched 2×2 table (Table 6.5). This table superficially resembles the ordinary (unmatched) table (Table 6.1), but each of the four cells of the table represents the results of matched pairs rather than individual subjects. Cells a and d represent those matched pairs in which both the exposed and the nonexposed members develop the same outcome. In a pairs, both develop the outcome; in d pairs, neither does. Cells b and c represent those matched pairs in

Table 6.5. Matched-pair analysis with dichotomous exposure and outcome (general case)

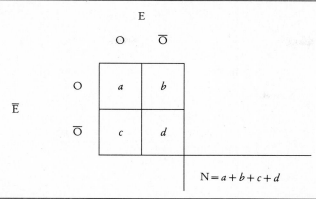

E, Exposed; $\overline{E}$, nonexposed; O, outcome; $\overline{O}$, absence of outcome; a, matched pairs in which both exposed and nonexposed members develop the outcome; b, matched pairs in which the nonexposed member, but not the exposed member, develops the outcome; c, matched pairs in which the exposed member, but not the nonexposed member, develops the outcome; d, matched pairs in which neither the exposed nor nonexposed members develop the outcome; N, total number of matched pairs; 2N, total number of study subjects.

which the members experience opposite results. In b pairs, only the nonexposed member develops the outcome; in c pairs, only the exposed member does. The matched-pair relative risk ($RR_{matched}$) is calculated as:

$$RR_{matched} = \frac{a+c}{a+b} \tag{6.5}$$

and the matched attributable risk ($AR_{matched}$) as:

$$AR_{matched} = \frac{c-b}{N} \tag{6.6}$$

The method is illustrated in Table 6.6 for our smoking-MI example. The 400 study subjects now consist of 200 matched pairs. For seven pairs, both the smoker and the nonsmoker developed an MI, and for 150 pairs, neither did. In 14 pairs, only the nonsmoker developed an MI, whereas in 29 pairs, only the smoker did. The matched-pair relative risk and attributable risk are 1.71 and 7.5% respectively.

Confounding bias due to exposure contamination is best dealt with at the design stage by blinding study subjects, their care-givers, and observers of the outcome to both the association under study (if feasible and ethical) and the subjects' exposure status. But contamination bias and other sources of confounding can also be controlled for in the analysis, assuming that differences in contaminating exposures and in susceptibility are measurable and have been formally assessed. Several multivariate statistical techniques are available for dealing with multiple confounders,

Table 6.6. Matched-pair analysis for smoking and myocardial infarction (MI)

		Smokers		
		MI	No MI	
	MI	7	14	21
Nonsmokers				
	No MI	29	150	179
		36	164	200

$$RR_{matched} = \frac{7+29}{7+14} = \frac{36}{21} = 1.71$$

$$AR_{matched} = \frac{29-14}{200} = \frac{15}{200} = 7.5\%$$

depending on the measurement scales used for expressing exposure and outcome. These will be mentioned briefly in Chapters 13–15.

When exposure, outcome, and confounding variables are all categorical and the number of confounding variables is small, stratification is usually the control procedure of choice. When a standard population exists (or can be created), then the rate of outcome in each exposure group can be standardized, using either the direct or indirect methods described in Chapter 3.

A more commonly used approach is the *Mantel-Haenszel procedure* [6], in which the results from each stratum are weighted approximately according to the sample size of the stratum to yield an overall relative risk. This procedure does not depend on any standard population. When both exposure and outcome are dichotomous, the Mantel-Haenszel relative risk (RR_{MH}) is defined as follows:

$$RR_{MH} = \frac{\sum a_i(c_i + d_i)/N_i}{\sum c_i(a_i + b_i)/N_i} \tag{6.7}$$

where a_i = the number of subjects in the ith stratum who are positive for both exposure and outcome

b_i = the number of subjects in the ith stratum who are positive for exposure but negative for outcome

c_i = the number of subjects in the ith stratum who are negative for exposure but positive for outcome

d_i = the number of subjects in the ith stratum who are negative for both exposure and outcome

and N_i = the total number of subjects in the ith stratum

The expressions are then summed ($\sum$) over all strata to arrive at the numerator and denominator.

Table 6.7. Success (S) and failure (F) for two medical treatments (T_1 and T_2): control for confounding (by sex) using Mantel-Haenszel procedure

A. Overall
("crude") results

	S	F	
T_1	40	60	100
T_2	60	40	100
	100	100	200

Relative "risk" (RR) of success
$$(T_1:T_2) = \frac{40/100}{60/100} = 0.67$$

B. Results stratified
by sex

♀

	S	F	
T_1	24	3	27
T_2	58	30	88
	82	33	115

Relative "risk" (RR) of
$$\text{success} = \frac{24/27}{58/88} = 1.35$$

♂

	S	F	
T_1	16	57	73
T_2	2	10	12
	18	67	85

Relative "risk" (RR) of
$$\text{success} = \frac{16/73}{2/12} = 1.32$$

Overall Mantel-Haenzel relative "risk" of success (RR_{MH}) =
$$\frac{\sum a_i(c_i + d_i)/N_i}{\sum c_i(a_i + b_i)/N_i} = \frac{24(58 + 30)/115 + 16(2 + 10)/85}{58(24 + 3)/115 + 2(16 + 57)/85} = \frac{20.62}{15.34} = 1.34$$

The procedures and calculations are illustrated in Table 6.7. The overall results of an observational cohort study comparing success (S) and failure (F) rates with two treatments (T_1 and T_2) are shown in 6.7A. T_1 clearly appears to be the less efficacious treatment, with a 40% vs 60% success rate, or a "relative success rate" (analogous to relative risk) of $\frac{40/100}{60/100} = 0.67$.

The overall crude results are confounded by sex, however. Women have a much higher success rate than men, irrespective of treatment, and women are less likely to receive T_1. Since sex does not lie on the causal path between treatment and outcome, it fulfills all three criteria for a confounding variable. The stratified analysis shows the clear superiority of T_1 in both men and women. Although the absolute rates of success are lower in men for both treatments, the relative success rates (T_1 relative to T_2) are similar in both sexes, i.e., 1.35 and 1.32. The Mantel-Haenszel analysis combines the stratum-specific results to yield an unconfounded overall result, with a relative success rate ($RR_{MH} = 1.34$) intermediate between the two sex-specific rates.

Fortunately, such extreme examples, in which the crude result is opposite in direction to the adjusted (unconfounded) one, are rare. This type of situation is often referred to as *Simpson's paradox*. More commonly, the crude exposure-outcome association is biased upwards or downwards to a lesser degree. As we shall see in Chapter 14, however, a small bias can sometimes spell the difference between statistical significance and nonsignificance. The Mantel-Haenszel procedure protects against such an eventuality and can be used for any number of strata.

6.4 Effect Modification and Synergism

Variables other than exposure and outcome can modify the exposure-outcome association without confounding it. In such cases, the overall crude measure of association is unbiased but represents the average effect of the modifying variables (so-called *effect modifiers*) [7], and the overall measure may "hide" important effects. More information can often be revealed by reporting the association measure within categories of the effect modifier.

This form of *uncombined* stratified analysis (also called *subgroup analysis*) is illustrated in Table 6.8. We return to our smoking-MI example but with the addition of age as an effect modifier. Part A of the Table represents the overall results (identical to Table 6.2). As shown in part B, smoking has only a small effect ($RR = 1.40$) on the risk of MI in the younger men (≤ 50 years) but a very large effect ($RR = 3.60$) in the older men (> 50 years). Because the older group is smaller than the younger one, the overall result ($RR = 2.13$) is "diluted".

This is *not* a confounding effect. Although age is associated with outcome independent of exposure, it is not associated with exposure (the proportion of smokers is 50% in both age groups). The important point is that the overall relative risk, though an unbiased weighted average of the two stratum-specific rates, hides important information revealed by the stratified, subgroup analysis.

This is in contrast to the example of confounding illustrated in Table 6.7, where the stratum-specific relative risks were similar to each other but very different from

Table 6.8. Effect modification (by age) in cohort study of smoking and myocardial infarction (MI)

A. Overall results

	MI	No MI	
Smokers	32	168	200
Nonsmokers	15	185	200
	47	353	400

$$RR = \frac{32/200}{15/200} = 2.13$$

B. Results stratified by age

Younger (≤ 50 years)

	MI	No MI	
Smokers	14	126	140
Nonsmokers	10	130	140
	24	256	280

$$RR = \frac{14/140}{10/140} = 1.40$$

Older (> 50 years)

	MI	No MI	
Smokers	18	42	60
Nonsmokers	5	55	60
	23	97	120

$$RR = \frac{18/60}{5/60} = 3.60$$

the overall crude measure. Although Tables 6.7 and 6.8 illustrate "pure" confounding and "pure" effect modification respectively, the two phenomena are not mutually exclusive and may coexist.

When two or more exposure variables are positively associated with outcome, their presence in combination will usually produce a greater effect than any will alone. This combined effect is called *synergism*. In our example of Table 6.8, older age can be considered a kind of "exposure," and the combined effects of smoking and old age appear to be synergistic. The statistical demonstration of such a com-

Table 6.9. Advantages and disadvantages of cohort studies

A. Advantages
    1. Can provide more accurate picture of baseline state
    2. Sample selection by exposure essential for rare exposures
    3. Can minimize losses to follow-up and assess their effect
    4. If concurrent, can protect against contamination and detection biases
B. Disadvantages
    1. Poorly suited to the study of rare outcomes
    2. If long latent period, prolonged follow-up required
    3. Careful follow-up is labor intensive and costly

bined effect is called *statistical interaction*. The quantification of statistical interaction depends on whether the underlying etiologic model (how the exposures combine to cause the outcome) is additive (the effects add arithmetically) or multiplicative (the effects multiply geometrically). A detailed discussion of this issue is beyond the scope of this text but is available in several references [7–10].

6.5 Advantages and Disadvantages of Cohort Studies

Cohort studies have several major advantages over other types of observational studies (Table 6.9). First, cohort directionality is the only directionality that permits identification of subjects prior to exposure, thereby providing a more accurate picture of the baseline state. This often enables better control for susceptibility bias than is possible with case-control or cross-sectional studies. Second, the possibility of sample selection by exposure (which is not available for case-control studies) is essential for studying the effects of rare exposures. Third, losses to follow-up can be minimized, and those that do occur can be assessed for their effect on the exposure-outcome association. This is not possible in case-control or cross-sectional studies. Fourth, concurrent cohort studies can protect against contamination and detection biases by standardizing exposure and follow-up procedures and by blinding subjects, observers, and care-givers.

    Cohort studies also have their disadvantages, however. They are not as suitable for studying rare outcomes as case-control or cross-sectional studies that select their samples by outcome. Huge cohorts would be required to ensure adequate numbers of outcome events to yield statistically meaningful results. For concurrent cohort studies, the existence of a long latent period between exposure and outcome requires prolonged follow-up. Finally, careful follow-up procedures (in concurrent studies) are expensive in terms of time and money. Thus, cohort studies are both difficult and costly when the outcome is rare and when prolonged follow-up is required.

    One disadvantage shared by cohort and other observational studies is the difficulty in controlling for exposure selection bias and other forms of confounding caused by unmeasured (and perhaps unknown) variables. When such sources of confounding are important, an experimental study (clinical trial) is far preferable. The following chapter discusses the design, analysis, and application of clinical trials.

References

1. Feinstein AR (1970) Clinical biostatistics. III. The architecture of clinical research. Clin Pharmacol Ther 11: 432–441
2. Feinstein AR (1971) Clinical biostatistics. XI. Sources of "chronology bias" in cohort statistics. Clin Pharmacol Ther 12: 864–879
3. Doll R, Hill AB (1964) Mortality in relation to smoking: ten years' observations of British doctors. Br Med J 1: 1399–1410
4. Levin ML (1953) The occurrence of lung cancer in man. Acta Unio Int Contra Cancrum 9: 531–541
5. Miettinen OS (1976) Estimability and estimation in case-referent studies. Am J Epidemiol 103: 226–235
6. Mantel N, Haenszel W (1959) Statistical aspects of the analysis of data from retrospective studies of disease. JNCI 22: 719–748
7. Miettinen OS (1974) Confounding and effect modification. Am J Epidemiol 100: 350–353
8. Rothman KJ (1974) Synergy and antagonism in cause-effect relationships. Am J Epidemiol 99: 385–388
9. Kupper LL, Hogan MD (1978) Interaction in epidemiologic studies. Am J Epidemiol 108: 447–453
10. Rothman KJ, Greenland S, Walker AM (1980) Concepts of interaction. Am J Epidemiol 112: 467–470

Chapter 7: Clinical Trials

7.1 Research Design Components

As discussed at the beginning of Chapter 6, a cohort study may use either an observational or experimental design. Having dealt with observational cohort studies in some detail in the last chapter, we shall now focus our attention on experimental cohort studies, or clinical trials. In clinical trials, exposure is assigned by the study investigators, rather than occurring naturally or being selected by the subject or his clinician. Consequently, exposure in clinical trials is often referred to as *treatment*.

7.1.1 Sample Selection

Assignment of treatment defines the method of sample selection for clinical trials. Sample selection is by exposure, and two or more groups defined by the treatments are compared for the development of the study outcome (Fig. 7.1).

7.1.2 Baseline State

Issues concerning the baseline state are similar to those in observational cohort studies, except that the study sample must, by definition, be assembled before exposure. In other words, the timing of a clinical trial is always concurrent. This is an advantage over historical and mixed-timing observational studies, in which the sample is assembled when exposure has already occurred and in which it may not be known, therefore, whether some subject characteristics might be a result, rather than a cause, of exposure. Depending on the method used for assigning treatment, baseline susceptibility factors may assume greater or lesser importance. As we shall see, random assignment markedly reduces the potential for confounding due to sus-

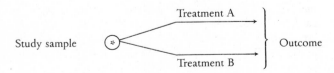

Fig. 7.1. The classical clinical trial design comparing two treatments (A and B). *Asterisk,* Randomization (or other mode of treatment assignment)

ceptibility bias, and particularly for confounding by indication. For this reason, the randomized clinical trial, or RCT, has become the design of choice in comparing two or more clinical treatments.

7.1.3 Exposure (Treatment)

Because it serves as the basis of sample selection in clinical trials, exposure is measured on a categorical scale, with each category representing an exposure (treatment) group. When a new treatment is compared with an existing standard treatment, the new one is often referred to as the *experimental treatment* and the standard as the *control treatment.* An inactive control treatment that is indistinguishable (regarding appearance, sensation, smell, and taste) from the experimental treatment is called a *placebo.* As with observational cohort studies, ordinal treatment groups (e.g., placebo, low-dose treatment, high-dose treatment) permit evaluation of a dose-response effect.

Issues of treatment potency are similar to those discussed for observational studies but with one important difference. Because treatments are assigned by the study investigators, many clinical trials have attempted to standardize treatment comparisons by using a rigid, fixed-dose treatment schedule. Good clinicians usually adjust the dosage regimen of a given treatment in individual patients in order to maximize benefits and minimize side effects. When fixed regimens dictated by the trial protocol prevent this flexibility, treatment potency may be insufficient to result in clinical benefit [1]. The result may be a false inference that a treatment is not efficacious. Consider, for example, the University Group Diabetes Program (UGDP) clinical trial comparing various treatments for diabetes [2]. Critics have suggested that the ineffectiveness of the two oral agents (tolbutamide and phenformin) might be explained by the fact that dosage was not optimized, i.e., not tied to attempts to control the blood or urine glucose concentration [3].

It is often a good idea to include, in the trial protocol, the measurement of variables that reflect the potency of the treatments studied. Such variables are called *intermediate outcomes* and permit the investigator to assess, for example, whether the treatment produced the physiologic effect required to achieve the study outcome. In the UGDP trial, for instance, measurement of the blood glucose concentration would have revealed whether the agents administered had actually produced the desired decrease. Failure to lower blood glucose would indicate inadequate potency.

Even if the potency of the *assigned* treatment is adequate, the treatment actually *received* by the study subjects may be too weak to affect the outcome because of poor *compliance.* A negative trial result may occur because a treatment is not taken, rather than because it is not efficacious. A drug cannot be expected to produce its desired clinical effect if it is not taken or is taken in inadequate dosage. It is generally advisable to measure treatment compliance in clinical trials, either directly or indirectly, e.g., by periodic "pill counts" or urine testing for presence of the study drug or some inert but easily detectable "marker," such as riboflavin. The importance of compliance should be stressed at the time of subject enrollment and periodically during treatment. When only "super compliers" are studied, however, the trial results may be poorly generalizable to the "real" clinical world. In any case, measurement of compliance is essential in interpreting a trial's results, be they positive or negative. I will return to this issue in Section 7.5.

Contamination bias is a danger as much in clinical trials as in observational cohort studies. Assignment of treatment, even if randomized, provides no protection against treatment "accompaniments" by the subjects' care-givers. Only blinding the latter to treatment assignment can prevent this potential source of confounding bias.

7.1.4 Follow-Up

Because of their cohort directionality, clinical trials include a period of follow-up in their design. As with observational studies, follow-up must be sufficiently long to include the latent period for the study treatments, i.e., to permit the biological expression of their effects. Losses to follow-up should be minimized both to maximize statistical efficiency and to avoid sample distortion bias, and those losses that do occur should be characterized well enough to permit estimation of bias that might have occurred.

As in observational cohort studies, the *potential* duration of follow-up (as distinct from its *actual* duration) should not vary according to treatment (see Section 6.1.5). Finally, detection bias can best be avoided by standardizing the frequency and extent of follow-up visits, examinations, and diagnostic tests, and by ensuring that the standard protocol is followed and maintained irrespective of treatment.

7.1.5 Outcome

The issues related to outcome for a clinical trial are identical to those in a cohort study. The outcomes are usually incident outcomes and develop de novo during follow-up in subjects free of the outcome at the time the cohorts were assembled.

The investigator has the usual difficult choice between "hard" (objective, easily measurable) and "soft" (subjective, not so easily measurable) outcomes. The latter in particular provide an opportunity for differential information bias in favor of a new experimental treatment, and appropriate blinding of both study subjects and observers of the outcome is necessary to protect against such bias.

7.2 Assignment of Exposure (Treatment)

7.2.1 Nonrandom vs Random Assignment

The main advantage of experimental studies over observational studies is the opportunity for reducing confounding bias due to exposure selection or other reasons for unequal susceptibility in the different exposure (treatment) groups. Such bias reduction can occur, however, only when neither the study subjects, nor their clinicians, nor the investigators control the treatment assignment. In observational studies, treatment is usually determined by some combination of subject and clinician preference. The mere substitution of investigator preference for subject or clinician preference in a clinical trial is insufficient to protect against bias, because the investigator's treatment allocations may be affected (consciously or unconsciously) by knowledge of the subject's underlying susceptibility. Thus, treatment assignment must occur according to a pre-established protocol that cannot be controlled by the investigators, the study subjects, or the subjects' clinicians.

Systematic assignment of treatment would, on the surface, seem to meet these requirements. If trial enrollment occurs sequentially over time, for example, alternate treatments could be assigned to subjects successively as they are enrolled. With alternate assignment, however, a subject might present himself (or be referred by his clinician) for enrollment only when the new or "preferred" treatment was next to be assigned. Similar opportunities for bias could arise if alternate enrollment dates are used instead of alternate subjects. Even the use of "unit" or "chart" numbers (e.g., odd vs even last digits) would not be totally immune from bias if such numbers could be influenced by the order in which subjects present themselves in the study institution.

Use of an alphabetic rule (e.g., the first letter of the last name) would, of course, place treatment assignment beyond control of subjects, clinicians, and investigators. But it is conceivable that the association of certain letters with certain ethnic groups could lead to an unequal distribution of ethnicity between the treatment groups. If ethnicity is independently (of the treatment) related to the outcome, confounding would then occur. Thus, systematic treatment assignment can lead to bias even when outside the influence of the relevant parties.

The best means of reducing susceptibility bias is by assigning treatment on a random basis, i.e., by ensuring that assignment occurs by the laws of chance. In this way, every subject will have the same probability of receiving a given treatment. Neither subjects, clinicians, nor investigators can affect the treatment received, and important susceptibility factors should distribute themselves randomly. To ensure that this has in fact occurred, investigators should always compare the treatment groups created by the randomization according to prognostically important sociodemographic and clinical factors. Such a comparison is often summarized in tabular form and is an essential part of the presentation of the report of the trial's results. The example shown in Table 7.1 is taken from the Veteran's Administration (VA) Cooperative Study Group placebo-controlled RCT of treatment with antihypertensive agents [4].

7.2.2 Methods of Randomization

The most common method of randomization makes use of published tables or computer-generated lists of random numbers. Instructions for using such tables (see Appendix Table A.1) or lists are identical to those for random sampling and were discussed in Chapter 4. If equal numbers are desired in both of two treatment groups, the random numbers corresponding to each subject can be arranged in numerical order. The first half of the group will then receive treatment A, the sec-

Table 7.1. Comparison of treatment groups (active vs placebo) created by randomization, VA anti-hypertensive trial [4]

Characteristic	Active		Placebo	
	(n)	*(%)*	*(n)*	*(%)*
Race				
White	31	42.5	35	50.0
Black	42	57.5	35	50.0
Family history of hypertension				
None	23	31.5	19	27.1
Present	49	67.1	48	68.6
Unknown	1	1.4	3	4.3
Cardiac symptoms				
None	52	71.2	48	68.6
Present	21	28.8	22	31.4
Heart size by chest roentgenogram				
Normal	44	60.3	39	55.7
Enlarged	29	39.7	31	44.3
Diabetes				
Absent	65	89.0	65	92.9
Present	8	11.0	5	7.1
Total randomized	73	100	70	100

ond treatment B. When three treatments are involved, the ordered subjects are divided into thirds, and so on.

Once the randomization schedule has been devised, the assigned treatments must, of course, be communicated to the clinicians who administer them. One of the best and most frequent methods for accomplishing this involves the use of opaque envelopes that must be opened to reveal the assigned treatment. Upon enrollment of each subject, the next envelope in numbered sequence is opened to determine the treatment for that subject. When the treatments involve look-alike tablets, capsules, or liquids, another method involves sequentially numbering each bottle or package. The treatment corresponding to each number is obtained from the random number table, and the code remains unknown to the personnel dispensing the treatments.

Coin flips, dice, or playing cards can also be used to randomize treatment assignment, but such methods are used far less frequently than random numbers. Regardless of which method of randomization (and communication) is used, that method should be indicated whenever the trial is described and reported. The mere use of the term "random assignment" is insufficient, because some authors have used the term "random" in a rather loose sense to indicate "without any pre-established order." As we have seen, however, assignment must be truly random to be immune from bias.

7.2.3 Stratified and Blocked Randomization

Unfortunately, even true randomization of treatment assignment does not *guarantee* that confounding will not occur. The only guarantee is that confounding factors will distribute themselves randomly. Randomly does not mean evenly. Ten coin flips do not guarantee 5 heads and 5 tails, or even that the result will not be more extreme than 4 and 6, or even 3 and 7. The chance occurrence of 0 heads and 10 tails is unlikely, but not impossible. In fact, the probability can be calculated as $P = (\frac{1}{2})^{10} = 0.00977$. Similarly, random assignment can occasionally result in the uneven distribution of important confounding variables. Since a chance occurrence of 1 out of 20 (i.e., $P = 0.05$) is the usual threshold for establishing its "statistical significance," a statistically significant difference in the distribution of a given confounding variable will occur once out of every 20 randomizations.

To protect against possible bias by the chance maldistribution of one or more important potential confounding factors, some trials use a *stratified randomization* in which subjects are first assigned to a stratum defined by the confounder(s). A separate randomization is then carried out for each stratum. This procedure is analogous to stratified random sampling (see Section 4.3.2).

To maximize statistical efficiency by ensuring that approximately equal numbers of subjects receive each study treatment, randomization is occasionally carried out within *blocks* of specified size. For example, in a two-arm RCT, randomization by blocks of ten will ensure that for every ten subjects enrolled, five will receive each of the two treatments. Blocking is often particularly helpful in the setting of multiple strata by preventing large within-stratum imbalances in treatment assignment.

7.2.4 Individual vs Group Randomization

Randomization of individual subjects is entirely appropriate for the classic drug-efficacy trial. In such a trial, subjects are treated individually, treatment groups remain distinct, and an unbiased comparison of drug vs placebo, or drug A vs drug B, is thus likely. For some types of treatment, however, random assignment by individuals can actually be detrimental, because interaction among subjects may lead to systematic errors in classifying the treatment actually received (i.e., the treatments actually received will be more similar than those allocated), and hence a biased comparison. Psychosocial, educational, and health care service interventions are particularly prone to this problem, since subjects are likely to interact with one another between administration of the intervention and measurement of the outcome. For such trials, treatment assignment by hospital room or ward, school, or geographic region may be preferable to randomization of individuals [1].

Group randomization appears preferable whenever relatively closed, naturally formed groups are capable of modifying the treatment allocated to individuals within those groups. For example, of the dozen or so controlled clinical trials assessing the effect of early maternal-infant contact on subsequent maternal attachment behavior (so-called bonding), most randomized individual women, rather than entire postpartum wards. Thus, mothers receiving different treatments (early contact vs usual "routine") were housed on the same ward, and often in the same room. Communication among these mothers might well be expected to reduce the difference between the treatments actually received and thereby reduce the difference in outcome [5]. Randomization by group (in this example, postpartum ward) can avoid this source of (information) bias.

Unfortunately, however, group randomization results in a markedly reduced sample size, because the unit of statistical analysis becomes the group, rather than the individual [6, 7]. One alternative, which provides the scientific advantages of group randomization while permitting the statistical advantages of analysis by individual, involves the use of a pretrial study period to demonstrate that individuals in different groups experience similar outcomes when exposed to the same treatment. Equivalent pretrial results increase the plausibility that any differences in outcome that occur when the same groups are exposed to different treatments during the trial are attributable to the treatments, rather than to potentially confounding differences between the groups.

7.2.5 Parallel vs Crossover Designs

In the clinical trial designs we have considered thus far, a group of subjects receiving a given treatment is compared with other groups receiving one or more different treatments. Such a design is called a *parallel design,* because the study groups receive their respective treatments simultaneously, i.e., in parallel. In a *crossover design,* however, each study subject receives each treatment in series by "crossing over" in sequence from one to the other. For example, patients with asthma might each receive, in sequence, two different treatment regimens to see which of the two treatments is more efficacious among the group as a whole.

Crossover trials have a major advantage over parallel trials in statistical efficiency, in that a given treatment difference is demonstrable with fewer subjects. There are two reasons for this: (a) each subject receives both treatments (in a two-treatment comparison) and thus "counts" twice, and (b) variability in treatment response due to individual subject characteristics is eliminated and the "signal-to-noise ratio" thus enhanced. Proper conduct of crossover trials, however, requires randomization of treatment sequence (A,B vs B,A), time-dependent (rather than outcome-dependent) crossover of treatments, and elimination of (or control for) carry-over effects from the first treatment [8].

The statistical analysis of crossover trials is similar to that of matched pairs and will be discussed in Chapters 13 and 14.

7.3 Blinding in Clinical Trials

Randomized treatment assignment is only one of the design features in clinical trials that help minimize analytic bias. By randomly distributing susceptibility factors, confounding bias from this source is rendered unlikely. Randomization can also reduce sample distortion bias, because even if the study sample is unrepresentative of the target population, the resulting distortion will be nondifferential with respect to exposure, and thus the treatment effects will be unbiased. Protection against information bias, however, as well as other sources of confounding bias, depends on adequate blinding of subjects, observers, and care-givers.

Blinding of study subjects is necessary to protect against contamination (confounding) of the true treatment effect by the so-called *placebo effect*. The placebo effect is the nonspecific effect that any treatment can have on the outcome, especially when the subject believes it to be efficacious. The main reason for providing look-alike, feel-alike, smell-alike, taste-alike placebo treatments when comparing an experimental treatment with no treatment is to facilitate subject blinding.

Blinding of observers is also necessary to prevent the information bias that would occur if the outcomes were determined by observers who are aware of the treatment received. As discussed previously, such awareness can influence the outcome assessment, either consciously or unconsciously, especially if the outcome is subjective.

When a clinical trial incorporates blinding of both the subjects and the observers, the trial is said to be *double-blind*. When care-givers other than the observers are aware of treatment status, however, even double blinding is insufficient, because the study treatment can be contaminated (confounded) by doctors, nurses, physical therapists, or others who may alter the quantity or quality of their care according to the study treatment received. Failure to protect against this source of bias was one of the major defects in the maternal-infant "bonding" trials alluded to earlier [5].

Unfortunately, blinding may be infeasible for some treatments. This is obviously true for most surgical procedures but also pertains to many behavioral (e.g., exercise vs no exercise in a trial to prevent myocardial infarction) and health care (e.g., care by nurse practitioner vs physician) interventions. Furthermore, unblinding can arise owing to differences in side effects that occur with different treatments, even if those treatments originally seem indistinguishable. This is especially likely to create a bias when the control treatment involves a placebo. One strategy for measuring potential bias due to unblinding involves asking subjects, after they have completed treatment, to guess whether they received the active treatment or placebo; bias should be suspected whenever treatment effects appear only in subjects who are unblinded. A good example of the use of this strategy was one of the RCTs of vitamin C in the prevention and treatment of the common cold [9]. Unblinded subjects who received vitamin C reported a shorter duration and lesser severity of colds; in subjects who remained blind, no such differences were found.

7.4 Analysis of Results

Because treatment assignment automatically creates categorical exposure (treatment) groups, the exposure-outcome association is assessed by comparing the outcome among the groups. For continuous outcomes, this involves a comparison of means. For categorical outcomes, the comparison is of rates, with relative and attributable risks applicable in the case of dichotomous outcomes. Statistical inference for means and rates will be discussed in Chapters 13 and 14 respectively.

Randomized treatment assignment and adequate blinding reduce the potential for confounding bias; consequently, stratified or multivariate statistical analyses are not usually required. In the absence of stratified randomization, however, any given confounding factor has a 1 in 20 chance of a statistically significant association with treatment. When one or more potential confounders are associated with treatment after simple (nonstratified) randomization, a stratified analysis or multivariate adjustment may be necessary to avoid confounding.[1] For continuous confounders and outcomes, such procedures may also help to improve the reproducibility of the resulting treatment difference (increase the signal-to-noise ratio) and thus to enhance its statistical significance. Furthermore, stratification may be desirable in assessing effect modification; i.e., treatment may affect outcome in some subgroups but not others.

7.5 Interpretation of Results

7.5.1 Efficacy vs Effectiveness

One of the major problems likely to arise during a clinical trial is that subjects either may not have received or complied with the treatment to which they were assigned or, having received it initially, may have switched to another. Another problem is that subjects may withdraw from participation in the trial before treatment or follow-up are complete. These realities of clinical research create major problems in interpreting the trial's results.

Such problems have led to two different ways of analyzing the results of a clinical trial and, consequently, to two different interpretations. Which of the two approaches is taken depends on whether one is interested in treatment efficacy or treatment effectiveness.

Efficacy refers to the potential effect of treatment under optimal circumstances, i.e., whether treatment *can* have an effect on outcome. Thus, an analysis for efficacy would compare subjects according to the treatment actually received (rather than the one assigned) and would exclude subjects who complied poorly, those who switched over (and thus received both treatments), and those who withdrew during the trial. An analysis for efficacy is also called an *explanatory* trial analysis [10–12].

Effectiveness refers to the actual effect of treatment in the "real world" of people who comply poorly, change treatment (owing to unsatisfactory results or side effects of initial treatment), or become lost to follow-up – i.e., whether treatment *does* have an effect on outcome. An effectiveness analysis compares all subjects according to their original, assigned treatment and thus includes poor compliers, switch-overs, and withdrawals. Other terms for effectiveness analysis include *pragmatic, management,* and *intention-to-treat* trial analysis [10–12].

Both efficacy and effectiveness may be important. Efficacy is usually of primary interest to biologists, physiologists, and (to some extent) pharmacologists, i.e., to those interested in biologic potency and mechanisms of action. It is also a sine qua

---

[1] It is important to emphasize that some variables are bound to distribute themselves asymmetrically by treatment. This will occur, on average, with 1 of every 20 variables examined. But control for all such asymmetrically distributed variables is unnecessary, since random differences between treatment groups are already taken into account in calculating the probability of an erroneous statistical inference. Thus, in-depth searches for such variables are not indicated. Control for confounding, whether by stratified randomization or by adjustment in the analysis, is necessary only for those *few* potential confounders identified a priori as important candidates.

non of effectiveness, since a treatment that cannot work under optimal circumstances will not work in clinical practice. Treatments can be efficacious without being effective, however, and it is effectiveness that is of primary concern to patients and clinicians. Nonetheless, efficacious but ineffective treatments may still be useful for certain patients (e.g., those without side effects and those with good compliance).

7.5.2 Selective Subject Participation

To an even greater extent than in observational studies, subjects (or their clinicians) may be unwilling to participate in clinical trials, and especially in RCTs. Treatment assignment by the study's investigators means that neither the subject nor his or her clinician can choose, and many subjects therefore decline to participate. Not only does this result in smaller numbers of participants, with consequent statistical limitations, but those who participate may be quite different from those who do not. The trial's external validity, or generalizability, thus may not extend beyond the narrow confines of a highly selective target population [1].

A common example of this type of problem arises whenever low-risk or high-risk patients are preferentially enrolled in a trial. A treatment comparison in one of these risk strata may not be generalizable to the other. In an RCT of a new cancer chemotherapeutic agent, for example, only patients with advanced disease resistant to conventional treatment may be enrolled. Failure of the agent among such high-risk cases does not indicate whether it is efficacious in lower-risk patients without previous treatment. The problem is even more insidious whenever motivational differences responsible for selective participation can also affect the study outcome, because the nature of these differences may not be known and, even if appreciated qualitatively, may be difficult to measure.

Trial investigators should keep track of, and include in all reports, both the numbers and relevant characteristics of all participants and nonparticipants. Such characteristics include any sociodemographic or clinical factors that can affect the outcome. Unless participation rates are exceptionally high (80%–90%), investigators should compare participants and nonparticipants and indicate characteristics of the target population to whom the results appear to apply.

7.5.3 The Hawthorne Effect

The *Hawthorne effect* refers to the tendency of study participation per se to affect outcome. The term originated in studies carried out in the 1920s at the Hawthorne Works of the Western Electric Company in Chicago. A variety of interventions (e.g., changing the light intensity) were used in an attempt to improve workers' productivity, but the investigators found that productivity increased regardless of what intervention was introduced. Although a Hawthorne effect can arise in any study concerned with behavioral outcomes or outcomes that can be influenced by behavioral changes, RCTs carry with them the sense of uncertainty and risk (randomization), which may be more potent behavior modifiers than mere observation.

If participation affects outcome equally in all treatment groups, no systematic bias is introduced in the treatment comparison, and internal validity is maintained. But because the potential magnitude of the treatment effect may be limited (the so-called *ceiling effect*), the end result may be either a smaller treatment difference or no significant difference, and thus an externally invalid inference concerning the treatment's effectiveness in a more general population.

To minimize the potential for a Hawthorne effect, trial subjects can be kept unaware that they are being studied, or at least unaware of the precise treatment comparison or the research hypothesis. For many types of treatments, however, such blinding is not ethically defensible. In such cases, the possibility of a Hawthorne effect should be acknowledged by the trial's investigators, and inferences concerning external validity modified accordingly.

7.6 Ethical Considerations

Ethical issues are of importance in all types of epidemiologic studies, because the sociodemographic and clinical data that constitute the primary products of such studies are often of a sensitive nature. Although the data are almost always analyzed and reported in the aggregate without identification of individual subjects, some persons are reluctant to be interviewed or examined for purposes other than their own health care, and a few object even to allowing investigators (other than their own clinicians) access to their medical records. Clinical trials pose even greater ethical problems, however, because their experimental design means that treatments are assigned by the trial's investigators, rather than by the subjects or their clinicians [13, 14]. When assignment is randomized, the problems are compounded by the aspect of risk or chance. And, when blinding of subjects, observers, and care-givers is further added, the ethical considerations often become more complex, and perhaps even more important, than the scientific ones.

In order for an RCT to be ethically justifiable, none of the trial treatments should be known to have superior efficacy, based on the available evidence at the time the trial begins. Even though convincing "proof" of superiority of one treatment may be lacking, however, prior equality of treatments is the exception, rather than the rule. In the routine development of new drugs, for example, manufacturers must present evidence of efficacy from small uncontrolled trials (so-called Phase II studies) before proceeding to an RCT (Phase III). For both legal and economic reasons, they often have good evidence of efficacy (vs no treatment) before instituting placebo-controlled RCTs. Yet the latter are required by the U.S. Food and Drug Administration, for example, before the drugs can be marketed.

Furthermore, the requirements of randomization and blinding often place clinicians in the conflicting role of attempting to care for an individual patient, on the one hand, and of wishing to contribute to the advancement of knowledge (and perhaps of their own careers), on the other. It is probably rare for a clinician to be neutral concerning treatment, and if he does indeed have a preference, can he support randomization of his patient? This becomes especially problematic when the trial is not the first to test a particular treatment. Although it is always preferable to base treatment preferences in clinical practice on more than a single study, it may be difficult for a subject or clinician to accept a 50–50 chance of receiving a new treatment when a previous trial, or even two or three previous trials, have shown the treatment to be superior to the existing "standard."

Nonetheless, many thoughtful (and ethical) scientists make the opposite argument. According to them, it is more ethical to allow subjects to receive a standard treatment before convincing evidence favors a new one than to allow unproven, potentially harmful and costly therapies to be adopted prematurely. We need only adduce the now-abandoned practices of purging and blood-letting to remind us that the annals of medical history are replete with ineffective and even harmful remedies staunchly defended over long periods by the best clinicians of their time. The difficulty comes in defining the threshold for "convincing" and "proven," which is likely to be lower for clinicians wishing to do the most good and least harm by their patients than for researchers wishing to establish scientific "truth."

Although these ethical dilemmas are not easily resolved, the recent insistence, in many developed societies, on informed consent and institutional review boards has provided important ethical safeguards. *Informed consent* is required by most research funding agencies and clinical journals whenever studies involve human experimentation and usually consists of a full disclosure of trial procedures, including randomization and blinding. Informed consent means that the subject is given a chance to ask questions, is under no pressure or obligation to participate, and is informed that his or her care will not suffer if he or she declines participation or later decides to withdraw. A signed statement of informed consent is often required. Despite these requirements, however, the complexities of modern medicine and other clinical disciplines, as well as those of trial design, often prevent the consenting subject from being fully informed.

Institutional review boards (IRBs), also called human investigation committees, usually consist of committees composed of lay persons, clinicians, administrators, lawyers, and ethicists and are based within a hospital, research institute, or academic institution. Their purpose is to review trial (and other human study) protocols, to ensure the protection and ethical treatment of study subjects, and to suggest appropriate changes in informed consent procedures or study design. The IRB may also request that the trial's data be analyzed periodically by an outside statistician or committee, so that a clear difference in treatment efficacy is recognized promptly, further enrollment is halted, and subsequent patients can receive the better treatment. IRB approval is often required by the institution at which the trial will be carried out, as well as by the agency providing the funding.

Variations in the classic RCT design (Fig. 7.1) have been proposed in an effort to overcome some of its inherent ethical difficulties. Zelen has proposed a design (Fig. 7.2) in which subjects are randomized to "consent not sought" vs "consent sought" groups. Those in the former group receive the existing standard treatment, while those in the latter are *offered* the new experimental treatment, with the standard treatment given if they decline [15]. This design retains the scientific benefits of randomization while allowing those subjects in the "consent sought" arm to choose whether or not they want the new treatment. In addition to preventing blinding, however, such a design also creates problems of statistical efficiency and interpretation, since the groups should be compared according to the randomization arms,

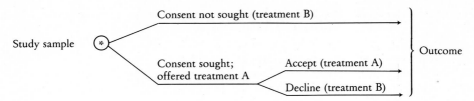

Fig. 7.2. Alternative clinical trial design comparing new (A) and conventional (B) treatments. *Asterisk,* Randomization

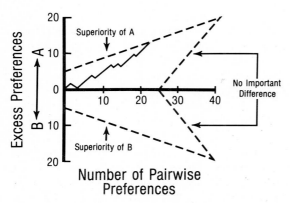

Fig. 7.3. Sequential analysis of clinical trial comparing two treatments (A and B)

and the "consent sought" arm contains subjects receiving both treatments, i.e., the effect of the new treatment is contaminated with that of the standard.

The sequential design differs from the classic design in that sample sizes are not fixed in advance but are determined by the cumulative trial results [16]. The results are analyzed in successive pairs in which the two subjects are assigned different treatments until either one of the two treatments is shown to be statistically superior or it becomes clear that the difference between the two is small enough to ignore. The method of analysis is illustrated in Fig. 7.3. The outcome in the first subject randomized to receive treatment A is compared with that of the first subject randomized to treatment B. A "step" is then taken off the line of equality (the x axis, corresponding to 0 excess preferences) toward the treatment favored in the first pairwise comparison. Subsequent pairs are compared similarly until the path defined by the cumulative "steps" crosses one of the lines indicating either superiority of A, superiority of B, or no important difference. Sequential designs were originally devised in World War II to minimize the sample size necessary to demonstrate a treatment difference, but they also have ethical advantages, because the trial is stopped as soon as the results are clear. Their advantages are limited, however, to treatments of short duration (so that many subjects are not enrolled needlessly while the results of previous enrollees are awaited). Furthermore, smaller trials, while beneficial in some respects, do not convey as much information as larger trials, both because the results

Table 7.2. Advantages and disadvantages of clinical trials

A. Advantages
1. Reduced potential for confounding bias
2. Reduced potential for sample distortion bias
3. Conducive to blinding of subjects, observers, and care-givers
B. Disadvantages
1. May be impracticable
2. May be unethical
3. Often expensive
4. May reduce generalizability

may not be as widely applicable (generalizable) and because limited numbers may prevent analysis of smaller subgroups or detection of rare adverse outcomes of treatment.

7.7 Advantages and Disadvantages of Clinical Trials

The main advantage of clinical trials (Table 7.2) over observational cohort studies is that trials, especially if randomized, allocate exposure (treatment) without respect to susceptibility factors or to how the study sample was selected. Trials thus provide considerable protection against confounding bias and sample distortion bias. Furthermore, the design of the RCT is more conducive to blinding of subjects, observers, and care-givers than is an observational study of patients whose treatments are discussed and prescribed by their own clinicians.

Practical or ethical considerations may render clinical trials infeasible. For example, it would be impossible to assign blood type or other genetic traits, impracticable to attempt to direct mothers to breast feed or bottle feed their newborn infants, and unethical to expose subjects purposefully to potential toxins or carcinogens. Another problem with clinical trials is their cost. An observational study of treatments occurring in clinical practice can usually be accomplished for a small fraction of the cost required by a clinical trial, because the costs of treatment and follow-up in a trial must usually be borne by the trial itself. A large-scale, multicenter RCT can thus cost hundreds of millions of dollars. Finally, as alluded to earlier in this chapter, the contrived setting in which treatment takes place can affect the external validity (generalizability) of a trial's results.

Despite their imperfections, clinical trials remain the "gold standard" for evaluating clinical treatments. They have contributed enormously to the evolution of more effective therapeutic and preventive measures for a variety of clinical conditions and are represented by an increasing proportion of articles published in leading medical journals [17]. Although use of a clinical trial design, even with randomized treatment assignment, does not confer certainty on the conclusions of a study, the RCT is the epidemiologic research design of choice whenever randomized assignment is feasible and ethical.

References

1. Kramer MS, Shapiro SH (1984) Scientific challenges in the application of clinical trials. JAMA 252: 2739–2745
2. University Group Diabetes Program (1970) A study of the effects of hypoglycemic agents on vascular complications in patients with adult-onset diabetes. I. Design, methods, and baseline results. II. Mortality results. Diabetes 19 [Suppl 2]: 747–830
3. Feinstein AR (1971) Clinical biostatistics. VIII. An analytic appraisal of the University Group Diabetes Program (UGDP) study. Clin Pharmacol Ther 12: 167–191
4. Veterans Administration Cooperative Study Group on Antihypertensive Agents (1967) Effects of treatment on morbidity in hypertension: results in patients with diastolic blood pressures averaging 115 through 129 mmHg. JAMA 202: 116–122
5. Thomson ME, Kramer MS (1984) Methodological standards for controlled clinical trials of early contact and maternal-infant behavior. Pediatrics 73: 294–300
6. Cornfield J, Mitchell S (1969) Selected risk factors in coronary disease: possible intervention effects. Arch Environ Health 19: 387–394
7. Buck C, Donner A (1982) The design of controlled experiments in the evaluation of nontherapeutic interventions. J Chronic Dis 35: 531–538
8. Louis TA, Lavori PW, Bailar JC, Polansky M (1984) Crossover and self-controlled designs in clinical research. N Engl J Med 310: 24–31
9. Karlowski TR, Chalmers TC, Frenkel LD et al. (1975) Ascorbic acid for the common cold: a prophylactic and therapeutic trial. JAMA 231: 1038–1042
10. Schwartz D, Lellouch J (1967) Explanatory and pragmatic attitudes in therapeutic trials. J Chronic Dis 20: 637–648
11. Sackett DL, Gent M (1979) Controversy in counting and attributing events in clinical trials. N Engl J Med 301: 1410–1412
12. Louis TA, Shapiro SH (1983) Critical issues in the conduct and interpretation of clinical trials. Annu Rev Public Health 43: 25–46
13. Schafer A (1982) The ethics of the randomized clinical trial. N Engl J Med 307: 719–724
14. Lebacqz K (1983) Ethical aspects of clinical trials. In: Shapiro SH, Louis TA (eds) Clinical trials: issues and approaches. Marcel Dekker, New York, pp 81–98
15. Zelen M (1979) A new design for randomized clinical trials. N Engl J Med 300: 1242–1245
16. Armitage P (1971) Statistical methods in medical research. Blackwell Scientific Publications, Oxford, pp 415–425
17. Fletcher RH, Fletcher SW (1979) Clinical research in general medical journals. N Engl J Med 301: 180–183

Chapter 8: **Case-Control Studies**

8.1 Introduction

In cohort studies (and clinical trials), subjects are followed in a forward direction from exposure to outcome. Inferential reasoning is from cause to effect.

In case-control studies, on the other hand, we start with the outcome and ask or find out about prior exposure. The directionality is backward, and the reasoning is inductive, from effect to cause. In some ways, therefore, case-control studies can be thought of as the chronological and logical inverse of cohort studies. Feinstein has coined the term *trohoc* (cohort spelled backwards) to illustrate this relationship [1]. Another frequently encountered synonym is *case-referent study*. The generally accepted term *case-control study* derives from the usual dichotomous categorization of outcome as present *(cases)* or absent *(controls)*.

8.2 Research Design Components

8.2.1 Sample Selection in Case-Control Studies

In case-control studies, prior exposure status is ascertained after the study subjects have been assembled. Thus, the study sample may be selected from the target population by either outcome status or other criteria. If the outcome is rare, random sampling or other mode of sample selection is far less efficient than selection by outcome, because many more subjects would be required to provide statistically meaningful results.

Regardless of which sample selection method is used, study subjects are usually classified (i.e., categorized) according to their outcome status. In the majority of case-control studies, outcome is dichotomously assessed as either present or absent, and subjects are classified as cases or controls respectively. (The terms *diseased* and *nondiseased* have also been applied to these two outcome categories but are best reserved for true diseases or other adverse health outcomes.)

Because the outcome has already occurred (among the cases) when study subjects are sampled, opportunities abound for sample distortion bias in case-control studies. Differential surveillance or selective loss to follow-up, which can usually be guarded against in the design and execution of cohort studies, have already occurred in case-control studies when the study sample is assembled. Sample distortion bias will be discussed in some detail in Section 8.4.1.

8.2.2 Outcome: Selection of Cases

When sample selection is based on outcome, the investigator can choose study subjects according to either incident or prevalent outcomes. *Incident* outcomes are those that develop de novo over time. Consequently, case-control studies with sampling by incident outcomes usually require the assembly of cases over a period of time. *Prevalent* outcomes include all subjects with the outcome at a given point in time, regardless of when they developed the outcome or how long they have had it at the time they are studied. When sample selection occurs by criteria other than outcome, outcome status is determined at the time the sample is assembled, and all outcomes are therefore prevalent.

The difference between incident and prevalent cases is entirely analogous to the difference between incidence and prevalence rates. The prevalence of an outcome depends on its average duration as well as its incidence and is thus influenced by mortality, treatment, and spontaneous resolution. Prevalent cases will thus underrepresent cases who died rapidly, those who were successfully treated, and those who recovered on their own. Incident cases will include all those newly occurring over a given period and will therefore be more representative of the entire spectrum of disease or other outcome under study.

Cases should be selected according to predetermined strict objective criteria, and they should be representative of cases in the target population. When prevalent cases are used, the resulting exposure-outcome association tends to become a measure of the relationship between exposure and nonfatal, chronic, and irremediable cases of the outcome. Although this is fine for outcomes such as birth defects (at least those not leading to spontaneous abortion or stillbirth) or conditions for which most or all cases are mild and permanent (e.g., male-pattern baldness, hay fever), it is often unsatisfactory in epidemiologic studies. Most health outcomes comprise a clinical spectrum of cases, and associations between exposure and the entire spectrum can often be sought only by using incident outcomes as the basis for case selection.

8.2.3 Outcome: Selection of Controls

As with cases, controls should be selected according to predetermined criteria to ensure the absence of the outcome ("nondiseased" status). Similarly, they should be representative of controls in the target population. The choice of controls, however, remains one of the thorniest methodologic issues in case-control studies. Although it might appear that normal, healthy subjects would constitute the best control group, it may be better to choose subjects with similar referral, surveillance, and other factors capable of distorting the study sample (see Section 8.4.1).

One approach that is sometimes taken is to have a healthy community control group, as well as another control group from a similar source as the case group (e.g., hospital-based). If the measure of exposure-outcome association is similar in both case-control comparisons, the investigator can have more confidence in the conclusions. If the two results differ, however, it is difficult to know which to believe.

Perhaps the best control group would consist of a representative sample of sub-jects free of the outcome who *would* have been included as cases *if* they had devel-oped the outcome [2]. Defining and locating such a sample, however, may be diffi-cult.

8.2.4 Exposure

As in other epidemiologic studies, definition of exposure requires an appreciation of the underlying biologic model for how exposure causes outcome. An exposure can cause an outcome only if it precedes it, of course. Consequently, the primary expo-sure of interest is *prior* exposure, rather than *contemporaneous* (exposure at the time outcome status is assessed). To the extent that contemporaneous exposure is a valid proxy for prior exposure, it may be substituted. Sex, race, blood groups, or inherited enzyme deficiencies are permanent characteristics that can be presumed to predate the outcome. Contemporaneous smoking, drinking, or dietary habits, however, may not validly reflect the prior habits that may have caused the study outcome.

The period and duration of exposure that is investigated should relate to the known or suspected latent period of the exposure factor. Cancer initiation and promotion are known to require years or even decades between exposure to a carcin-ogen and the clinical appearance of a cancer. Thus, a case-control study of asbes-tos exposure and lung cancer should focus on exposure to asbestos that occurred years or decades earlier, rather than in the immediately preceding months. On the other hand, oral contraceptives (OCs) are believed to augment the risk of myocar-dial infarction (MI) by increasing blood coagulation (clotting) factors. Thus, the relevant exposure in a case-control study of OCs and MI should include OC use occurring up to the time immediately before (or, for practical purposes, at the time) the MI occurred.

There is a theoretical danger that an outcome present in an unrecognized, early stage might actually provoke the exposure, and thus lead to a significant exposure-outcome association. The horse and cart would be reversed here, since the outcome would be the cause of the exposure, rather than the other way around. Failure to recognize such reverse causality bias can result in the erroneous inference that expo-sure has caused the outcome. For example, Horwitz and Feinstein have pointed out that endometrial (uterine) cancer may result in postmenopausal uterine bleeding before other symptoms develop. They argue that since estrogens are often pre-scribed for postmenopausal bleeding, the uterine cancer detected some time later may be falsely ascribed to the estrogen exposure [3]. (Other investigators, however, have argued that endometrial cancer is usually detected rather quickly [4]. Further-more, the association with estrogen exposure persists even when exposure is defined by past, discontinued estrogen use [5].)

If exposure is measured on a categorical scale, strict a priori criteria should be established for assigning cases and controls to exposure categories. This is particu-larly important when study subjects are classified dichotomously as exposed vs non-exposed, because substantial misclassification may result from nebulous or errone-ous criteria of exposure. The dose, duration, and period of exposure should therefore be specified ahead of time. Although different definitions of exposure can be used in the context of a single study to investigate several types of exposure-outcome causal models, multiple hypotheses increase the possibility of chance associations being declared "statistically significant" (see Chapter 12). In any case, the various definitions or criteria of exposure should be specified a priori to permit the testing, rather than the mere generation, of etiologic hypotheses.

Ascertainment of exposure provides the main source of information bias in case-control studies. This will be discussed, along with other aspects of bias assessment and control, in Section 8.4.

8.3 Analysis of Results

8.3.1 Relationship to Measurement Scales

The presentation and analysis of the results depends on the types of measurement scales in which exposure and outcome are expressed. As mentioned earlier, outcome is usually expressed categorically. A study of the relationship between the two continuous variables of infant birth weight and maternal cigarette smoking during gestation, however, would still qualify as a case-control study, if the directionality of the study was from outcome to exposure. The linear correlation between the average number of cigarettes smoked per day by the mothers and their infants' birth weights would nicely reflect the degree of exposure-outcome association. This type of case-control study is unusual, however, and would be similar (except for unknown losses to follow-up) to a cohort study in which pregnant women were followed forward to delivery.

When the outcome is continuous and the exposure is categorical, the results can be analyzed by comparing the mean outcomes in each exposure group. Although such an analysis *appears* similar to a comparison of mean outcomes in cohort studies, the exposure groups defined in a case-control study are not representative of exposure groups in the target population, and their corresponding means are difficult to interpret.

The use of ordinal outcomes is also rare in case-control studies but permits the assessment of dose-response effects. One recent example is a study of the relationship between adolescent adiposity (fatness) and a history of having been breast-fed as an infant [6]. Subjects were classified by outcome as either obese, overweight, or normal based on their weight-for-height and skinfold thicknesses. Their mothers were then interviewed about the type of feeding (breast vs bottle) the subjects received as newborns, and the major analysis was a comparison of breast feeding rates among the three outcome groups of normal, overweight, and obese subjects.

Categorical outcomes and continuous exposures yield a comparison of mean exposure. While the information conveyed by such a comparison does provide a test of exposure-outcome association, the result is difficult to interpret in the usual sequence of causal inference, because our primary interest is not the average level of exposure preceding a given effect. Rather, the major inference concerns the effect of a particular level of exposure in the target population. Since, for a continuous exposure variable, the *distributions* of exposures in cases and controls are likely to overlap, and since the distribution of exposure in the target population will be a mix of the case and control distributions, no inference can be made concerning the effect of a given level of exposure merely by comparing the mean exposures in cases and controls.

The usual method of analyzing the results of a case-control study uses dichotomous outcomes and categorical (usually dichotomous) exposures. Continuous exposures can be categorized to permit the use of this strategy. As we shall see, such a method does indeed provide a good estimate of the effect of exposure in the target population. When both outcome and exposure are dichotomous, the results can be displayed in a 2×2 table (see Table 8.1). At first glance, the table appears identical to the cohort study 2×2 table illustrated in Table 6.1. The cases and controls correspond to the presence and absence of the outcome respectively. The difference is in the directionality of the research design: backward from outcome to exposure in the case-control study, forward from exposure to outcome in the cohort study.

The backward directionality imposes a backward method of analysis. Thus, we cannot compare the "rate" of cases in the exposed and nonexposed subjects $\dfrac{a}{a+b}$ vs $\dfrac{c}{c+d}$, because the exposure groups were formed by the exposure histories ascertained in the study, not by sampling from the target population. Only the outcome

Table 8.1. Two-by-two table for analyzing results of a case-control study with dichotomous outcome and exposure

	Cases (O)	Controls ($\overline{O}$)	
E	a	b	$a+b$
$\overline{E}$	c	d	$c+d$
	$a+c$	$b+d$	$N=a+b+c+d$

E, Exposed; $\overline{E}$, nonexposed; O, outcome present; $\overline{O}$, outcome absent

Rate of exposure in cases $= \dfrac{a}{a+c}$

Rate of exposure in controls $= \dfrac{b}{b+d}$

Odds of exposure in cases $= \dfrac{a}{c}$

Odds of exposure in controls $= \dfrac{b}{d}$

Exposure odds ratio $(OR_E) = \dfrac{a/c}{b/d} = \dfrac{ad}{bc}$

groups (cases and controls) are representative of the target population, and thus the major comparison is the rate of exposure in cases vs controls: $\dfrac{a}{a+c}$ vs $\dfrac{b}{b+d}$.

Although such a comparison in itself provides a valid test of the exposure-outcome association, it shares the same difficulty in interpretation as a comparison (for continuous exposures) of mean exposures. That is, it does not allow a direct inference about the effects or risks of exposure in the target population. As we shall see, the use of odds, instead of rates, will allow us to estimate the *relative risk* of exposure in the target population.

8.3.2 Odds and Odds Ratios

As in horse racing or other forms of betting, the *odds* of a given event is the ratio of the probability of its occurrence to the probability of its nonoccurrence. In horse racing, the odds are usually given as the odds *against* a given horse's winning the race. Thus, 5:1 odds indicates that the horse is five times more likely to lose than to win; hypothetically, if the race were to be run six times, the horse would lose five and win one. Conversely, the odds *in favor* of the horse's winning is 1:5. Since ratios can also be expressed as fractions, these odds can be expressed as 1/5.

Similarly, in Table 8.1, the odds of exposure in the cases can be expressed as a/c and that in controls as b/d. We can also form a ratio of these two odds, called the

$$\text{exposure odds ratio (OR}_E) = \frac{a/c}{b/d} = \frac{ad}{bc}. \tag{8.1}$$

Why do we compare the odds, rather than the rates, of exposure in cases and controls? As we have seen, the risks of outcome in exposed and nonexposed subjects, which would provide direct information about the relative risk of exposure in the target population, cannot be directly derived from the data supplied by a case-control study. In fact, the "rates" of cases in the two exposure groups are uninterpretable quantities that reflect the proportion of cases and controls sampled from the target population rather than the true risks of the outcome among the exposed and nonexposed in that population. *The reason for using odds is that the odds ratio is a fairly good estimate of the true relative risk of exposure in the target population, provided the outcome is rare.* The algebraic proof of this assertion forms the basis of the following section. Readers not interested in seeing this proof may skip to Section 8.3.4 without loss of continuity.

8.3.3 The Relationship Between the Sample Odds Ratio in a Case-Control-Study and the Target Population Relative Risk

The best way to illustrate this relationship is by demonstrating the results in the entire target population (i.e., without sampling), and then seeing how a cohort study and a case-control study arrive at similar expressions for the relative risk of exposure in the target population. I will use capital letters to indicate the population values, lowercase letters to indicate values obtained in the cohort study, and lowercase letters with primes (') for values in the case-control study.

In the target population, a large group of individuals are followed up for a period of time for the development of the study outcome. The results in the population can be displayed in a 2×2 table (Table 8.2). Since everyone in the target population can be classified both by their exposure status and their outcome status at the end of follow-up, the same 2×2 table would be obtained if the population study were done as a cohort or case-control study, provided there is no loss to follow-up.

The relative risk in the target population is given by $\dfrac{A/(A+B)}{C/(C+D)}$. If the outcome is rare, then A is very small relative to B ($A \ll B$) and C is very small relative to D ($C \ll D$). Consequently, we can define the *estimated relative risk* (RR_{est}) as

$$RR_{est} = \frac{A/B}{C/D} = \frac{AD}{BC} \tag{8.2}$$

Table 8.2. Relationship between the relative risk and the odds ratio: target population

	O	$\overline{O}$	
E	A	B	A+B
$\overline{E}$	C	D	C+D
	A+C	B+D	N=A+B+C+D

E, Exposed; $\overline{E}$, nonexposed; O, outcome present; $\overline{O}$, outcome absent

Rate (risk) of outcome among exposed $= \dfrac{A}{A+B}$

Rate (risk) of outcome among nonexposed $= \dfrac{C}{C+D}$

Relative risk (RR) $= \dfrac{A}{A+B} \Big/ \dfrac{C}{C+D}$

If outcome is rare, then $A \ll B$ and $C \ll D$

Then $\dfrac{A}{A+B} \approx \dfrac{A}{B}$ and $\dfrac{C}{C+D} \approx \dfrac{C}{D}$

Estimated relative risk (RR_{est}) $= \dfrac{A/B}{C/D} = \dfrac{AD}{BC}$

Odds of outcome among exposed $= A/B$

Odds of outcome among nonexposed $= C/D$

Outcome odds ratio (OR_O) $= \dfrac{A/B}{C/D} = \dfrac{AD}{BC}$

Odds of exposure among those with outcome $= A/C$

Odds of exposure among those without outcome $= B/D$

Exposure odds ratio (OR_E) $= \dfrac{A/C}{B/D} = \dfrac{AD}{BC}$

We can also calculate odds and odds ratios in the target population. The odds of exposure among subjects with the outcome is A/C, the odds among those without the outcome is B/D, and the $OR_E = \dfrac{A/C}{B/D} = \dfrac{AD}{BC}$. We can also consider the odds of developing the outcome among the exposed (A/B) and the nonexposed (C/D), as well as the *outcome odds ratio* (OR_O):

$$OR_O = \frac{A/B}{C/D} = \frac{AD}{BC} \tag{8.3}$$

Note that RR_{est}, OR_E, and OR_O are equivalent.

Let us now consider what happens in a cohort study derived from this target population (Table 8.3). We may select the study sample either by exposure or by other criteria. If exposure is rare in the target population, we may wish to sample by exposure to ensure an adequate number of exposed subjects in the study sample. If exposure is common, representative (e.g., random) sampling will produce similar results. Since the sample is representative of exposed and nonexposed subjects in the target population and is obtained irrespective of (i.e., before) outcome, $\dfrac{a}{b} = \dfrac{A}{B}$. That is, the odds of outcome among the exposed is the same as in the target population. Similarly, $\dfrac{c}{d} = \dfrac{C}{D}$ for the nonexposed. In the sample, the exposure odds ratios (OR_E) can be calculated as $\dfrac{a/c}{b/d} = \dfrac{ad}{bc}$, and the outcome odds ratio (OR_O) as $\dfrac{a/b}{c/d} = \dfrac{ad}{bc}$. But,

Table 8.3. Relationship between the relative risk and the odds ratio: cohort study

		O	$\overline{O}$	
E		a	b	$a+b$
$\overline{E}$		c	d	$c+d$
		$a+c$	$b+d$	$N = a+b+c+d$

E, Exposed; $\overline{E}$, nonexposed; O, outcome present; $\overline{O}$, outcome absent

Outcome odds ratio (OR_O) = $\dfrac{a/b}{c/d} = \dfrac{ad}{bc}$

Exposure odds ratio (OR_E) = $\dfrac{a/c}{b/d} = \dfrac{ad}{bc}$

Since the sample is representative of exposed and nonexposed subjects in the target population, $\dfrac{a}{b} = \dfrac{A}{B}$ and $\dfrac{c}{d} = \dfrac{C}{D}$

Thus $\dfrac{ad}{bc} = \dfrac{AD}{BC}$

since $\dfrac{a}{b} = \dfrac{A}{B}$ and $\dfrac{c}{d} = \dfrac{C}{D}$, both of these expressions are also equivalent to $\dfrac{AD}{BC}$. Thus, in a cohort study without sample distortion, the exposure and disease odds ratios in the study sample are equivalent to the odds ratios and estimated relative risk in the target population.

Finally, let us consider what happens in a case-control study derived from the target population (Table 8.4). We may select the study sample either by outcome or by other criteria, with the former preferred whenever the outcome is rare. Since the sample is representative of cases and controls in the target population, and is obtained irrespective of exposure status, $\dfrac{a'}{c'} = \dfrac{A}{C}$ and $\dfrac{b'}{d'} = \dfrac{B}{D}$. In other words, the exposure odds among cases and controls is the same in the sample as in the target population. The exposure odds (OR_E) can be calculated as $\dfrac{a'/c'}{b'/d'} = \dfrac{a'd'}{b'c'}$. Since $\dfrac{a'}{c'} = \dfrac{A}{C}$ and $\dfrac{b'}{d'} = \dfrac{B}{D}$, $\dfrac{a'd'}{b'c'} = \dfrac{AD}{BC}$. $\left(\text{Similarly, the outcome odds ratio} = \dfrac{a'/b'}{c'/d'} = \dfrac{a'd'}{b'c'} = \dfrac{AD}{BC}.\right)$ In a case-control study without sample distortion, therefore, the sample odds ratio is equivalent to the odds ratio and estimated relative risk in the target population.

As we have seen, if the outcome is rare, all these expressions will be very close to the true relative risk. What is meant by "rare"? The rarer the outcome, of course, the closer the odds ratio will approximate the true relative risk. In general, if 10% or less of the target population develop the outcome during the period of follow-up,

Table 8.4. Relationship between the relative risk and the odds ratio: case-control study

	Cases (O)	Controls ($\overline{O}$)	
E	a'	b'	$a' + b'$
$\overline{E}$	c'	d'	$c' + d'$
	$a' + c'$	$b' + d'$	$N = a' + b' + c' + d'$

E, Exposed; $\overline{E}$, nonexposed; O, outcome present; $\overline{O}$, outcome absent

Exposure odds ratio (OR_E) $= \dfrac{a'/c'}{b'/d'} = \dfrac{a'd'}{b'c'}$

Since the sample is representative of cases and controls in the target population, $\dfrac{a'}{c'} = \dfrac{A}{C}$ and $\dfrac{b'}{d'} = \dfrac{B}{D}$

Thus $\dfrac{a'd'}{b'c'} = \dfrac{AD}{BC}$

the approximation is fairly good [7]. In fact, many authors use the term "relative risk" rather loosely to indicate the *estimated* relative risk or odds ratio determined in a case-control study. It is probably better, however, to restrict the term "relative risk" to the true relative risk determined in a cohort study. (Miettinen has shown that if incident cases are used, and controls are selected periodically over the same duration of study as the cases, the odds ratio is actually equivalent to the incidence density ratio (see Section 6.2.4) without requiring the rare disease assumption [8].)

8.3.4 An Illustrative Example

To illustrate the algebraic concepts discussed in the previous section, let us consider a hypothetical example. (Three decimal places are retained to demonstrate the magnitude of the "error" in using the odds ratio as an estimate of the relative risk.) Let us imagine that newly published laboratory experiments demonstrate that rats who are fed tea with their regular diets have an increased incidence of renal (kidney) cancer. Because tea consumption represents such a widespread exposure in humans, we decide to mount an epidemiologic study to test the hypothesis that tea drinkers have an increased risk for developing renal cancer.

Because the rats did not develop their renal cancers until late in life, because we know that carcinogenesis is a process that may require years or even decades, and because renal cancer is a rather rare disease, we decide that a case-control study would be the most feasible approach to this question. Table 8.5 shows the hypothetical results that we *would* have obtained had an entire birth cohort of 300 000 from a given community been followed to age 60. For simplicity, we shall assume a fixed population without migration or loss to follow-up and without other causes of mortality before age 60. Two out of three individuals in this population are tea drinkers.

The relative risk of renal cancer in tea drinkers is 2.000, and the attributable risk due to tea consumption is 0.001, or 1 per 1000. The exposure odds ratio and outcome odds ratio are both 2.002, which is very close to the true relative risk (2.000). This is exactly what we would expect, because renal cancer is a rare disease (cumulative incidence through age $60 = \dfrac{500}{300\,000} = 0.00167$, or 1.67 per 1000).

Now let us see what happens when we do a case-control study with sampling of 500 controls from this target population. Let us assume that the medical records for this entire population are available and that we can identify all 500 cases of renal cancer that have occurred up to the time of study, when all surviving subjects would be 60 years old. By using the medical records to identify all new cases, rather than assessing all surviving subjects at age 60 for the presence or absence of renal cancer, we are selecting incident cases and thus should be in a better position to make causal inferences about tea consumption and the entire disease spectrum of renal cancer.

The results of this case-control study are shown in Table 8.6. Because we expect the control group to be representative of controls in the target population (i.e., the sample is undistorted), we expect the same proportion of exposure in our sample of controls as we obtained in the population. Thus, the 500 controls are divided into 333 tea drinkers and 167 nontea drinkers. The exposure odds ratio (OR_E) is 2.006. This is quite similar to the OR_E, OR_O, and RR_{est} obtained in the target population.

Table 8.5. Tea drinking and renal cancer: target population

	RC	No RC	
Tea drinkers	400	199 600	200 000
Nontea drinkers	100	99 900	100 000
	500	299 500	300 000

RC, Renal cancer

Risk of RC among tea drinkers = 400/200 000 = 0.002 (2 per 1000)

Risk of RC among nontea drinkers = 100/100 000 = 0.001 (1 per 1000)

Relative risk (RR) = $\dfrac{400/200\,000}{100/100\,000}$ = 2.000

Attributable risk (AR) = 400/200 000 − 100/100 000 = 0.001 (1 per 1000)

Odds of RC among tea drinkers = 400/199 600 = 0.002004

Odds of RC among nontea drinkers = 100/99 900 = 0.001001

Outcome odds ratio (OR_O) = $\dfrac{400/199\,600}{100/99\,900}$ = 2.002

Odds of tea drinking among subjects with RC = 400/100 = 4.000

Odds of tea drinking among subjects without RC = 199 600/99 900 = 1.998

Exposure odds ratio (OR_E) = $\dfrac{400/100}{199\,600/99\,900}$ = 2.002

Estimated relative risk (RR_{est}) = $OR_E = OR_O$ = 2.002

Table 8.6. Tea drinking and renal cancer: case-control study

	RC	No RC	
Tea drinkers	400	333	733
Nontea drinkers	100	167	267
	500	500	1000

RC, Renal cancer

Odds of tea drinking among cases = 400/100 = 4.000

Odds of tea drinking among controls = 333/167 = 1.994

Exposure odds ratio (OR_E) = $\dfrac{400/100}{333/167}$ = 2.006

(The slight difference, 2.006 vs 2.002, occurred because our sampling resulted in a need to round off the proportion of tea drinkers to 333 of 500, or 0.6660 for the proportion of exposed controls. In the target population, however, 199 600 of 299 500, or 0.6664 of the controls were exposed.)

As alluded to earlier, there is one extremely important trap to be aware of when analyzing a 2×2 table from a case-control study. The unwary "cohort-prone" reader may be tempted to calculate a relative risk directly from such a table. For example, in Table 8.6 some persons might naively calculate a "risk" in the exposed as 400/733, or 546 per 1000. This is obviously a ridiculously high risk, nowhere near the 2 per 1000 in the target population. Similarly, they would calculate the "risk" in the nonexposed as 100/267, or 375 per 1000, which is also ridiculous. Such persons would then derive a direct "relative risk" as $\dfrac{400/733}{100/267}$, or 1.457. This is quite different from the population value of 2.000, but not as ridiculous as the individual "risks."

This entire procedure, of course, is totally incorrect. In a case-control study we do not begin with a representative sample of exposed and nonexposed individuals in the target population. Instead, we begin with a representative sample of subjects with and without the outcome (cases and controls). The only true rates or risks we can calculate, therefore, are the rates of exposure in cases and controls, not the rates of outcome in the exposed and nonexposed. (We use odds instead of rates, however, to derive an estimate of the true relative risk.)

8.3.5 Analysis of Ordinal Exposure Categories

If exposure is measured on a polychotomous ordinal scale, a case-control study can be analyzed for dose-response effects. This is analogous to the assessment of dose-response effects in cohort studies (see Section 6.2.4 and Table 6.4). Odds ratios are calculated by comparing each exposure category with the lowest exposure, or "base," category (e.g., nonexposed). Rising (or falling) odds ratios with increasing categories of exposure indicate a dose-response relationship between exposure and outcome and thus strengthen causal inferences.

To illustrate, Table 8.7 presents data from our hypothetical case-control study of tea consumption and renal cancer (Table 8.6), but with tea drinking measured on a three-category ordinal scale: heavy (≥ 3 cups/day), light (< 3 cups/day), and none. The exposure odds ratio for light vs nontea drinking is 1.61, and that for heavy vs nontea drinking is 2.76. Thus, the greater the tea drinking, the higher the estimated risk of renal cancer.

8.3.6 Interpretation of the Odds Radio

Since the odds ratio is an estimate of the relative risk, a value of OR > 1 indicates that exposure is associated with an increased risk of developing the outcome. The higher the value of OR, the greater the risk. Conversely, a value of OR < 1 indicates that exposure is associated with a reduced risk, i.e., it *protects* against developing the outcome. The closer the value of OR is to 0, the greater the protection.

Table 8.7. Tea drinking and renal cancer: case-control study with ordinal exposure

		Cases (RC)	Controls (no RC)	
	Heavy (≥ 3 cups/day)	190	115	305
Tea drinking	Light (<3 cups/day)	210	218	428
	None	100	167	267
		500	500	1000

RC, Renal cancer

Exposure odds ratio (OR_E) for light vs nontea drinking $= \dfrac{210/100}{218/167} = 1.61$

Exposure odds ratio (OR_E) for heavy vs nontea drinking $= \dfrac{190/100}{115/167} = 2.76$

The odds ratio will rarely equal exactly 1, even in the absence of true risk or protection. In particular, small increases or decreases from 1 may occur by chance; this is especially true if the sample size is small. In Chapter 14 we will see how the odds ratio can be tested for statistical significance, i.e., how to assess whether its difference from 1 could have occurred by chance.

8.3.7 Calculating Etiologic Fractions from Case-Control Studies

The etiologic fraction (EF) can be derived in an entirely analogous fashion to cohort studies (see Eq. 6.3):

$$EF = \frac{P_E(OR-1)}{P_E(OR-1)+1} \tag{8.4}$$

where P_E is the prevalence of exposure in the target population and OR is the odds ratio determined in the case-control study. The rate of exposure in the control group, $\dfrac{b}{b+d}$, can be used to estimate P_E under the assumption that this rate will be fairly close to the rate of exposure in the overall target population. For the tea drinking and renal cancer example (Table 8.6),

$$EF = \frac{333/500 \ (2.01-1)}{333/500 \ (2.01-1)+1} = 0.40$$

In other words, 40% of the cases of renal cancer in our (hypothetical) target population can be attributed to tea drinking.

8.4 Bias Assessment and Control

8.4.1 Sample Distortion Bias

Because case-control studies begin with the outcome, many of the sources of sample distortion bias are "hidden," in the sense that they have already occurred when the case and control subjects are assembled for study, rather than occurring during the course of follow-up. Thus mortality, migration, and referral that differ according to both exposure and outcome will lead to a biased sample, and unless the investigator knows the pattern of these differences, she can neither assess the magnitude of the bias nor protect against it in the design or analysis.

In cohort studies, unequal surveillance can lead to information bias through biased detection of the outcome, but standardized examination and testing procedures, as well as appropriate blinding, can be incorporated into the design to minimize this bias. In case-control studies, however, the outcome has already been detected, and any systematic difference in ascertainment of outcome according to exposure will result in a biased sample for which the investigator has no opportunity for control or reduction.

Referral is also a potential source of sample distortion bias in case-control studies, because the outcome is often the very reason for referrals that may, independently, be associated with exposure. This is most likely to occur if the cases are referred by a clinician who also prescribes the exposure agent. For example, if cases are referred by a gynecologist, whereas controls are not, cases may be more likely to be taking estrogen than controls, even if there is no true association between estrogen exposure and the study outcome.

Finally, as discussed in Chapter 5, case-control studies are prone to Berkson's bias, a form of sample distortion bias that occurs when both the exposure factor and the outcome are causes for referral [9, 10]. This is particularly likely to occur when the exposure factor is itself a disease or other adverse health state. The exposure-outcome association becomes falsely inflated because subjects with both exposure and outcome are more likely to be referred (they can be referred for either the exposure condition or the outcome), and therefore included in the study sample, than subjects with either or neither. For example, a hospital clinic-based case-control study of hypertension (high blood pressure) as a risk factor for breast cancer may reveal a false association (or an association of inflated magnitude) merely because patients with both conditions have a "double" chance of being referred (selected).

Sample distortion bias is best reduced by preventive planning in the study design. Use of incident outcomes as cases will reduce bias due to differential follow-up by including fatal cases. Choosing cases and controls from the same referral source will remove one source of referral bias but will not affect Berkson's bias. Control for the latter requires information about the rates of referral for both the exposure and outcome conditions, which unfortunately is rarely available to the investigator. Finally, detection bias can be reduced by ensuring that cases and controls had the same opportunity for detection of the outcome. For example, a study of the risk of gall-stones in patients taking cholesterol-lowering drugs might sample cases and controls by selecting patients with positive and negative ultrasound studies respectively.

8.4.2 Information Bias

Case-control studies are prone to information (misclassification) bias in the ascertainment of exposure, especially when exposure history is obtained directly from the study subjects, rather than from their medical records. The reason is that, unlike cohort studies, such case-control studies require the subjects to remember accurately their past exposures. Nondifferential (between cases and controls) errors in recall will result in random misclassification of exposure (i.e., "noise") and thus bias the exposure-outcome association toward a null result (OR = 1).

Differential recall bias is a graver concern, however. Theoretically, cases might be more likely to remember exposure than controls. It is often argued, for example, that the mother of a baby who has just been born with a severe congenital anomaly is more likely to search her memory for a history of past exposure to a drug or a potential toxin than a woman who has just given birth to a perfectly healthy baby. Empirical verification of the existence, frequency, and magnitude of this bias is sorely lacking, however [11].

Observers are another potent source of information bias in case-control studies. Knowledge of the case vs control status on the part of the person obtaining the exposure history (either from medical records or by personal interview) can affect the diligence with which positive or negative histories are obtained. If an investigator is under a strong impression that a certain exposure is associated with a given outcome, she may press (even if unconsciously) cases much harder for their recollection of exposure than she will controls.

Misclassification of outcome can occur when prevalent outcomes are selected as cases and the outcome is transient (may be cured or may resolve on its own). Subjects who experienced the outcome in the past but are free of it at the time of study will then be misclassified as controls. This is best avoided by selecting incident outcomes as cases.

Misclassification of exposure can be reduced considerably by establishing a priori criteria of exposure, by incorporating standardized methods for stimulating memory in all subjects (cases and controls), and by blinding observers to both the case vs control status of the subjects and (if possible) the exposure-outcome association under study. The latter can be accomplished by inquiring about prior exposure to a number of factors, with the study factor thus "hidden" among the rest.

8.4.3 Confounding Bias

Confounding bias arises whenever factors associated with exposure are independently associated with outcome (providing that such factors do not lie on the causal path from exposure to outcome). The principal sources of confounding in case-control studies are (a) exposure-associated differences in background variables with independent effects on outcome (susceptibility bias), and (b) exposure accompaniments with independent effects on outcome (contamination bias). Such sociodemographic and clinical factors as age, sex, and socioeconomic status, disease severity, and comorbidity (the coexistence of other diseases or conditions) are the types of baseline susceptibility factors that are particularly likely to confound the exposure-outcome association in case-control studies. Examples of accompaniments would include associated toxic exposures (e.g., cigarette smoking among asbestos miners) and medical treatments (e.g., radiation and chemotherapy).

As with cohort studies, confounding in case-control studies can be controlled at either the design or the analysis stage. Design features include restriction and matching (see Chapter 5). Restriction tends to limit the target population to which the results of the study may be applied. Matching is a powerful strategy for controlling confounding, provided the number of factors and levels of those factors are small enough to ensure "matchability" of all (or most) of the cases. As previously mentioned, matched designs should receive matched analyses to enhance statistical efficiency.

A matched analysis in case-control studies is similar to the analysis of matched cohort studies with dichotomous exposure and outcome (see Tables 6.5 and 6.6). Table 8.8 shows a matched analysis from a hypothetical case-control study of breast feeding as a possible protective factor against subsequent gastroenteritis (intestinal infection) in the first year of life in 100 pairs (200 total subjects) of infants matched for age, sex, and socioeconomic status. The matched odds ratio ($OR_{matched}$) is defined as the ratio of the number of pairs discordant for exposure history, i.e.,

$\frac{c}{b} = \frac{9}{26} = 0.35$. (The OR < 1 here indicates a protective effect of breast feeding.) The

reader is referred to other sources for analytic strategies pertaining to matched triplets, quadruplets, or variable numbers of controls per case [12, 13].

A stratified (Mantel-Haenszel) analysis [14] is another powerful analytic tool for controlling confounding and requires no adjustments in the design, providing that potentially confounding variables are recognized and measured reproducibly and

Table 8.8. Breast feeding and gastroenteritis case-control study: matched-pair analysis

		Cases	
		BF	Not BF
Controls	BF	6	26
	Not BF	9	59
			100

$OR_{matched} = \frac{c}{b} = \frac{9}{26} = 0.35$

validly. The analytic method is analogous to that shown for cohort studies (see Table 6.7):

$$OR_{MH} = \frac{\Sigma a_i d_i / N_i}{\Sigma b_i c_i / N_i} \tag{8.5}$$

where a_i = the number of exposed cases in the ith stratum,
  b_i = the number of exposed controls in the ith stratum,
  c_i = the number of nonexposed cases in the ith stratum,
  d_i = the number of nonexposed controls in the ith stratum,
and N_i = the total number of subjects ($a_i + b_i + c_i + d_i$) in the ith stratum.

The procedure is illustrated in Table 8.9. We return to our hypothetical case-control study of tea drinking and renal cancer. The crude results were shown in

Table 8.9. Tea drinking and renal cancer: Mantel-Haenszel analysis after stratification by cigarette smoking status

			Cases (RC)	Controls (no RC)	
Smokers	Tea drinkers		350	80	430
	Nontea drinkers		75	20	95
			425	100	525
			Cases (RC)	Controls (no RC)	
Nonsmokers	Tea drinkers		50	253	303
	Nontea drinkers		25	147	172
			75	400	475

RC, Renal cancer

$$OR_{smokers} = \frac{ad}{bc} = \frac{(350)(20)}{(80)(75)} = 1.17$$

$$OR_{nonsmokers} = \frac{ad}{bc} = \frac{(50)(147)}{(253)(25)} = 1.16$$

$$OR_{MH} = \frac{\Sigma a_i d_i / N_i}{\Sigma b_i c_i / N_i} = \frac{(350)(20)/525 + (50)(147)/475}{(80)(75)/525 + (253)(25)/475} = 1.16$$

Table 8.6 and suggested that tea drinkers have double the risk ($OR_{crude} = 2.01$) of developing renal cancer that nontea drinkers have. We suspect, however, that the effect may be confounded by cigarette smoking, since tea drinkers are more likely to smoke than nontea drinkers, and cigarette smoking is an independent risk factor for renal cancer. Table 8.9 shows the Mantel-Haenszel analysis when the data are stratified by smoking status (smokers vs nonsmokers).

The tea drinkers are indeed more likely to be smokers (430 of 733) than the nontea drinkers (95 of 267). The stratum-specific odds ratios are similar in both smokers and nonsmokers (1.17 vs 1.16), indicating no effect modification (interaction) by smoking status and little, if any, remaining association between tea drinking and renal cancer. The Mantel-Haenszel odds ratio (OR_{MH}) is the same, of course, since it is merely a weighted average of the two stratum-specific ORs.

The final approach to controlling confounding uses multivariate statistical adjustment techniques, which permit assessment of the exposure-outcome association while simultaneously adjusting for any number of confounding or interacting variables. The technique usually employed is *multiple logistic regression.* Although a full discussion of the method is beyond the scope of this text, it will be mentioned briefly in Chapter 14.

8.5 Advantages and Disadvantages of Case-Control Studies

In many situations, case-control studies have distinct advantages over cohort studies (Table 8.10). The ability to sample by outcome makes the case-control study ideally suited to investigating rare outcomes. When outcomes are rare, huge cohorts would be required to ensure that a sufficient number of subjects develop the outcome for significant differences to emerge. For example, suppose agent A leads to disease D with an attack rate of 0.6 per 1000, and that the natural (nonexposed) rate of occurrence of disease D is 0.2 per 1000. A cohort study would require over 38 000 subjects to detect a significant difference between subjects exposed and those not exposed to agent A. With a case-control study, we can start with a much smaller number of cases and controls and still achieve statistical significance (providing exposure to agent A is not rare among the cases).

Secondly, case-control studies offer an advantage whenever outcomes are delayed, even if they are not rare. Although a historical cohort study would theoretically get around this problem, many exposures (e.g., tea drinking) may not be

Table 8.10. Advantages and disadvantages of case-control studies (vs cohort studies)

A. Advantages
  1. Statistically more efficient when outcomes are rare
  2. Quicker when outcomes are delayed
  3. Less costly
B. Disadvantages
  1. Enhanced potential for sample distortion
  2. Exposure ascertainment more prone to error and bias

ascertainable in routine medical records. With a concurrent cohort study, we might have to wait many years for the development of an outcome before getting an answer to the question under investigation. With a case-control study, however, we start with the outcome, and the answer is available as soon as exposure histories are obtained. The only necessary waiting occurs when incident cases are being accumulated.

Finally, case-control studies are usually cheaper to carry out than cohort studies. This advantage follows logically from the first two, because large numbers of subjects and prolonged follow-up are usually expensive.

The disadvantages of case-control studies center on their higher potential for sample distortion bias and information bias. Although bias due to omission of fatal and transient cases can be avoided by using incident cases, the opportunities for referral, detection, and Berkson's biases, as well as biased ascertainment of exposure, require careful strategies for sample selection and study design and even then may not be entirely avoided. Confounding, however, can be controlled as in observational cohort studies, provided that potentially confounding variables are considered and their measurement is sufficiently reproducible and valid. A helpful approach for reducing bias in case-control studies is to model certain features of their design on the randomized clinical trial [15]. By using strict inclusion and exclusion criteria, standardized memory "probes," interviewer blinding, and unbiased procedures to detect the presence or absence of the outcome, case-control studies can come closer to the methodologic "gold standard" of the randomized experiment.

On balance, the case-control study represents an important investigative strategy in epidemiologic research. When outcomes are rare or delayed, it is often the only feasible approach. In other circumstances, it can often provide an interim answer to a question of exposure-outcome association while awaiting the results of more definitive cohort studies or clinical trials. Adequate attention to sources of bias in both the design and analysis stages of case-control studies should help maximize the validity of their results [16–18].

References

1. Feinstein AR (1973) Clinical biostatistics. XX. The epidemiologic trohoc, the ablative risk ratio, and "retrospective" research. Clin Pharmacol Ther 14: 291–307
2. Miettinen OS (1985) The "case-control" study: valid selection of subjects. J Chronic Dis 38: 543–548
3. Horwitz RI, Feinstein AR (1978) Alternative analytic methods for case-control studies of estrogens and endometrial cancer. N Engl J Med 299: 1089–1094
4. Jick H, Walker AM, Rothman KJ (1980) The epidemic of endometrial cancer: a commentary. Am J Public Health 70: 264–267
5. Shapiro S, Kaufman DW, Slone D, Rosenberg C, Miettinen OS, Stolley PD, Rosenshein NB, Watring WG, Leavitt T, Knapp RC (1980) Recent and past use of conjugated estrogen in relation to adenocarcinoma of the endometrium. N Engl J Med 303: 485–489
6. Kramer MS (1981) Do breast-feeding and delayed introduction of solid foods protect against subsequent obesity? J Pediatr 98: 883–887
7. Kleinbaum DG, Kupper LL, Morgenstern H (1982) Epidemiologic research: principles and quantitative methods. Lifetime Learning Publications, Belmont, CA, p 146

8. Miettinen OS (1976) Estimability and estimation in case-referent studies. Am J Epidemiol 103: 226–235
9. Berkson J (1946) Limitations of the application of fourfold table analysis to hospital data. Biometr Bull 2: 47–53
10. Walter SD (1980) Berkson's bias and its control in epidemiologic studies. J Chronic Dis 33: 721–725
11. Lippman A, Mackenzie SG (1985) What is "recall bias" and does it exist? In: Marois M (ed) Prevention of physical and mental congenital defects. Part C. Basic and medical science, education, and future strategies. Alan R. Liss, New York, pp 205–209
12. Breslow NE, Day NE (1980) Statistical methods in cancer research, vol 1. The analysis of case-control studies. International Agency for Research on Cancer, Lyon, pp 162–189
13. Schlesselman JJ (1982) Case-control studies: design, conduct, analysis. Oxford University Press, New York, pp 213–219
14. Mantel N, Haenszel W (1959) Statistical aspects of the analysis of data from retrospective studies of disease. JNCI 22: 719–748
15. Feinstein AR (1985) Experimental requirements and scientific principles in case-control studies. J Chronic Dis 38: 127–133
16. Ibrahim MA (ed) (1979) The case-control study: consensus and controversy. Pergamon, Oxford
17. Horwitz RI, Feinstein AR (1979) Methodological standards and contradictory results in case-control research. Am J Med 66: 556–564
18. Hayden GF, Kramer MS, Horwitz RI (1982) The case-control study: a practical review for the clinician. JAMA 247: 326–331

Chapter 9: Cross-Sectional Studies

9.1 Introduction

In cohort studies, subjects are followed in a forward direction from exposure to outcome, and inferential reasoning is from cause to effect. In case-control studies, subjects are investigated in a backward direction from outcome to exposure; inference
is from effect to cause. In cross-sectional studies, the exposure and outcome are
both determined at the same point, or cross section, in time [1]. (Hence, another
name for this design is *prevalence study*.) Cross-sectional studies share many of the
features of case-control studies. They carry an additional disadvantage, however;
since exposure is ascertained at the same point in time as the outcome, the investigator cannot be certain that exposure preceded outcome. As we shall see, this disadvantage has important implications for causal inference.

9.2 Research Design Components

9.2.1 Sample Selection

As discussed in Chapter 4, the study sample in cross-sectional studies can be selected
by exposure, outcome, or other criteria. Random sampling or some other form of
representative sample selection is often used in such studies. In fact, the use of the
term "representative cross section" to refer to how sample subjects are selected from
the target population has led to some of the confusion between sample selection and
directionality in the classification of epidemiologic research design (see Chapter 4).
But both cohort and case-control studies can also use this method of sample selection. Furthermore, cross-sectional studies may profit by basing subject selection on
either exposure or outcome if either is rare in the target population. When exposure
is rare, statistical efficiency is enhanced when selection is by exposure. Conversely,
selection by outcome is preferable when the outcome is rare.

9.2.2 Outcome

Cross-sectional studies usually measure prevalent outcomes. Fatal cases, dropouts,
and migrants are not counted, nor are cases that were successfully treated or that
resolved spontaneously. Consequently, cross-sectional studies are best suited to

chronic, nonfatal conditions. Incident cases could be investigated for simultaneous exposure, however, and such a design would still be considered cross-sectional. For example, new patients with myocardial infarction could be interviewed concerning their (then) current smoking habits.

9.2.3 Exposure

Exposure is measured at the same point in time as outcome. (As explained in Chapter 4, the "same point in time" is an approximation.) Since exposure and outcome have usually been present for some time prior to the study, the investigator cannot be certain that exposure preceded outcome. Consequently, any inference that exposure caused outcome rests on the unknown true temporal sequence of events.

When the exposure variable is a genetic, anatomic, or otherwise permanent attribute, the issue of temporal sequence becomes less problematic for the investigator. Thus race, sex, blood type, or glucose-6-phosphate dehydrogenase (G-6-PD) genotype, for example, can usually be assumed to precede the study outcome. For these kinds of exposures, cross-sectional studies are equivalent to case-control studies.

This is also true whenever exposure determined at a particular point in time is a valid proxy for exposure occurring in the past. To the extent that dietary, smoking, or drug-taking practices measured at one point in time accurately reflect such practices within a time range consistent with the latent period for the outcome, the results of a cross-sectional study should be similar to the results of a case-control study. Since such practices often change over time, however, and may even change in response to the study outcome (i.e., as effect rather than cause), use of the cross-sectional design is best suited to outcomes with short latent periods.

9.3 Analysis of Results

The analysis of the results of a cross-sectional study depends on the method of sample selection and on the measurement scales for exposure and outcome. When selection is by exposure, analysis is similar to that used for cohort studies. For continuous outcomes, mean outcomes are compared between the groups defined by exposure status. For incident categorical outcomes, the outcome rates are compared in exposure groups; if dichotomous, relative and attributable risks can be calculated. When selection is by exposure and outcomes are prevalent rather than incident, the relative risk derived from a cross-sectional study is often referred to as a *prevalence rate ratio*.

When sample selection is by outcome, analysis is similar to that used for case-control studies. Outcome is usually dichotomized (case vs control), and odds ratios can be calculated. The classification of outcome status as "case" vs "control" does not render the design truly case-control, however, since the exposure ascertained in cross-sectional studies is simultaneous with, rather than prior to, the outcome. As noted earlier, these two designs do in fact become equivalent when the exposure variables are permanent characteristics or when the latent period from exposure to outcome is very short. As with case-control studies, the outcome must be rare for the odds ratio to be a reasonable estimate of the relative risk (see Section 8.5.3).

When sample selection is by random, representative, or other criteria, the results of a cross-sectional study can be analyzed using either of the above strategies (cohort or case-control). In general, the cohort approach is preferred, because it usually permits a direct comparison of means or rates in groups defined by exposure, as well as calculation of true relative risks when the outcome is dichotomous.

9.4 Bias Assessment and Control

Cross-sectional studies are generally prone to the same sources of sample distortion bias, information bias, and confounding bias as case-control studies. Since ascertainment of exposure is based on contemporaneous exposure, however, there is less opportunity for information bias in the exposure measurement. Since cross-sectional studies do not rely on the subject's memory of exposure, its measurement is less likely to be randomly erroneous or differentially selective (those with the outcome being more likely to recall exposure) than in case-control studies. Adequate blinding of interviewers and clear, a priori criteria for exposure are usually sufficient to guard against this form of bias in cross-sectional studies.

Design strategies for reducing sample distortion bias are identical to those discussed for case-control studies in Chapter 8. Restriction, matching, stratification, or multivariate adjustment techniques can be used to control for confounding bias in cross-sectional studies. The choice of a statistical procedure depends on the method of sampling and on whether the results are analyzed by the cohort or case-control approach (see Section 9.3).

The potential for reverse causality bias is of crucial importance in cross-sectional studies and is the major reason why causal inferences are more tenuous than in cohort or even case-control studies. Imagine, for example, a cross-sectional study of obesity as a possible risk factor for osteoarthritis (degenerative joint disease) of the hips and knees. Without knowing that the obesity preceded the arthritis, an equally tenable inference (following demonstration of a statistical association) would be that osteoarthritis is a risk factor for obesity. Persons who develop painful hips or knees might limit their physical activity and secondarily become obese.

9.5 "Pseudo-Cohort" Cross-Sectional Studies

One type of cross-sectional study can be made to look like a cohort study. Instead of following one group over time, different age groups are studied cross-sectionally. Data are obtained as a function of age but are based on different subjects rather than on the same subjects over time. Such studies are called *pseudo-cohort studies* because the data look longitudinal (i.e., based on the same subjects followed over time) even though they are cross-sectional.

An example of this design is insurance company life tables; such tables list the number of people surviving for 1 year at each year of age. These data are then used to calculate the chances of dying or living for specific periods of time after any given age. The problem is that this approach assumes that risk factors, medical care, and other aspects of public health are also constant, so that current mortality trends will remain unchanged for decades to come. The assumption is of course untrue. With general improvements in health in developed societies over the past few decades, persons at any age today will (on average) live longer than did those of the same age 50 years ago. Since life insurance premiums are based on the current mortality experience of earlier birth cohorts, the insurance companies benefit from the lower future mortality of later birth cohorts.

This example illustrates the effect that a given age cohort (i.e., those persons born at the same calendar time) can have on the cross-sectional age distribution of a clinical attribute: the so-called *cohort effect*. Another example of a cohort effect is the apparent deterioration in measured intelligence with age demonstrated in several cross-sectional studies [2]. More recent cohort studies, however, have shown that intelligence does not diminish with aging. Since intelligence tests reflect education and since successive generations have received more and better education, the elderly appear less intelligent than the young at any cross section in time. Cohort effects thus represent a confounding bias of calendar time on age. Such a bias can be discovered (and thus removed) only by analyzing the data longitudinally by age cohort, a technique known as *cohort analysis*. Consider once again our example of age and intelligence. Repeated intelligence testing of the same individuals within each age cohort would show no decrease in scores over time, whereas members of earlier birth cohorts would have lower scores at any given age than members of later cohorts tested at the same age.

9.6 Advantages, Disadvantages, and Uses of Cross-Sectional Studies

The major advantages of cross-sectional studies (see Table 9.1) are their rapidity and low cost, compared with cohort studies, and their relative freedom (vis à vis case-control studies) from faulty or biased memory. Since exposure and outcome are both ascertained at a single point in time, no follow-up is required. Data can therefore be obtained quickly and at little expense to the investigators. Furthermore, the potential for information bias in ascertaining exposure is less than in case-control studies, since subjects do not have to rely on their memory of past exposure. If observers are adequately blinded, contemporaneous exposure is likely to be measured reproducibly and validly.

Perhaps the main contribution of the cross-sectional design is in descriptive, rather than analytic, epidemiologic studies. Disease or other clinical phenomena can be classified by person (age, sex, race, ethnicity, socioeconomic status), place (nation, region, province, city, neighborhood, dwelling), or time. Cross-sectional studies are also useful for describing the clinical spectrum (symptoms, signs, laboratory test results, pathologic findings) of a given disease entity. For example, an

Table 9.1. Advantages and disadvantages of cross-sectional studies

A. Advantages
   1. Useful for descriptive studies
     a. Clinical spectrum of disease
     b. Prevalence surveys (public health)
   2. Rapid, inexpensive analytic studies provide early "clues"
   3. Less prone (than case-control studies) to exposure recall error and bias
B. Disadvantages
   1. May be unable to sort out cart vs horse (temporal sequence of exposure and outcome)
   2. Enhanced potential (vs cohort studies) for sample distortion bias

investigator might carry out a cross-sectional study of a large defined group of diabetic patients to describe the proportion with retinal, renal, cardiac, or peripheral vascular complications. Much of what we know about the varied clinical manifestations of many diseases, especially rare diseases, is based on such descriptive cross-sectional "case series." Furthermore, as discussed in Chapter 3, ascertaining the prevalence of a variety of diseases and conditions is of great importance to public health personnel in making their decisions about allocation of resources and targets for preventive or other intervention strategies.

Cross-sectional designs also have a role in analytic studies. Because they can be done quickly and inexpensively, cross-sectional studies can often provide the first clue to an exposure-outcome association, which can serve as a stimulus for more definitive cohort or case-control studies. In addition, in situations involving permanent exposure characteristics, short latent periods, or exposure measures that are valid proxies for past exposures, cross-sectional and case-control studies become equivalent. In such situations, cross-sectional studies have the advantage of being less prone to random error and bias in measurement of exposure.

The major disadvantages of cross-sectional studies are their frequent inability to distinguish cause from effect and their potential for sample distortion bias. The latter problem is one shared by case-control studies. The problem of distinguishing the horse from the cart, i.e., whether exposure preceded outcome or vice versa, is unique to cross-sectional studies and constitutes their major limitation in analytic research. Unless the exposure variable is a permanent attribute or the latent period is very short, causality inferences are rather tenuous. The importance of temporal sequence in causal reasoning will be discussed further in Chapter 19.

References

1. Kramer MS, Boivin J-F (1987) Toward an "unconfounded" classification of epidemiologic research design. J Chronic Dis 40: 683–688
2. Susser MW (1969) Aging and the field of public health. In: Riley MW, Riley JW, Johnson M (eds) Aging and society. Russell Sage Foundation, New York, pp 137–146

Part II

Biostatistics

Chapter 10: **Introduction to Statistics**

10.1 Variables

In Chapter 2 I defined the different types (scales) of epidemiologic variables and discussed principles of their measurement. In particular, I classified variables as either continuous or categorical, subdividing categorical variables into dichotomous vs polychotomous and further subdividing polychotomous variables as either nominal or ordinal. This framework will be retained in our discussion of statistical analysis.

10.2 Populations, Samples, and Sampling Variation

As has been repeatedly emphasized, almost all epidemiologic studies are carried out on a sample that is presumed to be representative of a particular *target population*. Since investigators (and the public) are usually interested in applying the results of a study beyond the actual subjects participating in the study, they must make inferences about the target population based on the data from the sample. In Chapters 4 and 5 I discussed the extent to which such inferences depend on the representativeness of the sample selection procedure and the absence of subsequent distortion of the sample. Also considered were the various methods of sample selection, the use of random sampling (including simple, stratified, and clustered random sampling) being emphasized as providing the best assurance of representativeness.

Another aspect of samples and sampling is sampling variation. Assuming a purely *stochastic* (i.e., probabilistic) mechanism for obtaining a sample from its source population, statistics for that sample will differ from the corresponding population statistics in a predictable way. In fact, if repeated random samples were selected from the same source population after replacing such samples (so that the same individual could be sampled more than once), the distribution of sample statistics (e.g., mean, rate, relative risk, odds ratio) that would be obtained can be described. This distribution of sample statistics describes a phenomenon known as *sampling variation*. Although sampling variation is based on a theoretical process of repeated sampling, the reproducibility of a statistic from a single sample remains an important consideration.

Since individuals in a population do not all have the same value for a given variable but rather exhibit a distribution of values, a small sample (even if randomly selected) might, just by "the luck of the draw," have a mean or rate that differs considerably from that of the entire population. Consequently, small samples from the same population are likely to exhibit considerable sampling variation. On the other hand, repeated large samples would yield sample means or rates very close to the population value and, therefore, to each other. Thus, sampling variation is inversely related to the *sample size.*

10.3 Description vs Statistical Inference

Descriptive statistics are numbers intended to describe a study sample by summarizing and condensing a set of measurements on the individuals in that sample. They are analogous to, and often derive from, descriptive epidemiologic studies. Contrasts can be made between groups (e.g., a comparison of outcome in groups defined by exposure status), but no inferences are drawn about the unobserved source populations from which the groups derive. Rates (e.g., birth rates, death rates, rates of successful treatment) are used to describe categorical variables. Continuous variables are usually described by summary measures of central location and spread. Mean birth weight and median survival time are examples of central location statistics. Ranges, standard deviations, and percentile ranges are the kinds of statistics used to describe spread.

Statistical inference comprises a range of procedures and techniques that are used to draw conclusions about populations based on data from samples. Statistical inference can be classified under two main headings: (a) parametric estimation and (b) significance testing. In *parametric estimation,* inferences are drawn about *parameters*[1] (mathematical descriptors such as the rate, mean, relative risk, odds ratio, slope, correlation, or standard deviation) in the target population based on the analogous statistics (*estimators* of these parameters) obtained in the sample. Such inferences assume either a stochastic mechanism for generating the variable(s) being analyzed or a random sampling distribution. Parametric estimation includes the calculation of *confidence intervals* around sample statistics. In significance testing, probabilities (often called *P values*) are calculated based on hypotheses about the exposure-outcome association in the target population.

10.4 Statistical vs Analytic Inference

In Chapter 5 I distinguished between *statistical inference* and *analytic inference* as the two "arms" of internal validity in epidemiologic research. This distinction is worth re-emphasizing here and is analogous to that between measurement reproducibility and validity. Statistical inference applies various aspects of statistical theory, such as

---

[1] Many people use the term "parameter" as a synonym for "variable" or "factor." Although this is common in everyday parlance, I will avoid it in this text and restrict the use of "parameter" to its accepted statistical meaning.

parametric models of frequency distributions, to data obtained in a sample in order to draw conclusions about the existence and magnitude of exposure-outcome association in the target population from which it derives. Statistical inference assumes that the sample was randomly selected from the target population. In analytic inference, we also draw conclusions about associations in a target population based on evidence adduced in a sample, but the basis for inference is the absence of analytic bias.

In examining an exposure-outcome association demonstrated in a study sample, the "P value approach" of statistical inference addresses the following question: "How likely is an association at least as large as the one observed to have arisen solely as a result of sampling variation (i.e., by chance) from a target population in which no such association exists?" Alternatively, the confidence interval approach asks: "Based on the sample data, what is the likely range of estimates of association in the target population?" With both approaches, neither the specific research design (e.g., experimental vs observational cohort vs case-control vs cross-sectional) nor analytic bias are taken into account. The process is the application of statistical theory (a test of statistical significance), and the result is a mathematical probability.

Ensuring that chance alone is unlikely to explain an observed association is necessary, but not sufficient, for internal validity. In other words, once sampling variation has been dismissed as an explanation for the findings (because its probability is deemed sufficiently low), the exposure-outcome association must be demonstrated to be reasonably free of bias due to measurement error, sample distortion, confounding, and reverse causality. As we have seen, this depends largely on the careful design and execution of the study. Statistics and mathematics may be used in adjustment procedures to reduce confounding, but judgments about which factors require adjustment and which techniques should be used rest with the investigator.

Chapter 11: Descriptive Statistics and Data Display

11.1 Continuous Variables

11.1.1 Frequency Distributions

As outlined in Chapter 10, the major aim of descriptive statistics is to condense and summarize a set of measurements on a large number of individuals. Suppose we wished to describe the variable "age" (in completed years) in 250 patients who underwent cholecystectomy (gallbladder removal) at City Hospital during a 6-month period. Merely listing the 250 patients with their corresponding ages would convey very little useful information, because the number of individual measurements makes it difficult to discern any overall patterns in the data. In other words, it is difficult to see the forest for the trees.

Making sense out of so many numbers requires that the data be summarized. Perhaps the most informative method for summarizing and displaying a set of measurements for a continuous variable is by constructing a *frequency distribution.* This is accomplished by categorizing the continuous data (i.e., breaking down the range of observed values into a series of successive categories) and counting the number of study subjects whose measurements fall within each category. When proportions or percentages of the total group are given instead of counts, the resulting distribution is called a *relative frequency distribution.*

Once a frequency distribution has been constructed, it can be displayed in either tabular or graphic form. Table 11.1 summarizes both the frequency and relative frequency (percentage of total) distributions by age of the 250 postcholecystectomy patients described above. Figure 11.1 is the corresponding *histogram,* or *bar graph,* in which frequency (ordinate on left) and proportions (ordinate on right) are represented by the *areas* of the respective bars.

Several guidelines should be kept in mind in constructing frequency distributions and histograms:

1. The number of categories should be sufficient, but not excessive, relative to the total number of measurements. If too many categories are used, little data reduction (summary) is achieved; if too few are used, important information may be obscured.
2. Overlapping categories must be avoided, i.e., the limits (cutoff boundaries) for each category must be mutually exclusive. (For example, in a frequency distribution of systolic blood pressure measurements that included categories of 100–110

Table 11.1. Age distribution of 250 postcholecystectomy patients

Age (completed years)	Patients	
	(*n*)	(%)
16–20	2	0.8
21–25	2	0.8
26–30	5	2.0
31–35	9	3.6
36–40	17	6.8
41–45	31	12.4
46–50	83	33.2
51–55	46	18.4
56–60	35	14.0
61–65	20	8.0
Total	250	100

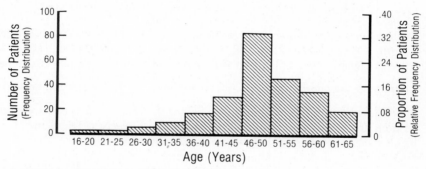

Fig. 11.1. Age histogram for 250 postcholecystectomy patients

and 110–120 mm Hg, one would not know in which of the two categories to place a subject with a systolic pressure of 110 mm Hg.

3. Although not an essential requirement, interpretation is aided by the use of equal category intervals (upper minus lower limits) and by the avoidance of open-ended intervals (e.g., ≥ 140 or 140+ mm Hg for systolic blood pressure).

Histograms provide a method for adjusting for unequal intervals in a frequency distribution. Because there are only nine total patients in the three youngest age categories in our example, it might seem advisable to "collapse" them into a single category, 16–30 years. In that case, however, the height of the corresponding histogram bar should be 3 (or .012), rather than 9 (or .036), so that the *total area* of the bar remains proportional to the overall frequency (or proportion) for the enlarged category. The area under a single bar spanning ages 16–30 would be (3)(15) = 45, which is the same total area as the sum of the areas for the first three bars in Fig. 11.1, i.e., (2)(5) + (2)(5) + (5)(5). Similarly, for the relative frequency distribution, (.012)(15) = .18 = (.008)(5) + (.008)(5) + (.020)(5).

11.1.2 Summary Statistics

In addition to tabular and graphic methods, continuous variables can often be summarized using simple statistics that describe the frequency distribution without actually displaying it. In the interest of parsimony (data reduction), we attempt to describe the essential attributes of a distribution using the fewest possible descriptors. Three major attributes of the distribution are usually described: *central tendency, shape,* and *spread.*

Three measures are in common use for describing central tendency: the mean, the median, and the mode. The sample *mean* or *average* $(\bar{x})$ is defined as follows:

$$\bar{x} = \frac{\Sigma x_i}{n} \tag{11.1}$$

where x_i = the value for the ith subject in the sample
$\qquad\ \Sigma$ = the Greek letter sigma, indicating a summation over all x_i's
and $\quad n$ = the number of subjects in the sample (also called the *sample size*).

The *median* is the midmost value of the distribution, i.e., the value for which 50% of the group have higher values and 50% have lower values. It is calculated by rank ordering (from lowest to highest) the values and then determining the value corresponding to the middle rank, i.e., the rank order $\frac{n+1}{2}$. Thus, if the group contains an odd number of subjects, the median will be the value of the subject with the middle rank. If the group contains an even number of subjects, the median will fall halfway between the values of the two midmost subjects.

The *mode* is the most common single value, i.e., the *peak* of the frequency distribution. It is the least used of the three measures of central tendency because it is not readily manipulated mathematically.

The calculation of each of the three central tendency descriptors is illustrated below for the following serum creatinine measurements (in mg/dl) in a group of 15 patients, arranged here in ascending order:

0.3, 0.6, 0.6, 0.7, 0.8, 0.8, 0.8, 0.9, 1.0, 1.0, 1.1, 1.3, 1.4, 1.6, 2.1

$$\text{mean} = \frac{\Sigma x_i}{n} = \frac{15.0}{15} = 1.0 \text{ mg/dl}$$

$$\text{median} = \frac{n+1}{2}\text{th value} = \frac{15+1}{2}\text{th value} = \text{8th value} = 0.9 \text{ mg/dl}$$

$$\text{mode} = 0.8 \text{ mg/dl (the only value that appears three times)}$$

The main characteristics of the shape of a frequency distribution are the number of peaks (modes) and the degree of asymmetry around its center. A distribution with two or more modes is referred to as *bimodal, trimodal,* etc. The asymmetry characteristic is called *skewness*. A distribution is said to be skewed to the right when the mean exceeds the median and the right "tail" is longer than the left. This type of distribution is typical of variables with a fixed lower bound but without upper bound, such as length of hospital stay. A distribution is skewed to the left when the mean is lower than the median and the left tail is longer than the right. An example is the age distribution in many developing countries, where high birth rates and short life expectancy result in a distribution skewed toward younger ages.

Three types of statistics are commonly used to describe the spread of a frequency distribution: range, percentile ranges, and standard deviation. The *range* is the interval between the lowest and highest value in the distribution (0.3–2.1 mg/dl in the above example of serum creatinine). A *percentile range* is an interval between two specified *percentile points*. The *inner 90 percentile range* includes all values between the 5th and 95th percentiles; the *interquartile range* includes those between the 25th and 75th percentiles.

To calculate a percentile point, we rank the values from lowest to highest and number each observation 1, 2, 3...*n*. The Pth percentile is the value corresponding to the $\left[\dfrac{(n+1)\,P}{100} \right]$ th rank. Thus, the median is equivalent to the 50th percentile point, since $\dfrac{(n+1)}{2} = \dfrac{(n+1)}{100}\dfrac{50}{}$.

Perhaps the most useful way of describing the spread of a distribution is to indicate the average or typical "distance" between the individual measurements and the center of the distribution. For example, one could subtract each individual value from the group mean. How could the resulting deviations (differences) then be summarized? Obviously, the average deviation would be zero, since the positive and negative differences around the mean would cancel. The average *absolute value* of the deviation would do nicely, but absolute values are difficult to manipulate mathematically. Squaring the deviations and then taking the average of the squared deviations also accomplishes the goal of eliminating the plus and minus signs. This is the basis of the formula for calculating a sample *variance*.

For a sample, the variance is denoted by s^2 and is defined as follows:

$$s^2 = \frac{\Sigma(x_i - \bar{x})^2}{n-1} \tag{11.2}$$

where x_i is the value for the ith subject in the sample, $\bar{x}$ the sample mean, Σ, the Greek letter sigma indicating a summation over all x_i's, and n the sample size. The quantity $n-1$ is called the number of *degrees of freedom*. (For a given mean $\bar{x}$, $n-1$ x_i's are considered "free" or independent. The nth value of x_i is determined by $\bar{x}$ and the previous $n-1$ x_i's.) The formula uses $n-1$ instead of n because the variance of the sample calculated in this way better approximates the variance of its source population.

Because the variance is based on squared deviations, it obviously does not represent the average or expected deviation of an individual from the sample. A better representation is achieved by taking the square root of the variance. The resulting quantity is called the *standard deviation* (abbreviated SD). The standard deviation for a sample is denoted by s and is defined as:

$$s = \sqrt{\frac{\Sigma(x_i - \bar{x})^2}{n-1}} \tag{11.3}$$

The standard deviation appears no easier to compute than the average absolute value of the deviations. Its justification lies in a computationally simpler formula that is algebraically equivalent to Eq. 11.3:

$$s = \sqrt{\frac{\sum x_i^2 - \frac{(\sum x_i)^2}{n}}{n-1}} \tag{11.4}$$

In other words, one sums the squares of each value, subtracts the quotient of the squared sum of the values divided by the sample size, divides the resulting difference by the degrees of freedom, and then takes the square root.

The sample standard deviation can also be expressed as a proportion, or percentage, of the mean value. This entity $\left[\frac{s}{\bar{x}} \text{ or } \frac{s}{\bar{x}}(100)\right]$ is called the *coefficient of variation* (abbreviated CV). It is useful for describing measurement variation, since its value is independent of the measurement units used. For example, the standard deviation of a set of height measurements will differ according to whether height is measured in inches or centimeters, whereas the coefficient of variation will be the same.

The range and percentile ranges can be used for describing the spread of any frequency distribution, regardless of its shape. The choice of which percentile range to report depends on the shape of the distribution. For example, the inner quartile range would poorly describe the spread of a bimodal distribution in which the two modes were widely separated. The standard deviation is best reserved for data that are distributed fairly symmetrically around the group mean (i.e., data with a non-skewed distribution), because it is affected by extreme (very high or very low) values. It is most appropriate when the distribution is what statisticians call *normal*. We shall have more to say about the normal distribution in Section 11.1.3.

There is one other sample statistic that is often erroneously used in the clinical literature as a descriptor of spread: the *standard error of the mean* (SEM). It is defined as:

$$\text{SEM} = \frac{s}{\sqrt{n}} \tag{11.5}$$

Because the SEM decreases with increasing sample size, however, it is *not* a good descriptor of the spread of a frequency distribution, despite its popularity. A large sample with a high standard deviation (i.e., a wide spread) may have a small standard error. Since the SEM is always smaller than the SD, it gives the impression that the spread of the data is less than it really is. Consequently, it may be favored by authors who wish to minimize, rather than summarize, the variability of their data. The use of so-called "error bars" (defined by ± 1 SEM) above and below mean values displayed on a graph is a common example of this practice.

The SEM is actually the standard deviation of a distribution of *means* obtained in repeated sampling from a source population. As we shall see in Chapter 13, it is important in making statistical *inferences* based on sample means. As a descriptor, however, it should be avoided.

11.1.3 The Normal Distribution

The *normal distribution* (the familiar "bell-shaped" curve) is the most important distribution in statistics. There are several reasons for this. First, although it is a *theoretical* distribution based on an infinitely large population (this is called a *probability distribution*), it describes the *empirical* distribution of certain measurements, such as height and weight, performed on subjects from actual populations. It also closely fits the distribution of repeated measurements obtained from the same individual (random measurement variation or error). In addition, the normal distribution serves as the basis of statistical inference for means (Chapter 13). Its theoretical basis and mathematical properties were first investigated by de Moivre, Laplace, and Gauss. In honor of the latter, the normal distribution is also called the *Gaussian distribution*. It must be emphasized that the term "normal" to describe this distribution has absolutely nothing to do with the usual clinical connotation of the word, indicating absence of disease or other adverse condition. We shall return to this point in Chapter 16.

The most important property of the normal distribution is that it is completely specified by two population *parameters:* the mean (μ) and standard deviation σ.[1] As shown in Fig. 11.2, the proportions of values lying within SD intervals of the mean are as follows:

  68.3% lie within ± 1 SD from the mean (i.e., $\mu \pm \sigma$)
  95.4% lie within ± 2 SD from the mean (i.e., $\mu \pm 2\sigma$)
  99.7% lie within ± 3 SD from the mean (i.e., $\mu \pm 3\sigma$)

For any probability distribution, the proportion (or percentage) of values lying within the interval defined by any two values of x is equivalent to the *area under the curve* subtended by those two values. The area under the entire curve is equal to 1 (or 100%), since the entire population is defined by the curve. The area under the curve above the median is 0.5. The area under any segment of the curve is also equivalent to the *probability* that any member of the group, chosen at random, will have a value of x lying between the two values defining that segment. Thus, the probability that any individual member of a population whose values are normally distributed will have a value within one, two, or three standard deviations from the group mean is 0.683, 0.954, and 0.997, respectively.

---

[1] Although I have tried to avoid excessive use of algebraic symbols, a certain minimum is required for clarity and economy of expression. In particular, formulas for statistical tests written out in text would be quite unwieldy. This text will follow the usual convention of using small Roman letters to indicate sample statistics and small Greek letters for the corresponding population parameters. Here is a table summarizing the symbols introduced thus far:

	Sample	Population
Mean	$\bar{x}$	μ
Standard deviation (SD)	s	σ
Variance	s^2	σ^2
Sample size	n	(usually infinite)

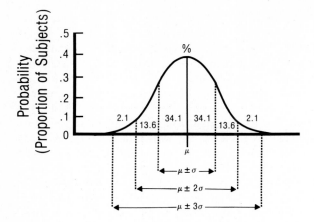

Fig. 11.2. The normal distribution

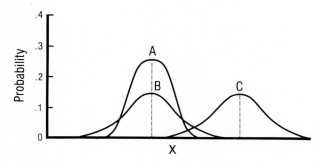

Fig. 11.3. Three different normal distributions

Since each normal curve is specified by its mean and standard deviation, different normal curves may differ from one another in either or both parameters (Fig. 11.3). Curves A and B have the same mean but different standard deviations. Curves B and C have the same standard deviation but different means. Curves A and C differ on both parameters. These differences can be eliminated, however, by transforming any normal distribution to a single *standard normal distribution* (also called the *z-distribution*). The transformation is called a *z-transformation* (or *z-score*) and is achieved by taking the *x* value, subtracting the population mean, and dividing by the standard deviation:

$$z = \frac{x - \mu}{\sigma} \tag{11.6}$$

Consequently, the *z*-score corresponds to the number of standard deviations that any value of *x* lies from the population mean. Hence:

1. If $x = \mu$, $\quad z = \dfrac{x - \mu}{\sigma} = \dfrac{\mu - \mu}{\sigma} = 0$

2. If $x = \mu + \sigma$, $z = \dfrac{x - \mu}{\sigma} = \dfrac{(\mu + \sigma) - \mu}{\sigma} = \dfrac{\sigma}{\sigma} = 1$

The areas under the curve of the z-distribution are thus:

0.683 between $z = -1$ and $z = +1$
0.954 between $z = -2$ and $z = +2$
0.997 between $z = -3$ and $z = +3$

Many times we need to calculate proportions or probabilities for values that lie other than exactly one, two, or three standard deviations from the mean. Such calculations are available in z-tables. These tables usually show the area under the curve for values of x that are *at least as far* from the mean as the value of x used in the z-transformation. These areas are called the *tails* of the standard normal distribution.

Some z-tables give one-tailed values and others give two-tailed values. The area in a one-tailed table is equivalent to the probability of obtaining (by random selection from the population) a value $\geq +z$ [*or*, equivalently, the probability of obtaining a value $\leq -z$]. The area in a two-tailed table shows the probability of getting a value at least as extreme as z in either the positive ($\geq +z$) or negative ($\leq -z$) direction. Two-tailed areas are therefore twice as large as one-tailed areas.[2]

Values of z are usually tabulated to two decimal places. Interpolation can be used to calculate z to three decimal places. One- and two-tailed z-tables are provided in Appendix Tables A.2 and A.3. You should examine and compare the two tables and confirm for yourself that two-tailed values are exactly twice the corresponding one-tailed values.

To illustrate the use of the z-distribution and z-tables, we shall consider the example of diastolic blood pressure in a sample of healthy adolescent boys. The distribution of these diastolic pressures in the source population of healthy adolescent boys is quite close to a normal distribution with $\mu = 70$ mm Hg and $\sigma = 10$ mm Hg. Using the normal approximation, first let us find the pressure that "cuts off" the upper 10% of the group (Fig. 11.4). We need to find the value of z corresponding to 0.100 in the one-tailed z-table, which is 1.28, and then solve for x:

$$z = \frac{x - \mu}{\sigma}$$

Therefore, $x = z(\sigma) + \mu = (1.28)(10) + 70 = 82.8$ mm Hg.

Next, let us consider the probability that a boy chosen at random from this population will have a diastolic pressure between 55 and 95 mm Hg (Fig. 11.5). We first must transform these x values into z-scores:

$$z_1 = \frac{55 - 70}{10} = \frac{-15}{10} = -1.50$$
$$z_2 = \frac{95 - 70}{10} = \frac{25}{10} = +2.50$$

---

[2] You should also be aware that some z-tables show the area between the two tails, i.e., between $-z$ and $+z$. This is just 1 minus the area in the two tails. All z-tables should contain a description of which areas are tabulated.

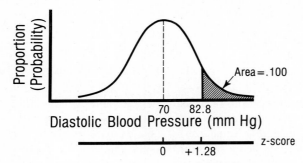

Fig. 11.4. Diastolic blood pressure in adolescent boys: finding the upper 10% "cutoff"

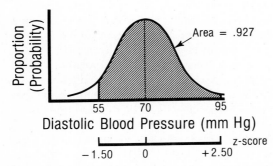

Fig. 11.5. Diastolic blood pressure in adolescent boys: probability of randomly choosing a boy with a value between 55 and 95 mm Hg

The corresponding areas in the tails beyond these two z values are:

  0.067 for z_1
  0.006 for z_2

The area between these two values is $1 - (0.067 + 0.006) = 0.927$. Thus, the probability is 0.927.

  Finally, to illustrate the use of the two-tailed z-tables, let us calculate the inner 95 percentile range of this distribution (Fig. 11.6). The total area in the upper and lower tails must be 0.05, which corresponds to $z = 1.96$ in the two-tailed table. Thus, the lower and upper z-scores will be -1.96 and $+1.96$ respectively. We then solve for the corresponding x's:

$$x_1 = z_1(\sigma) + \mu = (-1.96)(10) + 70 = 50.4 \text{ mm Hg}$$
$$x_2 = z_2(\sigma) + \mu = (+1.96)(10) + 70 = 89.6 \text{ mm Hg}$$

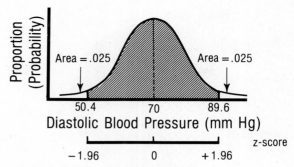

Fig. 11.6. Diastolic blood pressure in adolescent boys: finding the inner 95 percentile range

11.2 Categorical Variables

11.2.1 Rates (Proportions)

As discussed in Chapter 3, a categorical variable for a sample is best described by listing the rate or proportion of individuals in the sample within each category of the variable. Consider again the group of 250 postcholecystectomy patients whose age distribution was discussed in Section 11.1.1. Suppose we are interested in describing their outcome 6 months postoperatively in terms of the (dichotomous) presence or absence of right upper quadrant abdominal pain. The result can be expressed as a proportion (p) or percentage (100 p). If 140 patients are pain-free at 6 months, the overall rate for the group is $p = \frac{140}{250} = 0.56$, or 56%. Although such a result could be represented visually in a table or graph, a single rate or percentage usually suffices to convey the information. (The proportion of patients still experiencing pain is understood to be the *complement* (q) of the rate given, where $q = 1 - p$, i.e., $1 - 0.56 = 0.44$ or $100 - 56 = 44\%$.)

When describing rates for a polychotomous variable, more information must be provided. Suppose, for example, that the postoperative pain variable comprises the following four ordinal categories: more pain, no change, less pain, and no pain. (Assume that this scale has clear, specific criteria that yield reproducible, valid measurements.) The hypothetical results in the 250 study patients might then be described as follows: $\frac{15}{250}$ (6%) with more pain, $\frac{25}{250}$ (10%) with no change, $\frac{70}{250}$ (28%) with less pain, and the same $\frac{140}{250}$ (56%) with no pain. The sum of the proportions must equal 1, and that of the percentages, 100%.

When many categories are involved, the use of a table, histogram, or pie chart can often aid the reader in appreciating the relative magnitudes of the proportions in each category. The principles for constructing a table or histogram are the same as those discussed in Section 11.1.1, since continuous variables must first be catego-

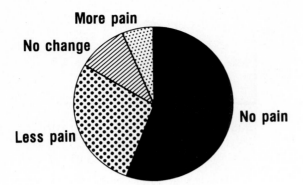

Fig.11.7. Pain outcome in 250 postcholecystectomy patients

rized in order to use these methods. The pie chart achieves the same effect by dividing a circle into "slices" whose size corresponds to the proportion or percent in each category. The size of each slice can be determined by calculating the angle formed by the two "edges" of the slice; each percent $= 360/100 = 3.6°$. For our postoperative pain study, the angles would be 6%, 10%, 28%, and 56% of 360°, or 21.6°, 36.0°, 100.8°, and 201.6°, respectively, for the four pain categories (see Fig.11.7).

11.2.2 Discrete Frequency Distributions

The number of sample subjects in each category constitutes the empirical frequency distribution for a categorical variable. Such a distribution is termed *discrete*, because the possible values of the variable are limited to the categories comprising the measurement scale. A histogram is an example of a discrete distribution. The shapes of discrete empirical frequency distributions will depend on the choice of categories chosen and the proportion of subjects in each category. Thus, unlike the normal distribution, which describes the empirical distribution of certain continuous attributes, these discrete distributions will not necessarily correspond to a symmetrical shape with definable mathematical properties.

Nonetheless, some discrete *probability* (i.e., for populations) distributions do have a mathematically definable shape. For example, for dichotomous variables whose value is determined by a pure stochastic mechanism (i.e., by chance), the resulting probability distribution is called the *binomial distribution.* It describes the number of target outcomes, t, that can be expected among a number of individuals, n, when the probability of achieving the target in any one individual is π. The probability (P) of any t can be calculated as follows:

$$P = \frac{n!}{t!(n-t)!} \pi^t (1-\pi)^{n-t}$$

where $n! = n$ factorial $[= n(n-1)(n-2)\ldots1]$
$t! = t$ factorial
$(n-t)! = (n-t)$ factorial
and $0! = 1$

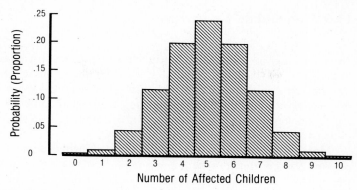

Fig. 11.8. The binomial distribution: expected numbers (and their probabilities) of affected children in families of ten children with one parent having Huntington's chorea

To illustrate, Fig. 11.8 depicts the binomial probability distribution for the expected number of affected children (t) in families of ten children ($n = 10$) in which one parent has Huntington's chorea, a fatal degenerative brain disorder. Because the inheritance pattern of Huntington's chorea is autosomal dominant, the probability of any one child eventually developing the disease is 0.5 ($\pi = 0.5$). Thus, the probability of having exactly three affected children in a family of ten children is:

$$P = \frac{10!}{3!\,7!}(0.5)^3\,(0.5)^7 = 0.117$$

Of all such ten-children families, 11.7% will have three affected children.

The binomial probability distribution shown in Fig. 11.8 is symmetrical. The highest probability is associated with having five affected children out of ten, with probabilities of having more or less than five affected children decreasing symmetrically on either side. This is the same distribution that would be expected for the number of "heads" in ten flips of a coin. Apart from its discrete nature (a histogram), it resembles the normal distribution. In fact, as the sample size (n) increases, the binomial distribution for $\pi = 0.5$ is very closely approximated by the normal distribution.

When $\pi \neq 0.5$, and the sample size is small, however, the binomial distribution is skewed, rather than symmetrical. It will be skewed to the right whenever $\pi < 0.5$ and skewed to the left whenever $\pi > 0.5$. When π approaches 0 (i.e., for rare events) and the sample size is large, the binomial distribution approaches another discrete probability distribution called the *Poisson distribution,* which has convenient mathematical properties that enable calculation of expected numbers and probabilities. The interested reader will find useful discussion of these properties and calculations in the references for this chapter [1, 2].

11.3 Concluding Remarks

For some descriptive studies, construction of frequency distributions and calculation of group means, medians, percentiles, standard deviations, or proportions are all the statistical analysis required. Often, however, an investigator wishes to make descriptive *inferences* about the target population from which his study group is a sample, e.g., estimation of the population mean or rate based on the mean or rate in the sample.

Most epidemiologic studies are analytic and involve an inference about the association between some exposure and outcome in the target population, based on the strength of association observed in the study sample. In addition to constructing confidence intervals around the observed estimate of association, that estimate is often tested for its plausibility under certain hypotheses about the true association in the target population. The next chapter discusses the principles of hypothesis testing and the interpretation of the "*P* values" that result from such testing.

References

1. Ingelfinger JA, Mosteller F, Thibodeau LA, Ware JH (1983) Biostatistics in clinical medicine. MacMillan, New York, pp 150–156
2. Bailar JC, Ederer F (1964) Significance factors for the ratio of a Poisson variable to its expectation. Biometrics 20: 639–643

Chapter 12: Hypothesis Testing and P Values

12.1 Formulating and Testing a Research Hypothesis

There are four stages in the execution of an analytic study. The first is the statement of a *research hypothesis*, i.e., the association that the investigator believes may exist between exposure and outcome in the target population. It can usually be posed in the form of a statement or question. Consider the example from Chapter 6 of cigarette smoking as a risk factor for myocardial infarction (MI), or heart attack. The research hypothesis might be expressed in terms of either a statement ("Cigarette smoking increases the risk of subsequent MI.") or a question ("Does cigarette smoking increase the risk of subsequent MI?").

The second stage is to *design* the study in such a way as to test the research hypothesis validly (without bias) and efficiently (using sufficient, but not excessive, resources). Research design and the reduction of analytic bias were the main topics of Chapters 4–9. The efficiency aspect relates primarily to calculation of required sample sizes and, for continuous outcome variables, reduction in variability (increase in reproducibility) by use of matching, stratification, and multivariate adjustment techniques. The latter issue was briefly discussed in Chapter 5; sample size calculations will be considered in Chapters 13 and 14.

After the design has been carefully laid out (and the necessary financial support has been secured), the study proper is begun and the *data* are *collected* (third stage). The final step is the *statistical analysis* of the data. The statistical analysis for an analytic study usually involves both descriptive statistics (data summary and display) and statistical inference, which includes both estimation of confidence intervals and hypothesis testing. The latter will be the focus of the remainder of this chapter.

In the conventional or *frequentist* approach to testing for statistical significance, the researcher usually examines the study data with respect to a *null hypothesis* (abbreviated H_o) that refers to the target population from which the study sample is assumed to be a random sample. The term "frequentist" arises from the frequency with which a particular sample statistic would be obtained by repeated random sampling (with replacement) from its source population. Although random sampling tends to be a rather infrequent method for subject selection in epidemiologic studies, study samples that are representative of their target populations should result in reasonably valid statistical inferences.

The null hypothesis is a theoretical construct that no association exists between exposure and outcome in the target population. Note that the null hypothesis is usually quite different from the research hypothesis. The investigator plans the research either because she thinks an exposure-outcome association exists, or because she or others are suspicious enough that it might exist to make such a study worthwhile. H_o, however, is an artificial "straw man" that provides a reference for examining the departure of the data actually obtained from the data that would be expected under H_o. For our smoking-MI example, the null hypothesis is that cigarette smoking is not a risk factor (i.e., does not alter the risk) for subsequent MI in the target population.

On occasion, the null hypothesis can be similar to the research hypothesis if the researcher believes that there is no exposure-outcome association in the target population. In general, however, the research and null hypotheses are entirely different and need to be kept separate. Once this distinction is clear, the testing of H_o then becomes the basis for assessing the "statistical significance" of an association observed in the study sample.

12.2 The Testing of H_o

12.2.1 Rejecting H_o

We begin testing the null hypothesis by assuming it to be true, i.e., that no exposure-outcome association exists in the target population from which the study sample is (hypothetically) randomly selected. We then calculate the probability under that assumption of obtaining, by *chance alone*, a degree of association between exposure and outcome at least as strong as that observed in the sample. In other words, we calculate the probability of obtaining such an association by chance if the study sample had been randomly chosen from a target population with no such association. This probability is called the *P value*. If *P* is less than a certain amount (by convention, 0.05), we consider H_o to be so unlikely that we *reject* it.

To recapitulate, we start out with the assumption that exposure and outcome are not associated (i.e., that H_o is true). If, under that assumption, the probability of obtaining, by chance, an exposure-outcome association at least as large as the one observed is very small, we then reject our initial assumption (H_o). Rejecting H_o means that we infer that the study sample is not a random sample from a target population in which H_o is true, but rather from a different target population in which exposure and outcome *are* associated.

Many investigators erroneously interpret the *P* value as the probability that the null hypothesis is true, which is actually the probability the investigator would like to know. Unfortunately, the frequentist approach to hypothesis testing is conditional on (i.e., assumes) the truth of the null hypothesis. The *P* value thus provides a very indirect measure of the probability that H_o is true. It represents the plausibility of the data *given* H_o, not the plausibility of H_o given the data. I will have more to say about the indirectness of this approach (and discuss an alternative approach) in Section 12.4.

The *P* value threshold for rejection of the null hypothesis should be established a priori. This threshold is called the *α-level* and, as indicated above, it is conventionally set at 0.05. We reject H_o if the probability of obtaining the observed or more extreme results by chance, under the assumption that H_o is true, is less than 0.05. Conversely, we are unwilling to reject H_o (i.e., we do not consider it sufficiently unlikely) if $P > 0.05$.

There is nothing "magic" about 0.05. It has come to be the accepted α-level for most studies in the medical and scientific literature. The difference, however, between a P value of 0.04 and 0.06 is very small; yet, this small difference can affect whether a scientific manuscript is accepted or rejected for publication or whether its results are believed or not. The sensible scientist will keep these artificial distinctions in their proper place and will not discard results if the P value is above 0.05, or automatically accept them as proven merely because the P value is below 0.05.

12.2.2 Type I Error

Even if $P < 0.05$, we may be wrong by rejecting H_o, but we consider that the probability of being wrong is acceptably low. A P value of 0.05 simply means that the results obtained in the study sample could have occurred by chance 5% of the time when the null hypothesis is true for the target population. Once out of every 20 samples, on average, rejecting a null hypothesis when $P = 0.05$ will result in an error. In other words, we will be rejecting the null hypothesis when, in fact, the null hypothesis is true. This type of error (erroneous rejection of the null hypothesis) is called a *Type I error* [1, 2]. Whenever we reject the null hypothesis, we run the risk of a Type I error. The lower the P value, the lower the risk. When we reject the null hypothesis with a P value of 0.001, we have only one chance in a thousand of making a Type I error.

Because clinical investigation is usually expensive and time consuming, studies are often used to answer several questions at once, that is, to test several hypotheses. Interventions may be compared for multiple outcomes, or a variety of clinical, sociodemographic, or treatment factors may be examined for their effects on one or more outcomes. When multiple tests of significance are performed, some significant exposure-outcome associations are likely to arise merely by chance. In fact, for every 20 independent tests of H_o, one (on average) will result in statistical significance just by chance. If 100 tests are carried out, and ten are associated with P values < 0.05, it is impossible to know which of the ten are mere chance findings and which represent "truly" significant associations. Similarly, in the usual situation of a single study on a single sample, there is no way to be certain whether an observed association represents a true (for the target population) finding or a Type I error.

To protect against a plethora of Type I errors, some statisticians advocate dividing the threshold α-level for rejecting H_o by the number of tests performed. Because many of the outcomes are associated with one another, however, the probabilities of their joint occurrence is usually greater then the product of their individual probabilities (i.e., they are not statistically independent). Thus, such a procedure may be overly conservative; it tends to attribute true differences to chance. At the very least, however, the investigator should indicate the number of tests performed in addition to the number achieving statistical significance and should modify his inferences accordingly.

Multiple testing becomes an even greater problem when the research hypothesis arises post hoc, i.e., after the data are collected, rather than a priori. When observed data are used to generate hypotheses for statistical testing, the calculated P values do not accurately reflect the true probability of an exposure-outcome association occurring by chance. After all, it is virtually certain ($P=1$) that *some* association will occur by chance. But betting on a horse after a race is not usually rewarded at the ticket window. Similarly, performing a statistical test of significance on an observed association because it "looks interesting" will result in significant P values that bear no relationship to the chance occurrence (given H_o) of an association hypothesized a priori.

12.2.3 Statistical Significance vs Clinical Importance

Regardless of whether we are correct or not in rejecting the null hypothesis, a *statistically significant* exposure-outcome association may or may not be *clinically important*. For example, suppose we wished to test the hypothesis that consumption of a new infant formula leads to a reduction in the serum sodium concentration. We might then compare the mean serum sodium concentration in a group of babies fed this formula with that in a group of babies fed a standard commercial formula. If the results were 139 and 140 mEq/l respectively, the association between the new formula and a lower serum sodium would be clinically trivial, despite the fact that with a large sample size such a difference might be statistically significant. As will be discussed in Section 12.3, the reverse situation can also arise; a clinically important association may not achieve statistical significance.

Thus, the clinical importance of an observed association or difference is a *clinical*, not a *statistical*, decision [3]. A clinical investigator should never let a consultant or journal editor convince him that a very low (highly significant) P value can compensate for a difference too small to be useful.

12.2.4 Directional vs Nondirectional Testing of H_o

I have already discussed the important distinction between the research hypothesis and the null hypothesis. I have also indicated that the research hypothesis can be put in the form of a statement or a question. What I shall now consider is the directionality or nondirectionality of the research hypothesis, and what that implies in terms of testing for statistical significance, i.e., testing of H_o.

In *directional* (or *unidirectional*) hypothesis testing, the research hypothesis implies not only that there is an association between exposure and outcome but also indicates the direction (positive or negative) of that association. In our smoking-MI example, the research hypothesis is that smoking *increases* the risk of myocardial infarction. In other words, we suspect that smoking might either increase the risk of MI or have no effect, but we have no suspicion whatsoever that it *protects* against MI. A directional test of H_o would thus be appropriate.

In *nondirectional* (or *bidirectional*) hypothesis testing, the investigator may have no a priori knowledge of the direction of the association under study. Consider, for example, a clinical trial of surgical (coronary artery bypass grafting) vs medical (drug) therapy for patients with coronary artery disease, in which the duration of survival is the principal outcome. We may have no way of knowing beforehand which treatment leads to a better outcome. Thus, a nondirectional test of H_0 will be indicated.

The P values listed in most statistical tables apply to nondirectional testing of H_0. This is called a *two-sided test* of the null hypothesis. It is also called a *two-tailed test*, because the distributions of the test statistics used to test H_0 often contain two tails, and the P value is equal to the area under the curve in these two tails.

When the research hypothesis is directional, however, and the observed exposure-outcome association is in the expected direction, a *one-sided (one-tailed) test* of H_0 can be used. To obtain a one-sided P value, the P value listed in a two-sided statistical table is simply divided by 2. It is essential that the observed association be in the expected direction, i.e., the direction hypothesized in the directional research hypothesis. If exposure is hypothesized to cause the outcome, but the data actually show a protective effect, the derived one-sided P value will be highly misleading. The investigator would then do better to refrain from reporting any P value and explain that the direction of the association was opposite to the one hypothesized.

The frequentist approach demands that if the research hypothesis implies a certain direction, that direction must be specified *before* the research is actually carried out, in other words, *before* the data are collected [1]. When in doubt, it is probably better to use a two-sided test. When the research hypothesis is nondirectional, a two-sided test *must* be used. When the research hypothesis is directional and the results are concordant with the direction hypothesized, a one-sided test can be justified. This distinction can be important, because dividing a P value by 2 (for example, $P=0.08$ to $P=0.04$) can create a "statistically significant" ($P<0.05$) result that can favorably alter the fate of a scientific paper.

12.3 Type II Error and Statistical Power

So far we have talked about what happens when $P<0.05$ and about the rejection of the null hypothesis. When $P>0.05$ (or some other chosen α-level), we do not reject H_0. The fact that the chance probability of obtaining an observed or greater exposure-outcome association is greater than 0.05 does not prove that the null hypothesis is correct, however. It merely indicates that the probability is not low enough to reject it.

Failure to reject H_0 does not confirm it. If $P=0.10$, for example, the probability of obtaining an association at least as large as the one observed, under the assumption that H_0 is true, is low. A P value of 0.10 is equivalent to a horse with 9:1 odds winning a race. By convention, however, we do not consider the observed result *sufficiently* unlikely to reject H_0. Whenever we accept the null hypothesis, i.e., whenever the P value is not low enough to reject it, we risk making another sort of error. This is called a *Type II error* or *beta error* [1, 2].

A Type II error can occur only when the null hypothesis is not rejected. This is important to remember. When we reject H_0, we run the risk of committing a Type I

Table 12.1. The two errors of hypothesis testing

		"Truth"	
		H$_o$ False	H$_o$ True
Inference	Reject H$_o$	Correct	Type I error
	Do not reject H$_o$	Type II error	Correct

error, the probability of which is equal to the *P* value. When we do not reject H$_o$, H$_o$ might still be untrue. In other words, exposure and outcome might indeed be associated in the underlying target population. The erroneous inference that H$_o$ is true when it is not is called a Type II error.

Thus, the decision either to reject or not reject H$_o$ is an inference, an inference that may be correct or incorrect. Depending on which inference we make, we are at risk for committing *either* a Type I *or* a Type II error. We are never at risk for *both* types of erroneous inference. These relationships are illustrated in the 2 × 2 table shown in Table 12.1.

The actual probability of a Type II error is signified by the Greek letter β (hence the alternative term, "beta error"). In the design phase of a study, β can be calculated by constructing an *alternative hypothesis*, H$_A$, which postulates a clinically important degree of association in the target population. The alternative hypothesis is usually directional and is often the same as the research hypothesis. β is the probability of failing to detect, by chance, a degree of association at least as large as the degree specified by H$_A$. "Detect" here indicates rejection of the null hypothesis, so β can also be defined as the probability of not rejecting H$_o$ when H$_A$ is in fact true. $1 - \beta$ is called the *statistical power* and is the probability of detecting the specified association in the study sample, i.e., the probability of rejecting H$_o$ when H$_A$ is true.

If a researcher wants to show that exposure and outcome are *not* associated to a clinically important degree (i.e., the research hypothesis is similar to the null hypothesis), the probability of failing to detect the degree of association specified by H$_A$ should be very low. H$_o$ can never be "proved," but the lower the plausibility of H$_A$, the higher the statistical power and the greater the assurance that exposure and outcome are not associated to a clinically important degree. Minimizing the potential for Type II error is essential to avoid missing such an association.

In designing a study, the probability of a Type II error is determined by three factors. β will be higher (and $1 - \beta$ correspondingly lower):

1. The *smaller* the hypothesized degree of association under H$_A$
2. The *smaller* the sample size *n*
3. The *larger* the sample variance s^2 (for continuous variables)

The first of these factors is based on judgment of the magnitude of an association that would be clinically important. The second factor is the only one over which the investigator has absolute control, since the sample variance (third factor) largely reflects the underlying variability of the measured attribute. (The component of sample variance due to measurement variation can often be reduced substantially by improving the reproducibility of the measurements; see Chapter 2.) Thus, sample size is an essential consideration for the investigator who wishes to minimize the possibility of a Type II error and maximize statistical power.

To illustrate these concepts, let us recall our clinical trial of coronary artery bypass surgery vs medical therapy in patients with coronary disease. Suppose the investigator planned to include only three patients in each group. Because sampling variation is very large with such small sample sizes (see Chapter 10), and because the duration of survival is likely to be highly variable from one patient to another, even a large, clinically important difference in mean survival time between the two groups is unlikely to be statistically significant. Any investigator who wants to "show" that exposure and outcome are *not* associated merely needs to restrict the number of study subjects to guarantee that no statistically significant association will be found. His argument remains unconvincing, however, because his risk of committing a Type II error is considerable.

The calculation of sample sizes required to detect a given association is one of the most important statistical considerations in the planning (design) stage of a research project. Because these calculations derive from the same theoretical framework and formulae used in inferential statistical analysis, they will be discussed in that context in Chapters 13 and 14.

12.4 Bayesian vs Frequentist Inference

The frequentist approach to hypothesis testing outlined in this chapter is the conventional one used today by most biostatisticians, epidemiologists, and clinical investigators. As we have seen, the approach is an indirect, and even backward, one. We calculate the probability of obtaining the data observed in the study sample, assuming that the sample has been randomly selected from a target population in which the null hypothesis is true (this is called *conditional on* the null hypothesis). In other words, if H_o is true in the target population, the probability of obtaining the sample data (or a more extreme result) is the P value. But what is the likelihood that the null hypothesis is in fact true? The frequentist approach provides no answer to this question.

The same problem arises in testing the alternative hypothesis. The frequentist approach enables calculation of a P value conditional on H_A being true, i.e., the probability of obtaining the sample data (or a result even more inconsistent with H_A) under the assumption that the sample was randomly selected from a target population in which H_A is true. The question the investigator would really like to answer is: What is the probability that the research hypothesis (often the same as H_A) is true? Once again, frequentist methods fail to provide a response.

Bayesian inference takes its name from Rev. Thomas Bayes, an eighteenth-century clergyman and mathematician who discovered an important relationship between conditional probabilities and expressed this relationship in what is now referred to as *Bayes' theorem.* Bayesian inference has two features that make it an attractive alternative to the frequentist approach. First, instead of the observed sample data being referred to *either* H_o or H_A, the data are *simultaneously* examined for their consistencies with *both* H_o *and* H_A [4]. The probability (called the *likelihood*) of obtaining the exact degree of observed exposure-outcome association given (i.e., conditional on) H_A is compared with the likelihood of those data given H_o by forming what is called a *likelihood ratio,* or LR:

$$LR = \frac{P \text{ (observed association} | H_A)}{P \text{ (observed association} | H_o)} \qquad (12.1)$$

where the vertical lines preceding H_A and H_o are read as "given" or "conditional on."

The second attractive feature of the Bayesian approach is that the likelihood ratio is combined with the ratio of the *prior probabilities* of H_A and H_o (i.e., before the study was carried out and the data were obtained) to yield the ratio of the *posterior* (after the data) probabilities. As discussed in Chapter 8, the ratio of a probability to its complement is called an *odds.* Thus, given that either H_A or H_o is true, the ratio of their probabilities, $\dfrac{P(H_A)}{P(H_o)}$, is the odds of H_A. According to Bayes' theorem, the posterior odds of H_A (which is what the investigator really wants to know) is the product of the prior odds and the likelihood ratio:

$$\frac{P_{\text{posterior}}(H_A)}{P_{\text{posterior}}(H_o)} = \frac{P_{\text{prior}}(H_A)}{P_{\text{prior}}(H_o)} \times \frac{P \text{ (observed association} | H_A)}{P \text{ (observed association} | H_o)} \qquad (12.2)$$

posterior odds = prior odds × likelihood ratio

The only difficulty in using the Bayesian approach is the need to estimate the prior odds. What were the probabilities of H_A to H_o before the study data were obtained? Sometimes the answer to this question can be addressed from previous investigations of the hypothesized association in similar study samples. Otherwise, evidence from animal studies or deductions from general physiologic or pathologic principles can be applied. Usually, however, some subjective judgment is required in estimating prior probabilities.

This requirement for subjectivity is the main reason why Bayesian inference is not used as often as it perhaps deserves to be. In fact, however, the frequentist approach to hypothesis testing and the Bayesian calculation of likelihoods also involve subjective judgment, because they depend on the choice of theoretical models (i.e., probability distributions for the population) used to examine the data obtained in a sample. The point is, all scientific inference includes subjective inference, even if the subjectivity is implicit, rather than explicit. No sensible scientist or clinician is going to suspend his critical judgment and all that he has learned from his training and previous research findings by making an inference based on the data from a single study, no matter how good that study may be.

If I tossed a coin five times and got five successive "heads," few people would conclude that the coin was unbalanced, despite the significant "P value" of $(1/2)^5 = 1/32 = 0.03$. Most would attribute the occurrence to chance, that is, a run of good (or bad) luck. Similarly, a single study that comes up with a very surprising finding should make the investigator or clinician alter his view of the world (at least to the extent of being less surprised if a similar result occurs in a subsequent study) but should not turn it upside down.

Since scientific inference inevitably involves incorporating new observations with prior beliefs, the only thing new about Bayesian inference is that the prior beliefs are made explicit and require quantification. Many researchers are uncomfortable with being forced to quantify their uncertainty, and this may be why the frequentist approach to statistical inference still predominates. Recent application of Bayesian principles to other aspects of clinical epidemiology, however, such as the interpretation of diagnostic tests (see Chapter 16), has resulted in an increased awareness and appreciation of the Bayesian approach [5]. It would not be surprising to see this approach applied increasingly in the future by clinical epidemiologists and statisticians.

References

1. Colton T (1974) Statistics in medicine. Little, Brown, Boston, pp 112–125
2. Feinstein AR (1975) Clinical biostatistics. XXXIV. The other side of statistical significance: alpha, beta, delta, and the calculation of sample size. Clin Pharmacol Ther 18: 491–505
3. Feinstein AR (1973) Clinical biostatistics. XXIII. The role of randomization in sampling, testing, allocation, and credulous idolatry (part 2). Clin Pharmacol Ther 14: 898–915
4. Miettinen OS (1985) Theoretical epidemiology: principles of occurrence research in medicine. Wiley, New York, pp 107–128
5. Browner WS, Newman TB (1987) Are all significant P values created equal? The analogy between diagnostic tests and clinical research. JAMA 257: 2459–2463

Chapter 13: Statistical Inference for Continuous Variables

13.1 Repetitive Sampling and the Central Limit Theorem

13.1.1 The Sampling Distribution of Means

Suppose, hypothetically, we chose a random sample of n subjects from some infinitely large population of known mean μ and standard deviation σ, determined the mean $(\bar{x})$ of that sample, replaced the same subjects back into the source population, then chose another random sample of the same size n, and repeated this process over and over again. What distribution would the repeated sample $\bar{x}$'s have? It turns out that if n is large enough, then the $\bar{x}$'s form a normal distribution, regardless of the distribution of the source population. The mean of this normal *sampling distribution* of $\bar{x}$'s is μ, the population mean; its standard deviation (called the *standard error of the mean*, or SEM) is $\dfrac{\sigma}{\sqrt{n}}$.

These interesting and useful facts derive from the *Central Limit Theorem*, one of the pillars of statistical theory. What requirements must be met for the Central Limit Theorem to apply? The main requirement is that n be large enough. How large is "large enough" depends on the distribution of the source population. If it is very close to normal, n can be as small as 2 or 3; if it is symmetric but not bell shaped, n should be 10 or 15; if it is quite non-normal (particularly if highly skewed in one direction), n may have to be 50 or even 100 [1].

These properties of the Central Limit Theorem would remain of only theoretical interest if their application depended on actual repetitive sampling. In the "real world" of clinical and epidemiologic investigation, research studies are carried out only once on a single sample of subjects, and the investigator has no chance to observe the distribution of $\bar{x}$'s of repeated samples. The Central Limit Theorem, however, tells us the mean and standard deviation of the normal distribution that *would* result from repetitive sampling.

By comparing the actual $\bar{x}$ obtained in a study sample with the mean (μ) and standard deviation $\left(\dfrac{\sigma}{\sqrt{n}} = \mathrm{SEM} \right)$ of the theoretical sampling distribution of $\bar{x}$'s, the investigator can determine how likely it is (i.e., the probability, or P value) that his sample originated from a source population with the same mean as the theoretical sampling distribution. This is equivalent to the probability that the sample mean observed $(\bar{x})$ would occur in random sampling from a source population with a given mean μ and standard deviation σ.

Calculating this P value is easily accomplished by constructing a *critical ratio* analogous to the z-score described in Chapter 11:

$$z = \frac{\bar{x} - \mu}{\sigma / \sqrt{n}}$$

In other words, the observed sample mean $\bar{x}$ is compared with its expected (under H_o) value μ by dividing its deviation from μ by its standard ("expected") deviation. The only difference in this critical ratio from the z-score introduced in Chapter 11 is that the probability distribution here is a sampling distribution of means ($\bar{x}$'s), rather than a distribution of individual values (x's). Thus, the SD of the distribution is $\dfrac{\sigma}{\sqrt{n}}$ rather than σ. Since this sampling distribution is normal (Gaussian) according to the Central Limit Theorem, the same z-tables can be used to interpret the resulting values of z (the critical ratio) and to calculate P values.

13.1.2 The *t*-Distribution

Unfortunately, the use of the standard normal z-distribution to test the statistical significance of $\bar{x}$, given a known μ, also depends on knowing σ, the population SD. When σ is unknown, a different probability distribution, the *t-distribution*, is required to test the significance of $\bar{x}$. The t-distribution was discovered by William S. Gossett, a statistician working at the Guinness Brewery in the early years of this century who published his observations under the pseudonym of "Student."

The t-distribution differs from the z-distribution in that, although its mean is the same (namely, μ), it uses the sample standard deviation s as an *estimate* of σ in the SEM. It is based on the following critical ratio:

$$t = \frac{\bar{x} - \mu}{s / \sqrt{n}}$$

Like the z-distribution, the t-distribution is bell shaped. Its two "tails," however, are higher than the tails of the normal distribution. Thus, the calculated P values (which correspond to the area under the curve of the tails) are higher, i.e., less significant, for a given difference between $\bar{x}$ and μ. Like the z-distribution, the t-distribution depends on the requirements of the Central Limit Theorem. The assumption that the underlying population distribution (of x values) is normal is particularly important for small samples.

The value of t is interpreted using the t-distribution with n-1 degrees of freedom, and P values can be calculated accordingly. Unlike the z-distribution, there is a different t-distribution according to the number of degrees of freedom. For small samples, the difference from the z-distribution is quite marked. For large samples ($n \geq 30$), the t-distribution becomes extremely close to the z-distribution, and the latter can be used for making inferences.

Although there is a different t-distribution for each different number of degrees of freedom *(df)*, it would be extremely cumbersome to have a separate t-table for each *df*. *t*-Tables, therefore, provide the various important *P* values (0.10, 0.05, 0.01, 0.001) in the columns. The *minimum* values of *t* necessary to yield those *P* values are listed in the rows according to the number of degrees of freedom. Such a table is Appendix Table A.4.

13.2 Statistical Inferences Using the *t*–Distribution

13.2.1 Estimating μ from x̄: Calculation of Confidence Intervals

As discussed in Chapter 10, one of the goals of statistical inference is parametric estimation, the estimation of a population parameter from data in a sample from that population. The parameter of interest to us here is the population mean μ. Given the sample mean $\bar{x}$ and sample standard deviation *s*, how can we estimate μ? The procedure is straightforward. We begin by constructing the critical ratio *t*:

$$t = \frac{\bar{x} - \mu}{s/\sqrt{n}}$$

We then solve for μ:

$$\mu = \bar{x} - t(s/\sqrt{n})$$

Since *t* can be either positive or negative, depending on whether $\bar{x} > \mu$ or $\mu > \bar{x}$, and since the *t*-tables list only positive values:

$$\mu = \bar{x} \pm t(s/\sqrt{n}) \tag{13.1}$$

$\bar{x} \pm t(s/\sqrt{n})$ is called a *confidence interval* around $\bar{x}$. Depending on how "confident" we want to be about the value of μ, the confidence interval will be more or less wide. A 95% confidence interval uses the value of *t* for $P = 0.05$ at $n - 1$ degrees of freedom. Using Eq. 13.1, we calculate the interval in which we are "95% confident" that μ would lie if the study sample were randomly selected from the target population.

To illustrate, suppose we have a random sample of 17 healthy adult male subjects with a mean hemoglobin concentration of 14.7 g/dl and a standard deviation of 1.12 g/dl. What would be the 95% confidence interval for the mean hemoglobin concentration in the population of healthy adult males? At $17 - 1 = 16$ degrees of freedom, the value of *t* required for $P = 0.05$ is 2.120. Thus:

$$\mu = \bar{x} \pm t(s/\sqrt{n}) = 14.7 \pm 2.120 \left(\frac{1.12}{\sqrt{17}}\right)$$
$$= 14.7 \pm 0.6 \text{ g/dl}$$
$$= 14.1 \text{ to } 15.3 \text{ g/dl}$$

If we wished to be 99%, instead of 95%, "confident" about μ, we would use the t required for $P=0.01$ in Eq. 13.1. For the above example, $t=2.921$, and the resulting confidence interval is:

$$14.7 \pm 2.921 \left(\frac{1.12}{\sqrt{17}} \right)$$
$$= 14.7 \pm 0.8 \text{ g/dl}$$
$$= 13.9 \text{ to } 15.5 \text{ g/dl}$$

When $n \geq 30$, we can use the standard normal (z-) distribution to calculate confidence intervals. We merely substitute z for t in Eq. 13.1. The "critical" values of z for 95% and 99% confidence are 1.96 and 2.58 respectively.

13.2.2 Inferences Based on a Single Sample Mean: The One-Sample t-Test

Suppose we know the mean μ_o of some reference population of interest. We have a study sample with mean $\bar{x}$ and standard deviation s. We want to know whether the difference between $\bar{x}$ and μ_o is statistically significant, i.e., whether there is only a small probability that a difference at least as large as the one observed could arise by chance if the sample was randomly selected from the reference population. If our research hypothesis is directional, i.e., if we expect a difference between $\bar{x}$ and μ_o in only one direction ($\bar{x} > \mu_o$ or $\bar{x} < \mu_o$), this should be specified beforehand.

To test whether $\bar{x}$ differs significantly from μ_o, we proceed as follows:

1. Construct a null hypothesis (H_o). H_o states that μ, the mean of the source population of which the study sample *is* a random sample, is the same as μ_o. In other words:

$$H_o: \mu = \mu_o$$

2. Set up a critical ratio,

$$t = \frac{\bar{x} - \mu_o}{s/\sqrt{n}} \tag{13.2}$$

and calculate the value of t.

3. Consult the t-tables to find the P value corresponding to the t calculated in step 2 at $n-1$ degrees of freedom. (The z-table can be used when $n \geq 30$.) A one-tailed P value can be used if the research hypothesis was directional and the observed data are concordant with the hypothesized direction.

4. If $P < 0.05$ (i.e., t is greater than the minimum value required for $P=0.05$), we reject H_o and conclude that $\mu \neq \mu_o$. If $P > 0.05$, we conclude that the observed difference ($\bar{x} - \mu_o$) could have arisen by chance, in other words, that the sample could be a random sample of the reference population, and we do not reject H_o.

This procedure is called the *one-sample t-test.*

To illustrate, let us return to our example of serum hemoglobin concentration. Suppose we have a representative sample of 30 healthy men living in the mountains between 2000 and 2500 m above sea level. Because the partial pressure of oxygen is lower at high altitudes, and because increased hemoglobin production is an adaptive physiologic response to hypoxia, our directional research hypothesis is that healthy men living at 2000–2500 m will have *elevated* serum hemoglobin. The study data show a mean hemoglobin concentration of 15.3 g/dl, with a standard deviation of 1.17 g/dl. We wish to know whether the mean of 15.3 is significantly higher than the known mean of 14.7 g/dl for the reference adult male population living at sea level. From Eq. 13.2,

$$t = \frac{\bar{x} - \mu_o}{s/\sqrt{n}}$$
$$= \frac{15.3 - 14.7}{1.17/\sqrt{30}}$$
$$= 2.809$$

By consulting the *t*-table at $n - 1 = 29$ degrees of freedom, we can see that the one-sided *P* value lies between 0.005 and 0.01. (If we had used *z* instead of *t*, the one-sided *P* value would have been 0.002. This is perfectly consistent with the results of the *t*-test, thus illustrating the equivalence of *z* and *t* with large sample sizes.[1]) We therefore reject the null hypothesis that our study sample is a random sample of the reference (sea-level) population and conclude that it derives from a different population having a *higher* mean hemoglobin concentration, i.e., that $\mu > \mu_o$.

13.2.3 Inferences Based on a Difference Between Two Independent Sample Means: The Two-Sample *t*-Test

The most common use of the *t*-distribution is in the significance testing of two independent sample means. If one were randomly to choose two simultaneous samples of sizes n_1 and n_2 from two infinitely large (hypothetical) source populations, replace the samples, choose two new samples of the same size, replace them, and so on, the differences (*d*'s) between the two sample means $\bar{x}_1$ and $\bar{x}_2$ would be normally distributed, provided the source populations and sample sizes did not grossly violate the assumptional requirements of the Central Limit Theorem.

In the "real world" of clinical and epidemiologic research, an investigator has a study sample selected (not necessarily randomly) to be representative of some target population. In a cohort study, for example, the two groups being compared are defined by their exposure status (e.g., exposed vs nonexposed, treatment A vs treatment B), and their outcomes are believed to be representative of similar exposed members of the target population. The investigator wants to know if the observed difference in the outcome means of the two study groups, $d = \bar{x}_1 - \bar{x}_2$, is "statistically significant."

---

[1] When the standard deviation σ of the reference population is known, *z* can be used even if *n* is small.

To translate this real-world situation to the hypothetical world of infinitely large source populations and random sampling, we assume that the exposure dichotomy defines two distinct subgroups of the target population, and that each of these sub-groups can be imagined to be an infinitely large source population of which the exposure groups selected in the study are a random sample.

The null hypothesis is that the mean outcomes in these hypothetical source populations are identical:

$$H_o: \mu_1 = \mu_2 \text{ (or equivalently, } \delta = \mu_1 - \mu_2 = 0)$$

Because of the relationship between these source populations and the two actual exposure subgroups in the target population, this is equivalent to saying that exposure has no "effect" on (is not associated with) outcome in the target population. The investigator then tests the observed difference d to calculate the probability (P value) of obtaining a difference at least as large as d under the null hypothesis that $\delta = 0$. If $P < 0.05$, she rejects H_o and concludes that $\delta \neq 0$, and thus $\mu_1 \neq \mu_2$, i.e., the source population outcome means are not equal. The corresponding epidemiologic inference is that exposure affects outcome in the target population.

To test H_o, the observed difference ($d = \bar{x}_1 - \bar{x}_2$) is compared with the difference under H_o ($\delta = 0$) by constructing a critical ratio, using the standard error of the observed difference:

$$z = \frac{d - \delta}{SE(d)}$$
$$= \frac{(\bar{x}_1 - \bar{x}_2) - 0}{SE(\bar{x}_1 - \bar{x}_2)}$$
$$= \frac{\bar{x}_1 - \bar{x}_2}{SE(\bar{x}_1 - \bar{x}_2)}$$

The only remaining difficulty is the calculation of $SE(\bar{x}_1 - \bar{x}_2)$. Now, the variance of a difference between two independent variables equals the *sum* of the variances of the two variables. Since the variance of the sampling distribution of means is σ^2/n, the variance of the sampling distribution of a difference between two means is:

$$Var(\bar{x}_1 - \bar{x}_2) = \frac{\sigma_1^2}{n_1} + \frac{\sigma_2^2}{n_2}$$

The standard error of the difference is the standard deviation of this sampling distribution, i.e., the square root of the variance:

$$SE(\bar{x}_1 - \bar{x}_2) = \sqrt{\frac{\sigma_1^2}{n_1} + \frac{\sigma_2^2}{n_2}}$$

Since we do not know σ_1 and σ_2, the respective source population SDs, we estimate the standard error of the difference using the SDs of the two study (exposure) groups:

$$\hat{SE}(\bar{x}_1 - \bar{x}_2) = \sqrt{\frac{s_1^2}{n_1} + \frac{s_2^2}{n_2}}$$

where the "^" (read "hat") indicates an estimate. The use of s_1 and s_2 instead of σ_1 and σ_2 obliges us once again, for small samples, to use the t-, rather than the z-, distribution. Thus

$$t = \frac{\bar{x}_1 - \bar{x}_2}{\sqrt{\frac{s_1^2}{n_1} + \frac{s_2^2}{n_2}}}$$

One more complication remains. Unfortunately, the conventional t-test for two independent means is based on a null hypothesis that assumes $\sigma_1^2 = \sigma_2^2$, as well as $\mu_1 = \mu_2$. Usually this is not a problem; unless the difference in means is large, the variances often tend to be similar. To provide the best estimate of σ^2 (which, under our assumption, $= \sigma_1^2 = \sigma_2^2$), we *pool* the two sample variances by weighting them according to their respective degrees of freedom. We then compute the *pooled variance* (s_p^2) as follows:

$$s_p^2 = \frac{(n_1 - 1)s_1^2 + (n_2 - 1)s_2^2}{(n_1 - 1) + (n_2 - 1)} = \frac{(n_1 - 1)s_1^2 + (n_2 - 1)s_2^2}{n_1 + n_2 - 2} \qquad (13.3)$$

Then $\hat{SE}(\bar{x}_1 - \bar{x}_2) = \sqrt{s_p^2 \left(\frac{1}{n_1} + \frac{1}{n_2}\right)}$

Finally, we have:

$$t = \frac{\bar{x}_1 - \bar{x}_2}{\sqrt{s_p^2 \left(\frac{1}{n_1} + \frac{1}{n_2}\right)}} \qquad (13.4)$$

Equation 13.4 is called Student's (after Gossett) t-test of two independent sample means. The corresponding P value is determined by interpreting the value of t at $n_1 + n_2 - 2$ degrees of freedom.

To illustrate, let us once again consider the effect of altitude on the serum hemoglobin concentration. Let us assume that no applicable reference population value exists, and that we randomly select a group of 17 healthy adult men living at sea level and 30 similar men living at 2000–2500 m above sea level. These are the same groups considered earlier in this section, and their respective means and standard deviations are as follows:

$$\bar{x}_1 = 14.7 \text{ g/dl} \quad s_1 = 1.12 \text{ g/dl}$$
$$\bar{x}_2 = 15.3 \text{ g/dl} \quad s_2 = 1.17 \text{ g/dl}$$

Our directional research hypothesis is that exposure to high altitude results in a higher hemoglobin concentration, i.e., $\mu_1 < \mu_2$ or $\delta < 0$. The null hypothesis is that the two groups are random samples from source populations with identical means, i.e., $\mu_1 = \mu_2$ and $\delta = 0$.

We first compute the pooled sample variance from Eq. 13.3:

$$s_p^2 = \frac{(n_1-1)s_1^2 + (n_2-1)s_2^2}{n_1 + n_2 - 2} = \frac{(16)(1.12)^2 + (29)(1.17)^2}{17 + 30 - 2} = 1.33$$

Then we solve for *t*, using Eq. 13.4:

$$t = \frac{\bar{x}_1 - \bar{x}_2}{\sqrt{s_p^2\left(\frac{1}{n_1} + \frac{1}{n_2}\right)}} = \frac{14.7 - 15.3}{\sqrt{(1.33)\left(\frac{1}{17} + \frac{1}{30}\right)}} = -1.714$$

(The negative sign is a consequence of our labeling the sea-level group as group 1; *t* would have been +1.714 had the labeling been reversed.) Consulting the *t*-table at $17 + 30 - 2 = 45$ degrees of freedom, the one-sided *P* value corresponding to $t = 1.714$ is $P < 0.05$. Consequently, we reject H_o and conclude that the groups are not random samples from source populations with the same mean hemoglobin concentration. We infer that $\mu_2 > \mu_1$ and, therefore, that high altitude results in a rise in serum hemoglobin. Of course, such a cross-sectional study cannot exclude the possibility that the elevated hemoglobin concentration in fact preceded the second group's living at high altitude. In fact, the statistical significance of the difference relates only to the role of chance in producing the study results. Any analytic bias or other problem in study design would, naturally, invalidate our inference.

It is worth re-emphasizing that the significant difference observed above is based on a one-sided test of significance. If the *t* of 1.714 had been interpreted in a two-sided fashion, the resulting *P* value would have exceeded 0.05, and we would have been unable to reject H_o. This illustrates the importance of stating a research hypothesis in directional terms, if appropriate. Had we carried out a two-sided test, we would have failed to reject H_o, and the probability of a Type II error would have been considerable. Stated in another way, the statistical power to exclude a clinically important difference would have been unsatisfactorily low.

Another important point can be gleaned by comparing the results of this test with the one-sample *t*-test shown in Section 13.2.2. The high-altitude group is the same in both examples: $n = 30$, $\bar{x} = 15.3$, and $s = 1.17$. In the one-sample test, however, this group is compared with a known reference population mean (14.7), whereas in the two-sample test, the same group is compared with a group of 17 subjects with the same mean. The corresponding values of *t* in the two tests are 2.809 and 1.714 respectively.

Assuming the reference population has the same SD $(= 1.12)$ as the 17 sea-level study subjects, we could, in fact, carry out a "mock" two-sample test, assuming an infinite sample size in the reference population $(n_1 = \infty)$. The "pooled variance" then becomes, essentially, the variance of the population $= 1.12^2 = 1.25$. Since $\frac{1}{n_1} = 0$, the value of *t* becomes:

$$t = \frac{14.7 - 15.3}{\sqrt{1.25\left(\frac{1}{30}\right)}} = -2.939,$$

i.e., a result very close to that obtained in the one-sample test (with the sign reversed). The result is quite different from that of the "real" two-sample test, however, owing to the marked increase in sample size in going from a study group of 17 subjects to an infinitely large population, and the consequent reduction in the standard error term in the denominator. This once again illustrates the critical importance of sample size in achieving the statistical power to detect a difference.

Although significance testing using the t-test is the most commonly encountered approach to statistical inference for comparing two means, estimating a confidence interval around an observed sample difference is often more helpful. No null hypothesis is required, and the resulting inference therefore allows greater flexibility than the all-or-none decision about whether or not to reject H_o. The confidence interval is calculated as follows:

$$\delta = (\bar{x}_1 - \bar{x}_2) \pm t \sqrt{s_p^2 \left(\frac{1}{n_1} + \frac{1}{n_2}\right)} \tag{13.5}$$

where t is the two-tailed t value required for the $100(1-\alpha)\%$ confidence interval at $n_1 + n_2 - 2$ degrees of freedom.

For our example, the 95% confidence interval ($\alpha = 0.05$) around the observed difference in hemoglobin concentration is:

$$\delta = (14.7 - 15.3) \pm 2.016 \sqrt{(1.33) \left(\frac{1}{17} + \frac{1}{30}\right)}$$

$$= -0.6 \pm 2.016(0.350)$$

$$= -0.6 \pm 0.7 \text{ g/dl}$$

$$= -1.3 \text{ to } +0.1 \text{ g/dl}$$

13.2.4 Inferences Based on a Difference Between Two Paired Sample Means

When the two means arise from a study of matched pairs, the *paired t-test* is a statistically more efficient technique than the t-test for independent sample means.[2] *Statistical efficiency* refers to the power to detect (i.e., demonstrate the statistical significance of) a difference with a given (fixed) sample size. The more efficient the technique, the smaller the sample required to detect a given difference, and the smaller the difference that can be detected with a given sample size.

As we discussed in Chapter 5, a matched-pair analysis is one method of reducing confounding. When comparing outcome in two exposure groups, pairwise matching renders each pair as similar as possible concerning variables independently (of exposure) associated with the study outcome, so that any difference in outcome is more likely to be attributable to exposure, rather than to potential confounders. In addition to this reduction in confounding bias, matching for variables that are independently associated with outcome, even if they are not differentially associated with exposure (and therefore not confounding), succeeds in reducing the variability in

---

[2] In fact, the matching creates variables that are no longer independent, thus violating an underlying assumption of the t-test for independent sample means.

the outcome due to such variables. Although the difference in means is unaffected, the standard error of the difference is thereby reduced, thus raising the value of t and lowering the corresponding P value. Statistical power is increased because variability is reduced, without increasing the sample size; i.e., the analysis is more efficient.

A matched-pair analysis of means is appropriate whenever (a) each subject from one exposure group is matched to a subject from the other exposure group, or (b) the same subject receives each of the two study exposures. In our example of the effect of high altitude on the serum hemoglobin concentration, the first type would be exemplified by 30 sea-level subjects, each matched (paired) with a high-altitude subject by such variables as age, race, and smoking habits. The second type of pairing would be typified by a crossover clinical trial in which 30 subjects had their serum hemoglobin measured both at sea level and after living for several weeks at high altitude. Differential treatment of paired organs represents another example of this second (self-pairing) type of study, e.g., the use of two different topical anti-glaucoma agents in the two eyes of patients with bilateral disease.

To carry out the paired t-test, the investigator merely calculates the difference (retaining the plus or minus sign) for each matched pair ($d_i = x_{1i} - x_{2i}$, where i represents each of n successive pairs). By computing the mean difference $(\bar{d})$ and the estimated standard error of the difference $(s_d/\sqrt{n})$, the null hypothesis ($\delta = 0$) can be tested. Thus:

$$t = \frac{\bar{d} - \delta}{s_d/\sqrt{n}} = \frac{\bar{d}}{s_d/\sqrt{n}} \tag{13.6}$$

The calculated value of t is then interpreted by comparing it with a reference t-distribution with $n-1$ degrees of freedom. Note that n here is the number of *pairs*, not the total number of subjects or observations. Despite the reduced number of degrees of freedom, the reduction in variability (s_d) achieved by pairing will usually result in a marked improvement in statistical efficiency.

This will be illustrated once again using our example of high altitude and hemoglobin concentration. We shall use the example of self-pairing by showing the results of a hypothetical crossover trial in which six healthy men have their serum hemoglobin concentration measured both at sea level and at 2000–2500 m. To control for possible temporal effects, we randomize the sequence of the two exposures. Thus, some of the six will first be tested at sea level, while the others will begin at high altitude. To allow time for physiologic response, we have them live at their respective altitudes for several weeks before testing. The results are summarized in Table 13.1 and have been chosen to resemble those in the independent sample t-test seen in Section 13.2.3: $\bar{x}_1 = 14.7$ g/dl, $s_1 = 1.12$ g/dl, $\bar{x}_2 = 15.3$ g/dl, and $s_2 = 1.17$ g/dl.

The mean difference is -0.6 g/dl, thus illustrating the mathematical equivalence between the mean of the differences and the difference in the means ($14.7 - 15.3 = -0.6$ g/dl). The SD of the differences is only 0.28, i.e., only one fourth of the two group SDs. Using Eq. 13.6:

$$t = \frac{\bar{d}}{s_d/\sqrt{n}} = \frac{-0.6}{0.28/\sqrt{6}} = -5.249$$

Table 13.1. Results of a crossover trial of the effect of high altitude on serum hemoglobin (Hb) concentration (in g/dl)

Subject no. (i)	Hb at sea level (x_{1i})	Hb at high altitude (x_{2i})	Difference ($d_i = x_{1i} - x_{2i}$)
1	13.8	14.1	−0.3
2	16.1	16.4	−0.3
3	14.6	15.1	−0.5
4	15.0	15.8	−0.8
5	13.1	13.8	−0.7
6	15.6	16.6	−1.0
			$\Sigma d_i = -3.6$

$$\bar{d} = \frac{-3.6}{6} = -0.6$$

$$s_d = \sqrt{\frac{\Sigma(d_i - \bar{d})^2}{n-1}} = 0.28$$

$$t = \frac{\bar{d}}{s_d/\sqrt{n}} = \frac{-0.6}{0.28/\sqrt{6}} = -5.249$$

at $n - 1 = 5$ df, $P < 0.001$

At $6 - 1 = 5$ degrees of freedom, a t of -5.249 corresponds to a one-sided P value <0.001.

The absolute value of this t is much higher than the 1.714 obtained in the independent sample test, despite identical means and SDs and despite a much smaller sample size. In fact, if the data in Table 13.1 are analyzed by the independent sample t-test, i.e., with the pairing ignored, the resulting value of t is only -0.907, which is far from being statistically significant. This is a striking illustration of the statistical efficiency of the paired design and analysis.

As with inferences about mean differences based on unpaired samples, confidence intervals can be estimated from the observed mean difference from two paired samples:

$$\delta = \bar{d} \pm t(s_d/\sqrt{n}) \tag{13.7}$$

For the above example, the 95% confidence interval around the observed mean difference is

$$\delta = -0.6 \pm 2.571(0.28/\sqrt{6})$$
$$= -0.6 \pm 0.3$$
$$= -0.9 \text{ to } -0.3 \text{ g/dl}$$

13.3 Calculation of Sample Sizes

In the planning (design) stage of any clinical or epidemiologic investigation, one of the most important questions that the investigator needs to ask himself (or his statistical consultant) is, "How many subjects do I need to study in order to test my research hypothesis?" When the main comparison of interest is a comparison of two group means, the Central Limit Theorem can usually be used to answer this question. The method to be described is approximate. For small samples, it will underestimate the required sample size because it is based on the z-distribution. The t-distribution cannot be easily used for such calculations, since the value of t required for, say, a P of 0.05 depends on the sample size (actually on $n-1$, the degrees of freedom), which is unknown.

The investigator will need to protect himself against a Type II error. In particular, he will need to avoid obtaining a difference that is clinically important but fails to achieve statistical significance. He must, therefore, specify in advance the smallest difference in means he considers clinically worth detecting, as well as the statistical power $(1-\beta)$ he wishes to detect this difference. He must also estimate the standard deviation, σ, he expects in the underlying source population. This may be pure guesswork, or it may be based on a sample standard deviation *(s)* reported in previous studies. When uncertainty is great, sample sizes can be calculated for a range of values expected to include the true σ.

The formula for the calculation of required sample size (N) when the primary statistical test of significance will be an unpaired *t*- or *z*-test is:

$$N = n_1 + n_2 = 4\left[\frac{(z_\alpha + z_\beta)\,\sigma}{\delta}\right]^2 \tag{13.8}$$

where n_1 and n_2 are the number of subjects in each exposure group (these are assumed to be equal, i.e., $n_1 = n_2$);

z_α is the value of z required for the chosen level of α (Type I error) for either a one- or a two-sided test. Since $P = 0.05$ is the conventional α level chosen for most studies, z_α will be 1.96 for a two-sided test and 1.65 for a one-sided test;

z_β is the value of z required for the chosen level of β (Type II error). Since $1-\beta$ is the probability of detecting a difference at least as large as that specified under the alternative hypothesis, z_β is inherently one-sided. Commonly chosen levels of β are 0.20 or 0.10, corresponding to statistical power $(1-\beta)$ of 0.80 and 0.90 respectively. The one-sided z values corresponding to β's of 0.20 and 0.10 are 0.84 and 1.28;

σ is the value of the source population SD ($\sigma_1 = \sigma_2$) and is best estimated from sample SDs in previous studies;

δ is the clinically important difference, under the alternative hypothesis, that the investigator wishes to detect (the difference will be statistically significant at $P \leq 0.05$) with probability $1-\beta$.

From Eq. 13.8, it can be seen that the higher the statistical power, or the greater the variability (σ), or the smaller the difference the investigator wishes to detect, the greater the required sample size.

To illustrate the use of Eq. 13.8, we return to our example of serum hemoglobin in healthy men living at sea level vs high altitude. Let us assume that a difference (δ) of 0.5 g/dl is clinically important. We want to be sure to have a sufficient number of study subjects to render such a difference statistically significant at $P \leq 0.05$ or, if the difference is smaller, be 80% sure ($\beta = 0.20$) that the true difference in the source population is not ≥ 0.5 g/dl; z_β is thus 0.84. Since we plan a one-sided test of H_o, z_α is 1.65. We estimate σ from our previous studies as the square root of the pooled variance ($s_p^2 = 1.33$), or 1.15 g/dl.
Then

$$N = 4 \left[\frac{(1.65 + 0.84)\ (1.15)}{0.5} \right]^2 = 131.2$$

Since N must be divided equally between the two exposure groups, and since we cannot study fractions of an individual, we would need 66 subjects in each group. (We probably should anticipate several "dropouts" and thus plan to enroll 70 or 75 subjects in each group.)

In general, a far greater (often two-fold or more) sample size is required to protect against both Type II and Type I errors than to protect against Type I error (demonstrate "statistical significance") alone. The temptation to ignore Type II error is thus strong, especially when patients are involved, because the calculated sample sizes are smaller and therefore easier to achieve at a single center over a reasonable period of time. Despite its attractions, however, such a practice is perilous for the investigator, because she may well find herself unable to reject H_o or H_A.

Consider the example of a clinical trial of arterioplasty (surgical arterial repair) vs medical (drug) therapy in patients with hypertension caused by renal artery stenosis (narrowing). Suppose the principal investigator specifies 10 mm Hg in diastolic blood pressure reduction as a clinically important difference worth detecting. She estimates the standard deviation and, ignoring Type II error (i.e., leaving z_β out of Eq. 13.6), calculates her required sample size.

But suppose when the study is actually carried out with the calculated sample size, the results show a 9-mm Hg difference favoring surgery over medical therapy. Because the sample size was calculated based on a 10-mm Hg difference, the 9-mm Hg difference will not be statistically significant. The investigator may not consider the 9-mm Hg difference clinically important, but how sure can she be that the true difference in the treatments is *not* 10 mm Hg or even larger? Not very sure, unfortunately. So she is left in a situation where she can infer neither that there is a clinically important difference nor that there is not. The danger of this Scylla and Charybdis can be avoided only by considering Type II error (i.e., including z_β) in the sample size calculation.

Many investigators faced with the above results ($d = 9$ mm Hg; $P > 0.05$) would be tempted to enroll additional patients in the study in an effort to achieve statistical significance. There are two problems with such an approach, however. First, repeated significance testing increases the risk of detecting a significant difference arising solely by chance, i.e., of committing a Type I error. If results are repeatedly analyzed, the *P* value calculated from the test will *underestimate* the true risk of a Type I error (see the discussion of multiple significance tests in Chapter 12). Second, if the null hypothesis is in fact true, subsequent results may show a difference smaller than 9 mm Hg, and the difference may fail to achieve statistical significance despite the larger sample size.

This example reveals one of the problems with the hypothesis-testing approach to data analysis: it is based on "dichotomous" thinking. The investigator must choose between H_o and H_A, even if the data are not very compatible with either. The use of confidence intervals, however, is often a more helpful approach to statistical inference. No H_o or H_A need be postulated. Instead, the confidence interval indicates the range of differences in the target population compatible with the difference observed in the study sample. In the above example, the confidence interval around the observed difference of 9 mm Hg would include both 0 and 10 (i.e., neither H_o nor H_A could be rejected with confidence). But it would be centered at 9, with an upper bound considerably higher than 10 and a lower bound just below 0.

13.4 Nonparametric Tests of Two Means

The *t*-test (paired or unpaired) is the significance test of choice in comparing two means, provided the requirements of the Central Limit Theorem are not grossly violated. Unless the sample size is quite small, the source population may exhibit considerable departure from a normal distribution without disturbing, to an important degree, the sampling distribution of means or differences in means [1]. In statistical parlance, we say that the *t*-test is *robust*. Many researchers who have had some exposure to statistics have the quite mistaken notion that the *t*-test can be used only when source populations are normally distributed. Such is not the case.

When the requirements of the Central Limit Theorem are violated, however, alternative analytic strategies are required. This is particularly likely to occur when source populations exhibit extreme skewness in their distributions, that is, with a much larger tail in one direction than in the other [1]. Variables with 0 as the obligatory lower boundary, but without an upper boundary, exhibit distributions skewed to the right, with many low values and fewer and fewer high values extending into a long tail. Examples include length of hospitalization and the dose of a drug required to produce a given effect. Length of gestation, on the other hand, is skewed to the left, with very few above 42 or 43 weeks, and decreasing proportions at shorter and shorter gestations.

Faced with a highly skewed distribution, the investigator has two main choices. Either he can *transform* the original data in a way that normalizes the distribution (e.g., by taking their logarithms), or he may use a *nonparametric test*. A nonparametric test differs from the *t*-test and other *parametric tests* that use a sampling distribution of statistics (such as $\bar{x}$) obtained in samples to make inferences about the corresponding population parameters (such as μ).

To use a nonparametric test of two means, the actual magnitudes are ignored, and only the ranks (i.e., the relative magnitudes) are used to determine statistical significance. In the unpaired test, called the *Mann-Whitney U-test*, the two groups are combined and ranks are assigned (the lowest value gets a rank of 1). Each member of both groups is then compared one by one with every member of the other group, and a "winner" is declared for each comparison. The total number of wins in each group (called the "U statistic") is then calculated and is interpreted by referring to the number that would be expected under the null hypothesis that the wins were distributed by chance. For two groups of sample sizes n_1 and n_2, the chance-expected value of U is $\frac{n_1 n_2}{2}$. When the sample size is so large as to make this one-by-one comparison unwieldy, the two values of U can be calculated by determining the sums of the ranks (R_1 and R_2) in the two groups. The two values of U are then:

$$U_1 = n_1 n_2 + \frac{n_2(n_2+1)}{2} - R_2 \text{ and} \tag{13.9}$$

$$U_2 = n_1 n_2 + \frac{n_1(n_1+1)}{2} - R_1 \tag{13.10}$$

To determine the *P* value, the smaller of the two values of U is referred to the tabulated values (see Appendix Table A.5) required for the usual thresholds of *P* (0.10, 0.05, 0.01, 0.001) with different sample sizes n_1 and n_2. The smaller the observed U compared with the chance-expected value, the lower the *P* value.

To illustrate, the results of a hypothetical study comparing length of hospitalization in stroke victims receiving or not receiving physical therapy (PT) are shown in Table 13.2. One subject from each group had a hospitalization lasting 55 days. Since these values occupy the eighth and ninth ranks, each subject receives the tied ranking of 8.5. The U statistic can be calculated for the PT group as follows. The first PT subject wins three head-to-head comparisons with members of the non-PT group (members 2, 4, and 5) and loses the rest; the result is thus three wins. The second PT subject wins one and loses seven. The third has three wins, one tie (non-PT group member 8), and four losses. (Total wins = 3.5, since each tie counts as half a win). The fourth PT subject has 0 wins; the fifth, six wins; the sixth, four wins; the seventh, three wins; and the eighth, four wins. The total number of wins among the eight PT subjects ($=U_1$) is thus $3+1+3.5+0+6+4+3+4=24.5$ wins. The total number of possible wins is $8 \times 8 = 64$, whereas the chance-expected number is 32. The reader may verify that the number of wins in the non-PT group is $U_2 = 39.5$. The same results for U could be obtained using the sums of the ranks R_1 and R_2, i.e., Eqs. 13.9 and 13.10:

$$U_1 = n_1 n_2 + \frac{n_2(n_2+1)}{2} - R_2 = 64 + \frac{8(9)}{2} - 75.5 = 24.5$$

$$U_2 = n_1 n_2 + \frac{n_1(n_1+1)}{2} - R_1 = 64 + \frac{8(9)}{2} - 60.5 = 39.5$$

The smaller of the two U values (24.5) is then referred to the U table (Appendix Table A.5) for $n_1 = 8$ and $n_2 = 8$. It can be seen that 24.5 is not low enough (U = 13) to reject the null hypothesis, and we conclude that PT does not lead to a shorter hospitalization in stroke victims. The potential for Type II error, however, is consid-

Table 13.2. The effect of physical therapy (PT) on length of hospitalization (in days) in stroke victims: Mann-Whitney U-test

Subject no.	PT group (days)	Rank	"Wins"	Non-PT group (days)	Rank	"Wins"
1	41	6	3	118	16	8
2	23	3	1	15	2	1
3	55	8.5	3.5	84	13	7
4	12	1	0	38	5	2
5	91	14	6	33	4	2
6	68	11	4	79	12	7
7	47	7	3	94	15	8
8	65	10	4	55	8.5	4.5
	$R_1 = 60.5$ $U_1 = 24.5$				$R_2 = 75.5$ $U_2 = 39.5$	

For $n_1 = 8$ and $n_2 = 8$, $P > 0.05$

Table 13.3. The effect of physical therapy (PT) on length of hospitalization (in days) in stroke victims: matched-pair analysis (Wilcoxon signed rank test)

Pair no.	PT group (days)	Non-PT group (days)	Difference	Rank
1	41	33	+ 8	2.5
2	23	38	− 15	4
3	55	79	− 24	6
4	12	15	− 3	1
5	91	118	− 27	8
6	68	94	− 26	7
7	47	55	− 8	2.5
8	65	84	− 19	5

Sum of + ranks = 2.5
Sum of − ranks = $4 + 6 + 1 + 8 + 7 + 2.5 + 5 = 33.5$
For $n = 8$ pairs, $P < 0.05$

erable, considering the small sample size and the fact that four of the five highest rankings are found in the non-PT group.

In the paired nonparametric test of two means, called the *Wilcoxon signed rank test,* the differences between each matched pair are ranked with the sign (+ or −) of the difference ignored, assigning the rank 1 to the smallest difference. The sums of the ranks with positive signs is then compared with the sum of the ranks with negative signs. Under the null hypothesis, these sums should be equal, and the actual results can be referred to the distribution of sums around a median of 0 that would be expected by chance. These are tabulated according to the number of matched pairs and the sum of ranks required to achieve a given P value (see Appendix Table A.6).

To illustrate using our physical therapy example, the data of Table 13.2 have been rearranged as matched pairs in Table 13.3. Each PT subject has been matched with a non-PT subject for age, sex, severity of stroke, and co-morbidity (the presence or absence of cardiovascular or other serious diseases in addition to the stroke). The matching is intended to reduce any bias due to these potential confounders, as well as to reduce other sources of variation in the length of hospitalization. The second and third ranked differences (pair numbers 1 and 7) are tied at 8, and thus each receives a ranking of 2.5. Seven of the eight differences are negative, and the sum of the negative ranks is $4+6+1+8+7+2.5+5 = 33.5$, while the sum of the positive ranks is 2.5. As can be seen in Appendix Table A.6, for eight pairs a sum of ranks of ≤ 3 or ≥ 33 is required for a P value of 0.05. Since $2.5 \leq 3$ and $33.5 \geq 33$, we reject the null hypothesis. This significant result once again demonstrates the enhanced statistical efficiency of the paired approach.

Another approach to the analysis of these data involves merely examining the signs of the differences for each matched pair. Since, under H_o, the probabilitiy of a positive (or negative) difference for any matched pair is 0.5, the probability of seven or more (i.e., seven or eight) negative differences out of eight pairs is $\dfrac{8!}{7!1!}(0.5)^8$

$+ \dfrac{8!}{8!0!}(0.5)^8 = 0.035$, which is statistically significant. This is called the *sign test*. (The P value of 0.035 is one-sided; the corresponding two-sided P value, corresponding to a nondirectional research hypothesis, is 0.070.)

Nonparametric tests of means have the advantage of requiring no assumptions about source population distributions. Although they can be cumbersome to calculate by hand for large sample sizes, most computer software packages now include these tests in their repertoire, and calculation difficulties have become less important. (With large samples, however, t- or z-tests can usually be used without grossly violating the assumptions of the Central Limit Theorem.) Another disadvantage of nonparametric tests is that their use of relative magnitudes (ranks) rather than actual magnitudes results in a slight loss of statistical efficiency. To maximize statistical efficiency, it may occasionally be preferable to use a t-test, even if prior logarithmic or other transformation of highly skewed data is required.

13.5 Comparing Three or More Means: Analysis of Variance

To compare the mean outcomes in three or more exposure groups, the investigator uses a procedure called a *one-way analysis of variance* (ANOVA). The assumptions underlying the one-way ANOVA are similar to those required for the t-test, and the null hypothesis is that the groups are equivalent, i.e., that they represent random samples from hypothetical source populations with identical outcome means. In essence, the procedure divides the total variance among all study subjects (with group membership ignored) into two portions: (a) the portion accounted for by the differences between the groups, the *intergroup variance;* and (b) the portion due to the differences among the subjects within the same group, the *intragroup variance.* The larger the former relative to the latter (this ratio of variance is called an *F-ratio,* and the corresponding test of significance, an *F-test*), the less likely the differences among group means are due to chance. The t-test for two independent group means is merely the special case of the one-way ANOVA F-test when the number of groups is two.

The primary result of a one-way ANOVA is a P value representing an overall test of the null hypothesis. If $P < 0.05$, we infer that the source population means are not equivalent. The investigator is usually interested in going further, however, to find out which group or groups are responsible for the overall difference. Different pairs of groups (or combinations of groups) can then be compared, but P values must be adjusted to account for multiple testing, unless all tests are statistically independent of one another and are decided upon a priori. Several procedures are available for carrying out such secondary analyses, and the interested reader may wish to consult one or more appropriate references [2, 3].

Sometimes an investigator may wish to study the effects of two or more exposures or treatments simultaneously. Suppose we wished to assess the effects of both gender (male vs female) and a new antidepressant drug on depression (as measured by a pretested depression score) 6 months after initiating treatment. Although we could carry out a separate t-test for treatment effect in men and women, a *two-way analysis of variance* (ANOVA) provides both greater statistical efficiency and an opportunity to test for a sex difference independent of treatment [2, 3]. (The analysis of the *main effect*, the treatment difference, is more statistically efficient because it uses data from both sexes simultaneously, instead of from just one at a time.)

When two main effects are being studied, both can be assessed simultaneously without requiring the doubling of sample size that would be necessary in two separate studies. If, for example, we wished to assess the effects of both our new antidepressant drug and psychotherapy, we could randomize both treatments, thus producing four treatment groups: drug alone, psychotherapy alone, both treatments, and neither treatment. In addition to providing an assessment of each treatment alone, the two-way ANOVA would also examine the effect of interaction (effect modification) between the two treatments. This type of study design is called a *two-way factorial design*. Provided that the sample size is sufficient to yield adequate numbers of subjects in each subgroup formed by the combinations of different exposures, ANOVA methods can be extended (three-way, four-way, etc.) for larger numbers of study effects.

13.6 Control for Confounding Factors

In many studies, a simple comparison of two or more group means may be biased by confounding differences between the groups. This is far more likely to occur in observational than in experimental studies, but, as we have seen, even randomized clinical trials are not immune. Consider once again the outcome of depressive symptomatology (score) at, say, 6 months after initiating treatment. If the group receiving the new antidepressant drug is younger on average than the control group, and young depressed patients are known to have a better prognosis independent of treatment, then a result favoring the drug group might be due to the confounding effect of age rather than to a benefit of the drug.

In Chapter 5 we discussed several strategies for controlling for confounding factors. Pairwise matching is one such strategy; each patient receiving the new antidepressant could be matched by age (e.g., ± 5 years) with a control patient, and a paired *t*-test could be used to test for a significant difference. A second approach would be to stratify all study patients according to age (e.g., <20, 21–30, 31–50, and >50 years) and compare the stratum-specific mean depression scores in the two treatment groups.

Perhaps the most convenient strategy, in this day of prepackaged computer programs, is to *adjust* the group means according to the outcome each subject *would have* if he had the mean value of the confounder. This adjustment assumes a linear correlation (see Chapter 15) between the confounder and the outcome (age and post-treatment depression scores, respectively, in our example). This procedure is called *analysis of covariance* (ANCOVA) or *covariate adjustment* and can be used for any number of continuous and dichotomous categorical variables [2–4]. It can be combined with an assessment of two (or more) study effects by using two- (or more) way ANCOVA.

Whenever extraneous variables (i.e., variables other than exposure or outcome) are being considered, it is important to distinguish effect modifiers from confounders. As discussed in Chapter 5, effect modifiers do not bias the overall estimate of exposure-outcome association. Instead, the magnitude of the estimate differs with different values of the effect modifiers. In that case, reporting and testing a single difference in means for the entire study sample is rather uninformative (i.e., it hides important information), even if unbiased. Suppose, for example, that in our randomized clinical trial of a new antidepressant drug, the drug is not efficacious in patients with bipolar depression (manic-depressive disease) but is extremely efficacious in those with unipolar depression. Assuming the unipolar and bipolar patients are distributed evenly in the drug and placebo group, the results should be tested and reported for the two subgroups separately. (If the possibility of this difference in efficacy is appreciated in the design stage, the investigator would do better to restrict the trial to unipolar patients.)

References

1. Ratcliffe JF (1968) The effect on the *t* distribution of non-normality in the sampled population. JR Stat Soc 17: 42–48
2. Armitage P (1971) Statistical methods in medical research. Blackwell Scientific, Oxford, pp 189–268, 288–301
3. Snedecor GW, Cochran WG (1980) Statistical methods, 7th edn. Iowa State University Press, Ames, pp 215–237, 255–273, 365–392
4. Kleinbaum DG, Kupper LL (1978) Applied regression analysis and other multivariate methods. Duxbury, North Scituate, MA, pp 209–226

Chapter 14: Statistical Inference for Categorical Variables

14.1 Introduction to Categorical Data Analysis

As discussed in Chapter 2, many variables are naturally measured on a categorical rather than a continuous scale. This is true for outcome variables as well as exposure variables. In the last chapter, we focused our attention on the comparison of two or more means, usually representing the mean outcomes in two or more exposure groups. In such cases, exposure is categorical (e.g., medical vs surgical treatment for renovascular hypertension), and the outcome is continuous (e.g., post-treatment blood pressure). The conventional approaches to comparing the mean outcomes include t- and z-tests, analysis of variance, and various nonparametric tests.

In many clinical studies, however, exposure and outcome are *both* categorical. Comparisons of survival, complication rates, or pain relief in patients treated with two or more different regimens are common examples. For such studies, the statistical methods discussed in the last chapter are not generally applicable. Although formulas exist for t-tests and related techniques to test for significant differences between simple proportions for dichotomous variables, such formulas depend on distributional assumptions about the source populations and cannot be extended to analyses of polychotomous variables. As we shall see, however, these techniques are commonly used for estimating confidence intervals around single proportions and differences between two proportions, and for computing required sample sizes.

The conventional approach to assessing an association between a categorical exposure and a categorical outcome involves (for cohort studies) a comparison of the observed distribution of subjects in each outcome category among the groups defined by exposure (or the reverse for case-control studies). The observed distribution is then compared with the distribution that would be expected under the null hypothesis (H_o) of no exposure-outcome association: a random distribution of outcome in each exposure group and vice versa. If the observed distribution differs sufficiently from that expected by chance under H_o, i.e., if the probability of the observed (or a more extreme) distribution is less than 0.05, H_o is rejected.

In most clinical and epidemiologic studies involving categorical exposure and outcome, both variables are dichotomous. In a cohort study, an exposed group and a nonexposed group, or two groups receiving different treatments, are compared for their rate of a given outcome, e.g., death, wound infection, or premature delivery. In case-control studies, two different outcome groups (cases and controls) are compared for a history of prior exposure to the agent or maneuver under investigation. Most of our attention in this chapter will center on the statistical analysis of the association between a dichotomous exposure and a dichotomous outcome. This major discussion will then be followed by a brief consideration of analogous methods applicable to polychotomous variables.

14.2 Comparing Two Proportions

14.2.1 Association in 2 × 2 (Fourfold) Tables

Suppose we wish to compare postoperative wound infection rates in laparotomy (abdominal surgery) patients treated with either a broad-spectrum antibiotic or a placebo. We have randomized treatment assignment in 500 consecutive patients, with 240 receiving the antibiotic and 260 receiving the placebo, and the resulting infection rates are $p_1 = \dfrac{t_1}{n_1} = \dfrac{7}{240}$ (2.9%) and $p_2 = \dfrac{t_2}{n_2} = \dfrac{21}{260}$ (8.1%), respectively, where n_1 and n_2 are the numbers of subjects in the first and second exposure groups and t_1 and t_2 are the numbers within those groups who experience the "target" outcome.

These data can also be displayed in a 2 × 2, or fourfold, table, as shown for our example in Table 14.1 and in general statistical notation in Table 14.2. The row totals r_1 and r_2 represent the total numbers of patients receiving antibiotic and placebo, while the column totals c_1 and c_2 represent the total numbers of patients with and without wound infections. Any two proportions being compared can be displayed in a 2 × 2 table; conversely, any 2 × 2 table can be "translated" into two corresponding proportions.

In the tabular format, the greater the difference between the two proportions, the greater the *association* between the columns and the rows (the outcome and the exposure, respectively, in the format used throughout this text). In our example, we are interested in testing for a statistically significant association between preoperative treatment (antibiotic or placebo) and postoperative wound infection (yes or no).

To carry out such a test, we first establish a null hypothesis of no association in the underlying target population and then assess the probability that the association

Table 14.1. Postlaparotomy wound infection in patients receiving antibiotic vs placebo

	Infection	No infection	
Antibiotic	7	233	240
Placebo	21	239	260
	28	472	500

Table 14.2. Statistical notation for data displayed in a 2×2 table

	Outcome present	Outcome absent	
Exposed	a	b	$a+b\,(=r_1)$
Nonexposed	c	d	$c+d\,(=r_2)$
	$a+c$ $(=c_1)$	$b+d$ $(=c_2)$	$N=r_1+r_2=c_1+c_2=a+b+c+d$

r_1, row total for 1st row; r_2, row total for 2nd row; c_1, column total for 1st column; c_2, column total for 2nd column.

observed in the study sample arose by chance, assuming that the sample was randomly selected from the target population. Stated in terms of the two proportions, the null hypothesis states that the source populations of which the two exposure groups represent random samples have equal outcome rates, i.e., H_o: $\pi_1 = \pi_2$, with the π's corresponding to the p's in the study sample. The H_o of no association indicates that the columns should be *statistically independent* of the rows. We thus calculate the frequency with which we would *expect* (under H_o) subjects to fall into each of the four cells of the 2×2 table. If the observed cell frequencies differ sufficiently from the frequencies expected under H_o, we reject H_o and conclude that the columns and rows are not independent, i.e., that they are associated, in the target population.

How do we calculate the expected cell frequencies? The probability that two independent events will both occur is the product of their individual probabilities. Under H_o, the probability of a subject being in a given row is $\frac{r_i}{N}$, the row total divided by the total sample size. Similarly, the probability of a subject being in a given colum is $\frac{c_j}{N}$. Thus, under H_o, the probability of being in a given cell (i.e., a given row *and* a given column) is $\left(\frac{r_i}{N}\right)\left(\frac{c_j}{N}\right) = \frac{r_i c_j}{N^2}$. The expected cell frequency, E_{ij}, is then simply the probability of being in that cell times the total sample size:

$$E_{ij} = \left(\frac{r_i c_j}{N^2}\right)(N) = \frac{r_i c_j}{N} \tag{14.1}$$

In each cell of the table we then have both an observed (O_{ij}) and an expected (E_{ij}) frequency. Now we require a statistical method for comparing the O_{ij}'s with the E_{ij}'s that will guide us in our inference to reject, or not reject, the null hypothesis. The usual method for carrying out this comparison is the χ^2 test.

14.2.2 The χ^2 Test: Definition and Calculation

Chi square is a statistic whose known frequency distribution under H_o enables us to calculate P values. It is defined as follows:

$$\chi^2 = \Sigma \frac{(O_{ij} - E_{ij})^2}{E_{ij}} \qquad (14.2)$$

It can be calculated by computing the expected frequency (E_{ij}) for each cell, subtracting it from the observed frequency (O_{ij}) in the table, squaring the resulting difference, dividing by the expected frequency, and then summing this ratio over all four cells in the table.

Because this method of calculating χ^2 can be computationally unwieldy, several algebraically equivalent formulas may be preferable. Using our customary a, b, c, d notation to depict the four cells of the 2×2 table, as shown in Table 14.2, $\frac{(O_{ij} - E_{ij})^2}{E_{ij}}$ for the first cell is:

$$\frac{[a - (a+b)(a+c)/N]^2}{(a+b)(a+c)/N}$$

If we repeat this for each of the four cells and then sum the algebraic terms, we end up with the following formula:

$$\chi^2 = \frac{(ad - bc)^2 N}{(a+b)(c+d)(a+c)(b+d)} \qquad (14.3)$$

(The denominator can be seen to be the product of the two row totals and the two column totals).

If the data are not already displayed in a 2×2 table, the easiest way to calculate χ^2 is to compare the two proportions, $p_1 = \frac{t_1}{n_1}$ and $p_2 = \frac{t_2}{n_2}$, directly:

$$\chi^2 = \left(\frac{t_1^2}{n_1} + \frac{t_2^2}{n_2} - \frac{T^2}{N} \right) \left[\frac{N^2}{(T)(N-T)} \right] \qquad (14.4)$$

where $N = n_1 + n_2$ and $T = t_1 + t_2$

Equation 14.4 is probably the easiest of the χ^2 formulas to compute using a handheld calculator.

To illustrate the mathematical equivalence of Eqs. 14.2–14.4, let us calculate χ^2 for our postlaparotomy wound infection trial (Table 14.1). To use Eq. 14.2, we must first calculate the expected frequencies $(E_{ij}'s)$ for each of the four cells according to Eq. 14.1. These are shown in Table 14.3. Next, using Eq. 14.2,

$$\chi^2 = \Sigma \frac{(O_{ij} - E_{ij})^2}{E_{ij}} = \frac{(7 - 13.44)^2}{13.44} + \frac{(233 - 226.56)^2}{226.56} + \frac{(21 - 14.56)^2}{14.56} +$$

$$\frac{(239 - 245.44)^2}{245.44} = 3.09 + 0.18 + 2.85 + 0.17 = 6.29$$

Table 14.3. Expected cell frequencies (E_{ij}'s)[a] for data shown in Table 14.1

	Infection	No infection	
Antibiotic	13.44	226.56	240
Placebo	14.56	245.44	260
	28	472	500

[a] $E_{ij} = \frac{r_i c_j}{N}$ (Eq. 14.1)

Using Eq. 14.3 and the notation shown in Table 14.2,

$$\chi^2 = \frac{(ad-bc)^2 N}{(a+b)(c+d)(a+c)(b+d)} = \frac{[(7)(239) - (233)(21)]^2 (500)}{(240)(260)(28)(472)} = 6.29$$

Using Eq. 14.4 and the two native proportions, $p_1 = \frac{7}{240}$ and $p_2 = \frac{21}{260}$,

$$\chi^2 = \left(\frac{t_1^2}{n_1} + \frac{t_2^2}{n_2} - \frac{T^2}{N}\right)\left[\frac{N^2}{(T)(N-T)}\right] = \left(\frac{7^2}{240} + \frac{21^2}{260} - \frac{28^2}{500}\right)\left[\frac{500^2}{(28)(472)}\right]$$
$$= 6.29$$

Thus, the three equations yield precisely the same result for the value of χ^2. Regardless of which method is used to calculate χ^2, however, we need to know how to interpret the value calculated. In other words, how can we determine a P value from a given value of χ^2? This is discussed in the following section.

14.2.3 The χ^2 Test: Statistical Inferences

On inspection of Eq. 14.2, it is evident from the squared term in the numerator that χ^2 is always ≥ 0. The minimum value of $\chi^2 = 0$, which is the value obtained when $O_{ij} = E_{ij}$ (observed = expected) for each cell of the table. The maximum value will depend on the sample size, since larger numbers in each cell will permit greater absolute values for $O_{ij} - E_{ij}$, and hence for $(O_{ij} - E_{ij})^2$. The empirical frequency distribution for χ^2 is discrete; only certain values of χ^2 are possible, depending on the specific O_{ij}'s and E_{ij}'s for each cell. With larger sample sizes, however, the discrete distribution is closely approximated by the smooth curve representing the theoretical probability distribution for the source population.

Since large values of χ^2 indicate a large deviation of observed from expected, the higher the χ^2, the less likely it is that the study sample represents a random sample from a target population (represented by the expected frequencies) in which no association exists between exposure and outcome. In other words, the higher the value of χ^2, the lower the P value, and the greater our confidence in rejecting the null hypothesis.

The P value is the area under the curve of the smoothed χ^2 probability distribution above the obtained value of χ^2. In order to determine this P value we need one further piece of information: the number of degrees of freedom.

In calculating the degrees of freedom, marginal (row or column) totals are considered to be fixed. In fact, we have already made use of these fixed marginals in calculating the expected cell frequencies (E_{ij}'s) according to Eq. 14.1. In a 2×2 table, having fixed marginals means that any one cell automatically determines the other three, and thus the number of degrees of freedom equals 1.

This can be illustrated by considering Table 14.1 with only the marginal totals provided:

	Infection	No infection	
Antibiotic			240
Placebo			260
	28	472	500

Now let us see what happens when we are given the value of 21 in the left lower cell. Because of the fixed marginals, this 21 automatically determines the values of the three other cells, yielding the entire Table 14.1:

	Infection	No infection	
Antibiotic	7	233	240
Placebo	21	239	260
	28	472	500

The general formula for determining the number of degrees of freedom is:

$$df = (r-1)(c-1) \tag{14.5}$$

where r = the number of rows
c = the number of columns

Thus, for a 2×2 table, $df = (2-1)(2-1) = 1$

As with the t probability distribution, the shape of the χ^2 distribution varies according to the number of degrees of freedom. Unlike t, however, χ^2 is always positive, and the P values always corresponds to the area in the upper tail of the distribution above the obtained value of χ^2. This P value will change for a given value of χ^2 according to the number of degrees of freedom, increasing (becoming less significant) with increases in df.

Because of this dependence of P on both the obtained value of χ^2 and the number of degrees of freedom, χ^2 tables have been constructed in which the minimum value of χ^2 is given for a given df and the usual "threshold" P values (0.10, 0.05, 0.01, 0.001). In this regard, it is set up like the t-table. A representative χ^2 table is provided in Appendix Table A.7.

As we have mentioned, the P value determined from a χ^2 test corresponds to the area in the upper tail of the smoothed χ^2 probability distribution. But since $(E_{ij}-O_{ij})^2$, and hence χ^2, is always ≥ 0 regardless of whether $p_1 > p_2$ or $p_2 > p_1$, i.e., regardless of which proportion is larger, the χ^2 test is inherently two-sided. (In other words, there is no equivalent to the negative value of t obtained when $\bar{x}_2 > \bar{x}_1$. See Eq. 13.3.) In comparing two proportions, therefore, the P value obtained from a χ^2 test represents the probability of obtaining the observed difference in the two proportions $(p_1 - p_2)$ by chance under H_o, regardless of whether $p_1 > p_2$ or $p_2 > p_1$. Although one-sided P values are rarely reported for χ^2 tests, a research hypothesis that was stated a priori as clearly unidirectional ($\pi_1 > \pi_2$ or $\pi_2 > \pi_1$) and was subsequently supported by the data could justify a one-sided test. The one-sided P value is obtained by dividing the tabulated (two-sided) P value by 2.

To illustrate the use of the χ^2 table, let us determine the P value corresponding to the χ^2 of 6.29 obtained in our wound infection trial. At 1 df, a χ^2 of 6.29 yields a (two-sided) P value between $P = 0.05$ and $P = 0.01$. By convention, this is sufficiently small to reject the null hypothesis, and, if the design and execution are adequate to exclude analytic bias as an explanation for the findings, we conclude that the study antibiotic is indeed efficacious in reducing postlaparotomy wound infection.

14.2.4 The Continuity Correction for Small Samples

As mentioned above, the (theoretical) χ^2 probability distribution is a smooth, continuous curve. Observed frequencies, however, are discrete and so, therefore, are the possible calculated values of χ^2 from any study. When N is very large, many more values are possible for the O_{ij}'s and E_{ij}'s (and thus for χ^2), and the frequency distribution of possible χ^2 values begins to approach the smooth, theoretical probability distribution. For example, the wound infection rate in our antibiotic-treated patients of 7 out of 240 might represent theoretically any number from 6½ to 7½, i.e., a similar group of 2400 antibiotic-treated patients could have a rate anywhere from 65 to 75 out of 2400.

When N is small, many statisticians advocate the use of a *continuity correction* to compensate for the fact that the discrete possible values are not closely approximated by the continuous theoretical distribution. In 1934, Yates decided to subtract ½ from the absolute value of each $O_{ij} - E_{ij}$ to provide a better approximation. The resulting χ^2 with continuity correction (χ_c^2) is defined as follows.

$$\chi_c^2 = \Sigma \frac{(|O_{ij} - E_{ij}| - \frac{1}{2})^2}{E_{ij}} \tag{14.6}$$

where the symbol $|\ \ |$ indicates absolute value.
The equivalent form of Eq. 14.3 is:

$$\chi_c^2 = \frac{(|ad - bc| - N/2)^2 N}{(a+b)(c+d)(a+c)(b+d)} \tag{14.7}$$

The continuity correction is used only for comparing two proportions (i.e., for 2×2 tables), and χ_c^2 is interpreted at 1 df in the same way as the uncorrected χ^2. The continuity correction results in smaller values for χ^2, and resulting statistical inferences will thus be more conservative. In other words, H_o is less likely to be rejected. The lower risk of Type I error must, as always, be balanced against a greater risk of Type II error. For large samples, the continuity correction is probably unnecessary, but for small samples the P values calculated using χ_c^2 are closer to the exact probability (see following section) obtained using a pure stochastic (chance-generated) model.

14.2.5 The Fisher Exact Test

When the expected cell frequency in one or more cells of a 2×2 table is below 5, the smoothed χ^2 probability distribution, even with the continuity correction, does not provide a sufficiently accurate approximation of the true P value. In such cases, many statisticians recommend using the *Fisher exact test*. The Fisher test is based on the *hypergeometric distribution*, which is produced when two independent binomials (i.e., the two sample proportions) are inserted in a 2×2 table with fixed marginal totals. The test provides the probability of obtaining, by chance, an association between the columns and rows at least as large as the one observed, under the null hypothesis of no association and the condition of fixed marginals.

Given a hypergeometric distribution, the probability of the observed cell frequencies a, b, c, and d, given the row totals r_1 and r_2 and the column totals c_1 and c_2, is:

$$P = \frac{r_1! r_2! c_1! c_2!}{N! a! b! c! d!} \tag{14.8}$$

This formula, however, provides only the probability of the table obtained. As with the t and χ^2 tests, we are usually interested in calculating the probability (P value) of getting the results obtained *or* results more deviant from H_o, i.e., the area in the entire "tail" of the probability distribution of tables beyond the observed one.

To compute the P value for the Fisher exact test, we construct further 2×2 tables having more extreme cell frequencies than the observed one, while keeping the marginal totals constant. We then calculate the probability associated with each of these tables, using Eq. 14.8, and add these probabilities to that of the observed table. The resulting sum is the exact P value. Because the "more extreme" tables are those deviating from H_o in the *same direction* as the observed table, the calculated P value is, by definition, one-sided. To get the two-sided P value, the result is usually multiplied by 2.

As an example, consider the evaluation of a new cancer chemotherapeutic regimen in the treatment of advanced acute lymphoblastic leukemia (ALL) in children. In a randomized trial of 27 patients, 12 received the new treatment and 15 the existing standard regimen, and the results are shown in Table 14.4 in terms of "successes" (here defined as elimination of tumor cells from the bone marrow after treatment)

Table 14.4. Results of a clinical trial of two chemotherapy regimens for advanced acute lympho-blastic leukemia (ALL) in children

	Success	Failure	
New regimen	6	6	12
Standard regimen	2	13	15
	8	19	27

and failures. The success rate in children receiving the new regimen is $\frac{6}{12}$, or 50%, compared with $\frac{2}{15}$, or 13%, with the standard treatment. Could these results have occurred by chance if the two treatment groups are random samples from hypothetical source populations in which the two treatments are equally efficacious?

Using Eq. 14.8 we can calculate the probability of Table 14.4 as:

$$P = \frac{r_1!\,r_2!\,c_1!\,c_2!}{N!\,a!\,b!\,c!\,d!} = \frac{12!\,15!\,8!\,19!}{27!\,6!\,6!\,2!\,13!} = \frac{3.072 \times 10^{42}}{7.030 \times 10^{43}} = 0.0437$$

Maintaining the fixed marginals, there are only two possible tables with more extreme distributions favoring the new treatment:

	Success	Failure	
New regimen	7	5	12
Standard regimen	1	14	15
	8	19	27

	Success	Failure	
New regimen	8	4	12
Standard regimen	0	15	15
	8	19	27

The probabilities for these tables are calculated as follows, using the expression $\frac{r_1!\,r_2!\,c_1!\,c_2!}{N!} = 2.821 \times 10^{14}$, which remains constant for all tables:

$$P = \frac{2.821 \times 10^{14}}{7!5!1!14!} = 0.0054 \text{ and } P = \frac{2.821 \times 10^{14}}{8!4!0!15!} = 0.0002$$

The one-sided P value associated with the observed table is thus:

$$P = 0.0437 + 0.0054 + 0.0002 = 0.0493,$$

which just barely qualifies for conventional statistical significance. Because, however, we could not be sure, a priori, that the new treatment would not be *worse* than the existing standard, a one-sided test is probably inappropriate. The two-sided P value is $2 \times 0.0493 = 0.0986$, and we should not reject H_o. Consequently, we conclude that the observed difference in results might have arisen by chance.

If we had (inappropriately) used the χ^2 test to analyze the data from this trial, we would have calculated

$$\chi^2 = \frac{(ad - bc)^2 N}{(a+b)(c+d)(a+c)(b+d)} = \frac{[(6)(13) - (6)(2)]^2(27)}{(12)(15)(8)(19)} = 4.299,$$

which corresponds to $P < 0.05$, and we would have erroneously rejected the null hypothesis.

Although the calculations required for the Fisher exact test are fairly straightforward using hand-held calculators and factorial tables, the construction of additional 2×2 tables, and the computation of the probability for each, can entail considerable time and effort when the results are less extreme than those in our example. Fortunately, most standard software computer packages include the Fisher exact test in their "menus," and thus this calculational inconvenience pertains only to data analyzed by hand.

14.2.6 Matched-Pair Design

As discussed in Chapter 5, pair matching is often used in observational studies to reduce confounding. If pair matching is used in the design, the statistical analysis will be more efficient (i.e., have greater statistical power) if the matching is retained. The matched-pair χ^2 test, also called the *McNemar χ^2 test*, is the test generally used for comparing proportions in two pair-matched groups. It is the analog for categorical data of the paired *t*-test for continuous variables.
Using the notation given in Table 6.5, the formula is as follows:

$$\chi^2_{McNemar} = \frac{(b-c)^2}{b+c} \tag{14.9}$$

or, using the continuity correction:

$$\chi^2_{c, McNemar} = \frac{(|b-c|-1)^2}{b+c} \tag{14.10}$$

The value of χ^2 depends only on the observed frequencies in the two "discordant" cells b (nonexposed pair member with the outcome, exposed member without the outcome) and c (nonexposed member without the outcome, exposed member with the outcome). It is interpreted in the same way as the usual χ^2 (Appendix Table A.7) with one degree of freedom.

I shall illustrate the calculation of $\chi^2_{McNemar}$ using the data of Table 6.6, which shows the results of a cohort study of myocardial infarction (MI) in 200 smoking and 200 nonsmoking men matched by age, blood pressure, and serum cholesterol concentration. Of the 200 matched pairs, both members experienced an MI in seven pairs, neither member in 150 pairs, only the nonsmoking member in 14, and only the smoking member in 29. Thus,

$$\chi^2_{McNemar} = \frac{(14-29)^2}{14+29} = \frac{(-15)^2}{43} = 5.233,$$

which corresponds to a P value <0.05. The null hypothesis is therefore rejected, and we conclude that the smokers are indeed at greater risk for subsequent MI.

14.2.7 Testing the Statistical Significance of the Relative Risk and Odds Ratio

As discussed in Chapters 6 and 7, relative risks or odds ratios above 1 indicate that exposure is associated with an increased risk of developing the study outcome. Conversely, relative risks or odds ratios less than 1 indicate that exposure protects against development of the outcome. It is rare to obtain an RR or OR of exactly 1, however, and values less than or greater than 1 may well occur by chance even if the null hypothesis is true.

By performing a χ^2 test (matched or unmatched) on the same 2×2 table used to generate the RR or OR, the statistical significance of the observed value of RR or OR is automatically assessed. If RR (or OR) >1 and $\chi^2 \geq 3.84$, then exposure is associated with a significantly increased risk of the outcome. If RR (or OR) <1 and $\chi^2 \geq 3.84$, the exposure is associated with a significantly decreased risk of, i.e., protection against, developing the outcome.

Another approach to testing the significance of an observed RR or OR is to construct a confidence interval (usually 95% or 99%) around the observed value. If the interval excludes 1, then the RR or OR is declared statistically significant at the chosen level (α) of significance. There are several methods for calculating the confidence interval, but the easiest computationally is that proposed by Miettinen [1]:

$$CI = RR^{1 \pm (z_\alpha / \chi)} \text{ or } OR^{1 \pm (z_\alpha / \chi)} \tag{14.11}$$

where z_α is the two-sided z value corresponding to the chosen width of the confidence interval (1.96 for 95% and 2.57 for 99%), and χ is the square root of the observed value of χ^2.

For example, the relative risk of MI in smokers vs nonsmokers based on the nonmatched cohort study whose results are shown in Table 6.2 is 2.13. The calculated value of χ^2 is

$$\chi^2 = \frac{(ad-bc)^2 N}{(a+b)(c+d)(a+c)(b+d)} = \frac{[(32)(185)-(168)(15)]^2(400)}{(200)(200)(47)(353)} = 6.968,$$

which corresponds to a P value <0.01. Thus, we conclude that the relative risk of 2.13 is significantly greater than 1.

Using the confidence interval approach of Eq. 14.11,

$$95\% \ CI = RR^{(1\pm1.96/\chi)} = 2.13^{(1\pm1.96/\sqrt{6.968})} = 1.21 \ to \ 3.73$$

Since this interval excludes 1, we again conclude that the relative risk of 2.13 is statistically significant.

The confidence interval derived from Eq. 14.11 is often called "test-based," because it is based on the calculated value of χ^2. This fact also leads to another marginal advantage (besides computational ease) of the test-based method, namely, that conclusions about statistical significance are always identical to those achieved using the χ^2 test. The major disadvantage of the method is that it yields narrower confidence limits than those obtained using more exact (and computationally far more difficult) methods. The computational disadvantages of the other methods have been largely overcome by many statistical software packages, which provide standard errors for RRs and ORs that can be used to estimate confidence intervals. Readers interested in exploring these other methods are referred to Fleiss [2] and Kleinbaum et al. [3].

14.2.8 Control for Confounding Factors

As with comparisons of means, comparisons of proportions can be biased by confounding differences between the study groups. A fair test of the statistical significance of an association between exposure and outcome should always control for potentially important confounders. One such method of analysis has already been mentioned in Section 14.2.6, namely, the matched-pair (McNemar) χ^2 test. A matched-pair analysis, of course, either depends on pair matching in the design or wastes data already collected on subjects who cannot be matched. Furthermore, a matched-pair design is not always feasible when many confounders are involved and may not be worth the effort if large numbers of potential subjects are rejected because they do not meet the matching criteria.

Another method of controlling for confounding is stratification, which requires that the confounders be categorical variables or, if continuous, that they be categorized. In Chapters 6 and 8 we described the Mantel-Haenszel procedure for computing the summary relative risk and odds ratio, respectively, for stratified 2×2 tables. Mantel and Haenszel [4] also provide a formula for computing the stratified χ^2 for i strata:

$$\chi^2_{MH} = \left(\Sigma \frac{a_i d_i - b_i c_i}{N_i}\right)^2 / \Sigma \frac{r_{1i} r_{2i} c_{1i} c_{2i}}{(N_i - 1)(N_i^2)} \qquad (14.12)$$

The resulting χ^2 is interpreted at 1 degree of freedom. This formula can be applied to either cohort or case-control studies and is the appropriate test of significance for Mantel-Haenszel relative risks and odds ratios, respectively.

To illustrate the use of the Mantel-Haenszel χ^2, let us return to the stratified analysis presented in Table 6.7, which displays the results of an observational cohort study comparing success (S) and failure (F) rates with two treatments (T_1 and T_2). The overall ("crude") relative "risk" of success of T_1 vs T_2 is 0.67, which is biased by the confounding effect of sex. In the stratified analysis, the RR for women is 1.35, and that for men is 1.32. The Mantel-Haenszel RR is 1.34. The Mantel-Haenszel χ^2 can then be calculated as follows:

$$\chi^2_{MH} = \frac{\left[\dfrac{(24)(30)-(3)(58)}{115} + \dfrac{(16)(10)-(57)(2)}{85}\right]^2}{\dfrac{(27)(88)(82)(33)}{(114)(115)^2} + \dfrac{(73)(12)(18)(67)}{(84)(85)^2}} = \frac{27.974}{6.005}$$

$$= 4.658, \text{ which corresponds to a } P \text{ value } < 0.05.$$

We thus should reject the null hypothesis and conclude that the higher success rate of T_1 observed in the sample did not arise by chance from a target population in which T_1 and T_2 are of equal efficacy.

The Mantel-Haenszel procedure just described is the most appropriate and widely used technique for controlling for a small number of categorical (or categorized) confounding factors. It can be readily appreciated, however, that as the number of confounding factors increases, the computation becomes unwieldy (when done by hand). Furthermore, there may be some loss of control when continuous confounding variables are arbitrarily categorized.

Two multivariate statistical techniques are commonly used to adjust for multiple confounding variables: *discriminant function analysis* and *multiple logistic regression*. Both techniques provide simultaneous control for any number and combination of continuous and categorical confounders; both can be used for cohort, case-control, or cross-sectional designs; and both are commonly available in many standard statistical software packages. Logistic regression is usually preferred over discriminant function analysis, because the latter depends, to some extent, on the assumption of normally distributed predictor variables (exposure and confounders) in the source populations. Logistic regression has the further advantage that the resulting coefficient for each factor (exposure and all potential confounders) is the natural logarithm of the odds ratio for that factor's association with the study outcome. Most computer software packages also provide standard errors for the logistic coefficients that permit estimation of confidence intervals around the odds ratios. Both discriminant function analysis and multiple logistic regression are beyond the scope of this text, but the interested reader will find excellent discussions in several references [5–8].

As was discussed for differences in means, effect modification must be distinguished from confounding. If the difference between two proportions (or the relative risk or odds ratio) differs substantially in two or more subgroups of the study sample, reporting a single difference for the overall study sample will hide relevant information, even though no bias is introduced. For example, in comparing the difference in rate of myocardial infarction in smoking vs nonsmoking men, it might be found that the difference is far greater among older men than younger men. Data demonstrating modification of the smoking effect by age were shown in Table 6.8. In this case, the investigator would do better to test and report the smoking effect separately for the two age subgroups, even though the sample size (and hence statistical power) would be reduced for the separate subgroups.

14.2.9 The Dovetailing of Categorical and Continuous Data Analysis

So far, I have separated the approaches to analysis of continuous and categorical data. In particular, I have described the use of z- and t-tests for comparing two means, and the χ^2 and Fisher exact tests for comparing two proportions. But the two approaches can actually be shown to be quite similar.

For example, in studies with a dichotomous outcome variable, consider the "target" (e.g., "success") to have a value of 1, and the absence of the target ("failure") to have a value of 0. Then the mean outcome will be:

$$\bar{x} = p, \text{ where } p \text{ is the proportion of successes} = \frac{t}{n} = \frac{\text{number of successes}}{\text{number of subjects}}$$

and the standard deviation will be:

$$s = \sqrt{pq}, \text{ where } q = 1 - p$$

Using these formulas for the mean and SD, z- and t-tests can be constructed just as if the data were continuous. This is considered legitimate as long as the number of expected (under H_o) successes and failures, i.e., np and nq, are both ≥ 5, because then the binomial distribution (representing the exact probability for any given proportion) can be closely approximated by a t- or normal (z-) distribution. Formulas for these z- and t-tests are given in several standard texts [2, 9].

In fact, there is a direct mathematical relationship between the normal approximation of the binomial distribution and the χ^2 distribution: $z^2 = \chi^2$. For example, for $P = 0.05$, a z value of 1.96 is required. If we square 1.96, the result is 3.84, which is the χ^2 value necessary for $P = 0.05$. Similarly, $t^2 = \chi^2$ at an infinite number of degrees of freedom.

When the data are continuous to begin with, they can be converted to categorical data by choosing a "cutoff" point to define the two categories. We can then carry out a χ^2 test on the resulting proportions instead of a t-test on the native continuous data. For example, instead of doing a t-test for measuring a difference in systolic blood pressure between two groups, we could dichotomize the variable into "normal" (< 140 mm Hg) vs hypertensive (≥ 140 mm Hg). There are three problems with this approach, however:

1. Transforming continuous to categorical data involves some "waste." We are substituting a "lower-order" scale, and this is statistically inefficient (i.e., has less statistical power).
2. There is a greater opportunity for misclassification. A pressure measurement that is "off" by 1 mm Hg will have very little impact on a mean or a t-test, but it could

result in a change in category, and hence a change in the group proportion and χ^2 test, if a true systolic pressure of 139 is measured as 140.

3. The result of the statistical analysis depends on the choice of the cutoff point, thus leading to a potential for bias. In other words, the χ^2 test could lead to a different conclusion from the t-test, depending on where we draw the category boundaries. It is thus essential that these boundaries be decided a priori, i.e., before calculation of the χ^2 test, so that the investigator is not at liberty to pick a cutoff point that optimizes his chances for demonstrating statistical significance.

14.2.10 Confidence Interval Around a Difference in Two Proportions

Although significance testing is the most frequently encountered aspect of statistical inference when two proportions are compared, estimating a confidence interval around the observed difference is often more informative. Instead of testing how consistent the observed difference is with a "true" state of no difference, the confidence interval demonstrates how big the "true" difference is likely to be.

The estimation of such a confidence interval is based on the normal approximation of the binomial distribution. As discussed in Section 14.2.9, the sample standard deviation of a proportion p is given by $\sqrt{pq}$, where $q = 1 - p$. Consequently, the standard error $= \dfrac{\sqrt{pq}}{\sqrt{n}} = \sqrt{pq/n}$. Hence, the standard error for the difference

between two proportions p_1 and p_2 is $\sqrt{\dfrac{p_1 q_1}{n_1} + \dfrac{p_2 q_2}{n_2}}$. The $100(1-\alpha)\%$ confidence interval is then computed as follows:

$$\pi_1 - \pi_2 = p_1 - p_2 \pm z_\alpha \sqrt{\frac{p_1 q_1}{n_1} + \frac{p_2 q_2}{n_2}} \tag{14.13}$$

For our postlaparotomy wound infection trial (Table 14.1), the 95% CI

$$= p_1 - p_2 \pm 1.96 \sqrt{\frac{p_1 q_1}{n_1} + \frac{p_2 q_2}{n_2}}$$

$$= 0.029 - 0.081 \pm 1.96 \sqrt{\frac{(0.029)(0.971)}{240} + \frac{(0.081)(0.919)}{260}}$$

$$= -0.052 \pm 0.039$$

$$= -0.091 \text{ to } -0.013$$

14.2.11 Calculating Sample Sizes for Comparing Two Proportions

Although several of the formulas for the χ^2 test can be used for calculating approximate sample sizes required for achieving statistical significance when comparing two proportions, such formulas take no account of Type II error. Instead, sample sizes are usually calculated using the normal approximation of the binomial distribution.

Assuming an α-level of 0.05, the investigator must specify three additional components: π_1 and π_2, the proportions he estimates in the hypothetical source populations, such that $\pi_1 - \pi_2$ represents the minimum threshold for a clinically important difference; and $1 - \beta$, the statistical power he wishes to ensure that a difference as large as $\pi_1 - \pi_2$ will be detected. Assuming two study groups of equal size ($n_1 = n_2$), the total required sample size (N) is then:

$$N = n_1 + n_2 = 2\frac{\left[z_\alpha \sqrt{2\bar{\pi}(1-\bar{\pi})} + z_\beta \sqrt{\pi_1(1-\pi_1) + \pi_2(1-\pi_2)}\right]^2}{(\pi_1 - \pi_2)^2} \tag{14.14}$$

where $\bar{\pi} = \dfrac{\pi_1 + \pi_2}{2}$, and z_α and z_β are the z values corresponding to the chosen levels of α and β. As an alternative to this equation, Fleiss [2] has published sample sizes (for each group, i.e., n_1 or n_2) in the form of tables for specified values of π_1, π_2, α, and $1 - \beta$.

A "shortcut," approximate equation is the following:

$$N = n_1 + n_2 = \frac{4(z_\alpha + z_\beta)^2[\bar{\pi}(1-\bar{\pi})]}{(\pi_1 - \pi_2)^2} \tag{14.15}$$

As an example, suppose we were planning a case-control study of parental divorce before a child's tenth birthday as a risk factor for adolescent suicide. Suppose the divorce rate in the overall population is known to be 30%. Assuming an equal number of cases and controls, we wish to be 90% ($1 - \beta = 0.90$) certain of detecting a divorce rate of 40% among the parents of cases. (Note that this is based on a directional research hypothesis, and one-sided z values are indicated.) Thus:

z_α (one-sided) $= 1.65$ for $\alpha = 0.05$
z_β (one-sided) $= 1.28$ for $\beta = 0.10$
$\pi_1 = 0.30$
$\pi_2 = 0.40$
$\bar{\pi} = 0.35$

Using Eq. 4.14,

$$N = 2\frac{\left[1.65 \sqrt{2(0.35)(0.65)} + 1.28 \sqrt{(0.30)(0.70) + (0.40)(0.60)}\right]^2}{(0.30 - 0.40)^2} = 777.5$$

Rounding up to 778, we require 389 cases and 389 controls.
Using the shortcut equation (Eq. 14.15):

$$N = \frac{4(1.65 + 1.28)^2[(0.35)(0.65)]}{(0.30 - 0.40)^2} = 781.2,$$

or 391 cases and 391 controls.

Thus, the shortcut method comes quite close to the more mathematically correct procedure.

In case-control studies with dichotomous exposure and outcome, the measure of association of primary interest is the odds ratio (OR). Based on an equal number $(=n)$ of cases and controls, a known rate of exposure in the controls (π_1), and the OR considered to represent a clinically important effect, the formula $OR = \dfrac{ad}{bc}$ can be used to solve for π_2. For our adolescent suicide example, the 2×2 table would look like this:

	Suicides	Controls
Divorce	$\pi_2 n$	$\pi_1 n = 0.30n$
No divorce	$(1-\pi_2)n$	$(1-\pi_1)n = 0.70n$
	n	n

$$OR = \frac{ad}{bc} = \frac{(\pi_2 n)(1-\pi_1)n}{(\pi_1 n)(1-\pi_2)n} = \frac{\pi_2(1-\pi_1)}{\pi_1(1-\pi_2)}$$

If we chose 1.5 as a clinically important OR, we could then solve for π_2 as follows:

$$1.5 = \frac{\pi_2(0.70)}{(0.30)(1-\pi_2)}$$
$$0.45(1-\pi_2) = 0.70\pi_2$$
$$0.45 - 0.45\pi_2 = 0.70\pi_2$$
$$0.45 = 1.15\pi_2$$
$$\pi_2 = \frac{0.45}{1.15} = 0.39$$

We then calculate N using Eq. 14.14 or 14.15. Schlesselman has provided tables based on this approach that indicate the number of cases and controls required to detect a given OR once α, β, and π_1 have been specified [10].

A similar approach can be used for cohort studies using the relative risk (RR). π_1 and π_2 would then represent the proportion of nonexposed and exposed subjects, respectively, developing the outcome, and $RR = \dfrac{\pi_2}{\pi_1}$. Thus, if π_1 is known, π_2 can be computed directly from the chosen value of RR.

14.3 Statistical Inferences for a Single Proportion

14.3.1 Testing the "Significance" of a Single Proportion

Suppose we know the proportion π_0 of some reference population. We have a study sample measured on the same variable with proportion p. We want to know the probability that a difference at least as large as $p - \pi_0$ could have arisen by chance, under the null hypothesis that the sample was randomly selected from the reference population (H_o: $\pi = \pi_o$). If the probability is less then 0.05, we will reject H_o, and conclude that the observed difference $p - \pi_o$ is statistically significant. This procedure is exactly analogous to testing the significance of a single sample mean from a known population mean (see Section 13.2.2).

To accomplish this test of H_o, we merely calculate, for each of the two categories of the variable, the frequencies expected under H_o and then compute χ^2 as $\sum \frac{(O_{ij} - E_{ij})^2}{E_{ij}}$ over the two "cells." This χ^2 test for a single proportion is thus similar to the usual χ^2 test, except that it uses only two observed and two expected frequencies, instead of the four seen with the 2×2 table for comparing two proportions.

To illustrate, suppose the prevalence of hypertension among white men in the United States is known to be 15%. An investigator believes that industrial effluent from a certain factory may be contaminating the water supply of a nearby town, and that some of the components of this effluent are capable of raising the blood pressure. In a random sample of 100 white men from this town, 21 are found to be hypertensive. Is the prevalence of hypertension truly elevated, or could the difference (21% vs 15%) have arisen by chance?

The observed frequencies of hypertensive and nonhypertensive are 21 and 79, respectively, compared with the expected frequencies of 15 and 85. Then

$$\chi^2 = \sum \frac{(O_{ij} - E_{ij})^2}{E_{ij}} = \frac{(21 - 15)^2}{15} + \frac{(79 - 85)^2}{85} = \frac{36}{15} + \frac{36}{85} = 2.824,$$

which, using the conventional two-sided P value, corresponds to $P > 0.05$. Therefore, we should not reject the null hypothesis.

This procedure of comparing an observed proportion with an expected one can also be used to test theoretical models. The procedure is called "testing for goodness of fit" and can be expanded to an entire distribution (instead of just two) of observed and expected frequencies. If the difference between the observed distribution and that expected under the model is small, as indicated by a nonsignificant value of χ^2, the model is thereby "supported" (provided the sample size is adequate to protect against an important Type II error).

For example, suppose we believed a given disease to be inherited as an autosomal recessive. This hypothesis could be tested by observing the frequency of the disease among full siblings of patients known to have the disease. In the absence of any bias of ascertainment, selective abortion or mortality, etc., the proportion of affected siblings should be 0.25. If a large sample of siblings could be studied, a test of the difference between the observed and expected rate should provide a good test of the theory. If carriers could also be identified, then the distribution of normal, carrier, and diseased frequencies could be tested against the expected ratio of $1:2:1$ (0.25, 0.50, 0.25).

14.3.2 Confidence Interval Around a Single Proportion: Estimating π from p

When we have a single sample from a target population of interest, we may wish to calculate the range in which the population rate is likely to fall. This parametric estimation of π from p is analogous to estimating μ from $\bar{x}$ (see Section 13.2.1) and is the activity usually engaged in by opinion pollsters; a certain number of subjects are (preferably randomly) sampled for their political preference or their opinion about a prominent issue, and the result is expressed as a 95% or other confidence interval (often around a percentage, rather than a proportion).

To estimate such a confidence interval, we rely on the normal approximation of the binomial distribution. As discussed in Section 14.2.10, the standard error of a proportion $= \dfrac{\sqrt{pq}}{\sqrt{n}} = \sqrt{pq/n}$, where $q = 1 - p$. The $100(1-\alpha)\%$ confidence interval can then be calculated as follows:

$$CI = p \pm z_\alpha \sqrt{pq/n}, \tag{14.16}$$

where z_α is the two-sided z value required for the desired confidence interval. For a 95% CI, $z = 1.96$; for a 99% CI, $z = 2.58$.

To illustrate, let us return to the random sample of 100 men in our suspect town, 21 of whom were determined to be hypertensive. What is the 95% CI for the prevalence of hypertension among the town's men?

$$
\begin{aligned}
95\% \ CI = p \pm 1.96 \sqrt{pq/n} &= 0.21 \pm 1.96 \sqrt{(0.21)(0.79)/100} \\
&= 0.21 \pm 0.08 \\
&= 0.13 \text{ to } 0.29
\end{aligned}
$$

14.4 Comparison of Three or More Proportions

The χ^2 test is easily extended to comparison of three or more proportions, i.e., dichotomous outcome with polychotomous exposure. χ^2 is still defined as $\sum \dfrac{(O_{ij} - E_{ij})^2}{E_{ij}}$ and is interpreted at $(r-1)(c-1) = r-1$ degrees of freedom, where the data are displayed in 2 columns ($c = 2$) and r rows. The easiest formula for computing χ^2 is a modification of Eq. 14.4:

$$\chi^2 = \left[\sum \frac{t_i^2}{n_i} - \frac{T^2}{N} \right] \left[\frac{N^2}{T(N-T)} \right] \tag{14.17}$$

As an example, suppose our postlaparotomy wound infection trial included three treatments, two different antibiotics and a placebo, with infection rates of $\dfrac{10}{250}$, $\dfrac{7}{240}$, and $\dfrac{21}{260}$, respectively. Then

$$\chi^2 = \left[\frac{10^2}{250} + \frac{7^2}{240} + \frac{21^2}{260} - \frac{38^2}{750}\right]\left[\frac{750^2}{38(712)}\right] = 7.796,$$

which at 2 *df* corresponds to a *P* value between 0.01 and 0.05.

The $r \times 2$ χ^2 test is analogous to a one-way analysis of variance. The result is the extent of overall departure from equivalence of proportions. The overall χ^2 can be partitioned, however, to allow testing of pairs of proportions and other post hoc comparisons. On inspection of our example, it is evident that the wound infection rates in patients receiving either antibiotic are similar, but both are lower than the placebo rate. This "visual test" can easily be confirmed by comparing the contributions to the total χ^2.

When the exposure variable is ordinal, however, the usual χ^2 test does not take into account the inherent order among the categories. It merely tests the overall departure of observed from expected across the $r \times 2$ cells of the table. A test of mere association between columns and rows will be statistically inefficient, because it fails to distinguish between one- and two-category differences.

A preferable alternative is the χ^2 *test for linear trend.* Several versions of this test exist, but the most convenient is that given by Armitage [11]:

$$\chi_L^2 = \frac{N(N\Sigma t_i w_i - T\Sigma n_i w_i)^2}{T(N-T)[N\Sigma n_i w_i^2 - (\Sigma n_i w_i)^2]} \tag{14.18}$$

where n_i is the number of subjects in the *i*th exposure category, t_i is the number of subjects within the *i*th category who experience the "target" outcome, w_i is the "weight" (or "score") assigned to the *i*th category, N is the total number of subjects, and T is the total number who experience the outcome. Although somewhat arbitrary, the w_i's are usually assigned whole integers with equal intervals symmetrical around 0. Thus, for three ordinal groups, the weights would be -1, 0, and $+1$; for four groups, -3, -1, $+1$, and $+3$; and so on. The value of χ^2 is then interpreted at 1 *df.*

To illustrate, let us calculate χ_L^2 for the data shown in Table 14.5, which summarizes the results of a cohort study in which children with otitis media (middle-ear infection) were treated with oral amoxicillin in either the dosage range recommended by the manufacturer, a dosage above that recommended ("high dose"), or a dosage below the recommended dose ("low dose"). The children were followed for the duration of their 10-day course of treatment for the occurrence of diarrhea, a well-known side effect of oral amoxicillin. The ordinary χ^2 test yields a χ^2 value of 5.53, which at 2 *df* is not statistically significant. The χ^2 for linear trend (χ_L^2) of 5.16 at 1 *df,* however, yields a *P* value <0.05, indicating a significant dose-response relationship. Failure to consider the ordinal nature of the exposure variable in the analysis would thus have led to a loss of statistical efficiency.

Another approach to analyzing these data without losing the ordinal nature of the exposure would be to compare the *ranks* of exposures (dosage ranges) in the two outcome groups (children with and without diarrhea) using the Mann-Whitney U-test (see Section 13.4). Although such a procedure would be tantamount to analyzing the data like a case-control study, the test would be an appropriate test of association between exposure and outcome.

Table 14.5. Diarrhea occurring in children with otitis media treated with three different dosages of amoxicillin (see text)

		Diarrhea	No diarrhea	
$w_1 = +1$	High dose	12 $= t_1$	38	50 $= n_1$
$w_2 = 0$	Recommended dose	13 $= t_2$	87	100 $= n_2$
$w_3 = -1$	Low dose	4 $= t_3$	46	50 $= n_3$
		29 $= T$	171 $= N - T$	200 $= N$

Using Eq. 14.17:

$$\chi^2 = \left[\frac{12^2}{50} + \frac{13^2}{100} + \frac{4^2}{50} - \frac{29^2}{200} \right] \left[\frac{200^2}{(29)(171)} \right] = 5.53 \text{ At 2 } df, P > 0.05$$

$\Sigma t_i w_i = (12)(+1) + (13)(0) + (4)(-1) = +8$

$\Sigma n_i w_i = (50)(+1) + (100)(0) + (50)(-1) = 0$

$\Sigma n_i w_i^2 = (50)(+1) + (100)(0) + (50)(+1) = +100$

Using Eq. 14.18:

$$\chi_L^2 = \frac{200[(200)(8) - (29)(0)]^2}{(29)(171)[(200)(100) - (0)^2]} = 5.16 \text{ At 1 } df, P < 0.05$$

When the axes of the table are reversed, i.e., the outcome is ordinal and the exposure is dichotomous (a $2 \times c$ table), the Mann-Whitney test is even more appropriate [12]. The χ^2 for linear trend can be used here too, however, provided the analyst makes the following "substitutions":

1. t_i now becomes the number of subjects in the index exposure groups in each outcome category
2. n_i now becomes the total number of subjects in each outcome category
3. w_i now applies to the weights assigned to the outcome categories

14.5 Analysis of Larger ($r \times c$) Contingency Tables

When exposure and outcome are each measured on a polychotomous nominal scale containing three or more categories, the ordinary χ^2 test summing $\frac{(O_{ij} - E_{ij})^2}{E_{ij}}$ over all cells in the $r \times c$ contingency table can be used to test the null hypothesis at

$(r-1)(c-1)$ degrees of freedom. A significant value for χ^2, however, will indicate only an overall tendency for deviation of observed frequencies from those expected under H_o. It will not indicate which exposure and outcome categories are most responsible for the overall association.

Although visual inspection of the $r \times c$ table can often provide an impression, that impression can be confirmed by *partitioning* the overall table into smaller tables such that the degrees of freedom among all these "subtables" sum to $(r-1)(c-1)$. The χ^2 value in each subtable can then be assessed for statistical significance. Armitage [11] provides a good discussion of this procedure.

When exposure and outcome are both ordinal, the most appropriate test of association involves a test of linear correlation using ranks. Rank correlation will be discussed, along with other forms of linear correlation and regression, in Chapter 15.

References

1. Miettinen OS (1974) Simple interval-estimation of risk ratio. Am J Epidemiol 100: 515–516
2. Fleiss JL (1981) Statistical methods for rates and proportions, 2nd edn. John Wiley & Sons, New York, pp 23–24, 71–75, 260–280
3. Kleinbaum DG, Kupper LL, Morgenstern H (1982) Epidemiologic research: principles and quantitative methods. Lifetime Learning Publications, Belmont, CA, pp 296–307, 332
4. Mantel N, Haenszel W (1959) Statistical aspects of the analysis of data from retrospective studies of disease. JNCI 22: 719–748
5. Kleinbaum DG, Kupper LL (1978) Applied regression analysis and other multivariable methods. Duxbury, North Scituate, MA, pp 414–446
6. Anderson S, Auquier A, Hauck WW, Oakes D, Vandaele W, Weisberg HI (1980) Statistical methods for comparative studies: techniques for bias reduction. Wiley, New York, pp 161–177
7. Breslow NE, Day NE (1980) Statistical methods in cancer research, vol. 1. The analysis of case-control studies. International Agency for Research on Cancer, Lyon, pp 191–279
8. Hanley JA (1983) Appropriate uses of multivariate analysis. Annu Rev Public Health 4: 155–180
9. Colton T (1974) Statistics in medicine. Little, Brown, Boston, pp 153–174
10. Schlesselman JJ (1982) Case-control studies: design, conduct, analysis. Oxford University Press, New York, pp 293–313
11. Armitage P (1971) Statistical methods in medical research. Blackwell Scientific, Oxford, pp 353–368
12. Moses LE, Emerson JD, Hosseini H (1984) Analyzing data from ordered categories. N Engl J Med 311: 442–448

Chapter 15: Linear Correlation and Regression

15.1 Linear Correlation

15.1.1 Introduction

The main objective in most epidemiologic studies is the measurement of the association between exposure and outcome. Chapter 13 focused on testing the difference in outcome measured on a continuous scale in two (or more) exposure groups. The difference between the group means reflects the extent of association between the continuous outcome and the categorical exposure, and the corresponding P value derived from a t- or z-test indicates the probability of obtaining the observed or stronger degree of association by chance under the null hypothesis. In Chapter 14, both outcome and exposure were categorical (often dichotomous). The usual measures of association between a dichotomous exposure and a dichotomous outcome are the difference in proportions in those subjects with and without the outcome in the two exposure groups and the relative risk (RR) for cohort studies and the odds ratio (OR) for case-control studies. These measures are then usually tested for statistical significance using the χ^2 test or Fisher exact test.

How do we measure the association between exposure and outcome when both are continuous variables? One of the variables (usually exposure) could be dichotomized, and the means of the other variable (outcome) in the groups defined by that dichotomy could be compared by means of a t- or z-test. But as we saw in Chapter 14, categorization of continuous data may be statistically inefficient. The initial strategy for measuring the association between two continuous variables is usually to examine the extent to which the relationship between the two can be described by a straight line, i.e., the extent of their *linear correlation*.

Linear correlation measures the degree to which an increase in one of the variables is associated with a proportional increase or decrease in the second variable. Consider a cross-sectional study of the effect of impairment in renal function on the hemoglobin concentration. The investigator hypothesizes that progressive decrements in renal function (as measured by rises in the serum creatinine concentration) will be associated with a proportional fall in hemoglobin. The data on ten patients with chronic renal failure are shown in Table 15.1, and the corresponding *scatter diagram* is displayed in Fig. 15.1. If every point fell exactly on a straight line, the two variables would be said to be perfectly correlated.

It should be emphasized that linear correlation is strongly influenced by a few extreme values of the two variables whose correlation is being assessed. Suppose, for

Table 15.1. Serum creatinine and hemoglobin concentrations in ten subjects with chronic renal failure

Subject no.	Creatinine (mg/dl)	Hemoglobin (g/dl)
1	4.1	9.0
2	2.8	9.5
3	6.5	8.4
4	2.4	11.7
5	3.7	10.8
6	8.0	8.2
7	5.3	8.8
8	7.9	8.9
9	4.4	10.1
10	3.2	11.5

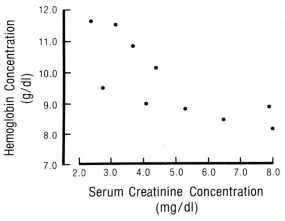

Fig. 15.1. Hemoglobin and serum creatinine concentrations in ten patients with chronic renal failure

example, the scatter diagram shows that most of the data points lie in a circle (indicating no correlation) but that a few lie bunched together in an area on a "diagonal" from, i.e., above or below *and* to the left or right of, the circle representing the majority of the points. The linear correlation may then be fairly high and may be a poor summary of the relationship between the two variables. A good rule of thumb, therefore, is to plot the data and examine them visually before reporting the linear correlation.

15.1.2 Dependent and Nondependent Correlation

In examining the relationship between exposure and outcome, we are testing the research hypothesis that the outcome *depends* on exposure. In our creatinine-hemoglobin example, hemoglobin is being tested for its dependence on renal function (as measured by the serum creatinine concentration). Even though the study is cross-sectional, the temporal relationship between the two seems clear on biologic grounds. Renal failure may cause anemia, but anemia does not usually (short of massive hemolysis) cause renal failure. Serum creatinine is the exposure variable, and hemoglobin is the outcome.

In the parlance of linear correlation and regression, exposure is usually called the *independent variable,* and outcome the *dependent variable.* In our example, it is as if the creatinine were "allowed" to vary independently, and the hemoglobin then depended on the observed value of creatinine. By convention, the independent variable is usually represented by x and the dependent variable by y. Thus, in Fig. 15.1, the serum creatinine concentration is indicated by the x-axis (abscissa), and hemoglobin by the y-axis (ordinate).

By way of contrast to the obviously dependent relationship between hemoglobin and creatinine, consider the relationship between blood urea nitrogen (BUN) and creatinine concentrations. The two are usually highly positively correlated, because they represent two different tests of renal function, even though other factors (e.g., state of hydration for BUN and muscle mass for creatinine) prevent the correlation from being perfect. In a cross-sectional study of these two variables, it would be difficult indeed to label one as "exposure" and the other as "outcome." Because both depend on renal function and neither depends on the other, their relationship with each other is nondependent. In a graphical display of the relationship, either one could be represented by the y-axis.

The decision that a relationship is dependent or nondependent thus arises from clinical reasoning, not from statistical inference. Because most clinical and epidemiologic studies are based on a hypothesized association between exposure and outcome, our major focus here will be on dependent relationships.

15.1.3 Measuring the Extent of Linear Correlation

The *Pearson correlation coefficient,* which is abbreviated by the letter r, is a descriptive statistic indicating the extent of linear correlation between two continuous variables. It is defined mathematically as follows:

$$r = \frac{\Sigma(x_i - \bar{x})(y_i - \bar{y})}{\sqrt{\Sigma(x_i - \bar{x})^2 \Sigma(y_i - \bar{y})^2}} \tag{15.1}$$

where x and y are the two continuous (independent and dependent, respectively) variables being correlated on each of the i study subjects.

The correlation coefficient r can range in value from -1 to $+1$, with 0 representing no correlation, -1 a perfect inverse correlation (negatively sloping line), and $+1$ a perfect positive correlation (positively sloping line) between the two variables. For our hemoglobin-creatinine example, $r = -0.779$, indicating a strong inverse correlation.

Since the linear correlation between two variables is rarely perfect (i.e., r rarely equals $+1$ or -1), we are often interested in measuring the *extent* to which the relationship between the two is explained by a straight line. To do this, we make use of a concept known as *explained variance.* As will be recalled from Chapter 11, the total variance of any continuous variable is the square of its standard deviation and is a measure of the spread of a group's set of values around its mean.

We can interpret r in these terms by measuring the proportion of total variance in one (usually the dependent) variable that is due to its linear relationship with the other (independent variable). Using our example of hemoglobin and creatinine, we can thus divide the variance in hemoglobin into two components: (a) that component due to the linear relationship between hemoglobin and creatinine and (b) that component due to sampling (random) variation or other sources. It can be shown that r^2 equals the proportion of variance in either variable due to its linear correlation with the other. In our example, $r = -0.779$, and thus $r^2 = 0.607$. Our interpretation of this value of r^2 is that approximately 61% of the variance in hemoglobin is "accounted for" by the serum creatinine.

The interpretation of r requires some further discussion. The correlation between two continuous variables x and y, as expressed by the correlation coefficient, refers to the degree of *linear* relationship between x and y. Now, there might be a very close relationship between the two variables but one that is not well described by a straight line. In that case, linear correlation might be very poor, despite the close mathematical relationship.

For example, consider the following equation:

$$y = 1 + (x - 3)^2$$

which is graphically depicted in Fig. 15.2. In this example, y is a perfect quadratic function of x (all points lie on the curve), but not a linear one (at least, not over the range of x's shown in the figure). Despite the obvious closeness of the relationship, $r = 0$.

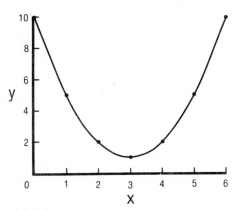

Fig. 15.2. Graphic representation of $y = 1 + (x - 3)^2$

15.2 Linear Regression

Linear regression is the process of fitting a straight line to two continuous variables x and y. Specifically, we wish to determine the statistics a and b in the equation:

$$\hat{y} = a + bx$$

where $\hat{y}$ (y "hat") indicates the fitted estimate of y based on a, b, and x. This is the general equation for a straight line, in which a is the intercept (the average value of y when $x = 0$) and b is the slope (the average change in y per unit change in x). Another name for b is the *regression coefficient*.

Mathematically, a and b can be computed as follows:

$$b = \frac{\Sigma(x_i - \bar{x})(y_i - \bar{y})}{\Sigma(x_i - \bar{x})^2} \tag{15.2}$$

$$a = \bar{y} - b\bar{x} \tag{15.3}$$

In our example of hemoglobin (y) and creatinine (x),

$$\hat{y} = 12.042 - 0.487x$$

This means that, on average, for every increase in serum creatinine concentration of 1 mg/dl, the decrease in hemoglobin concentration is 0.487 g/dl, at least over the range of measurements shown in Fig. 15.1. (It is hazardous to extrapolate the linear relationship between x and y beyond the observed measured ranges of x and y.)

As discussed in Section 15.1.2, the relationship between hemoglobin and creatinine is a biologically dependent one, in the sense that we believe that renal function (as measured by the serum creatinine) affects the hemoglobin concentration, rather than the reverse. It is for this reason that we have *regressed* hemoglobin (y) on creatinine (x). This follows the usual convention of regressing the dependent variable (y) on the independent variable (x).

Mathematically, however, we could regress x on y:

$$\hat{x} = a' + b'y$$

where the "primes" are used to indicate the intercept and slope of the "inverted regression" and are computed as follows:

$$b' = \frac{\Sigma(x_i - \bar{x})(y_i - \bar{y})}{\Sigma(y_i - \bar{y})^2} \tag{15.4}$$

$$a' = \bar{x} - b'\bar{y} \tag{15.5}$$

For our creatinine-hemoglobin example,

$$\hat{x} = 16.900 - 1.246y$$

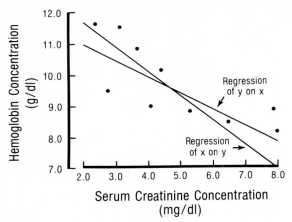

Fig. 15.3. Regression of hemoglobin concentration *(y)* on serum creatinine concentration *(x)* and vice versa

The two different regression lines are illustrated in Fig. 15.3. As we have seen, the regression of *y* on *x* is the biologically sensible one reflecting our hypothesis regarding exposure (renal failure) and outcome (anemia). The other regression line, though mathematically correct, is biologically nonsensical. The choice would have been more difficult, however, in our example of BUN and creatinine. In that (nondependent) case, either regression line would have been appropriate for displaying the relationship.

15.3 Correlation vs Regression

We now have two different descriptive statistics, or coefficients, to describe the extent of linear relationship between two continuous variables *x* and *y*. The correlation coefficient *r* is useful for describing the degree of linear "closeness," i.e., linear correlation, between *x* and *y*, irrespective of which is the dependent variable and which is the independent variable. A major advantage of *r* is that its value is the same regardless of the units in which *x* and *y* are measured. In our example, *r* = −0.779 no matter whether creatinine is measured in mg/dl or mmol/l. The one disadvantage of *r* is that it is not useful for *predicting* the value of *y* from a value of *x*.

To predict *y* from *x*, regression is required. The value of the regression coefficient *b*, however, will change with changes in the units in which *x* and *y* are measured. The value of *b* in our example would be entirely different from −0.487 if creatinine were measured in mmol/l instead of mg/dl.

The correlation coefficient *r* indicates the extent to which a relationship between *x* and *y* can be described by a straight line, whereas *b* is the rate of rise in *y* for every unit rise in *x*. The contrast in interpretation between the two coefficients is illustrated by the three regression lines shown in Fig. 15.4. Each of the three regressions

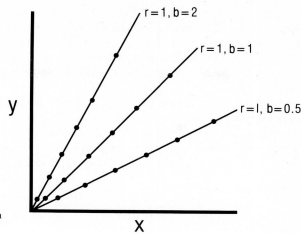

Fig. 15.4. The distinction between r and b

is represented by a perfect straight line. In other words, $r = +1$ for all three. The slope of b differs considerably among the three, however.

The invariable nature of r, irrespective of which variable is regressed on which, is easily appreciated from the mathematical relationship between r, on the one hand, and b and b', on the other. As can be seen from inspection of Eqs. (15.1), (15.2), and (15.4):

$$
\begin{aligned}
r &= \frac{\Sigma(x_i - \bar{x})(y_i - \bar{y})}{\sqrt{\Sigma(x_i - \bar{x})^2 \Sigma(y_i - \bar{y})^2}} \\
&= \sqrt{\frac{\Sigma(x_i - \bar{x})(y_i - \bar{y})\Sigma(x_i - \bar{x})(y_i - \bar{y})}{\Sigma(x_i - \bar{x})^2 \Sigma(y_i - \bar{y})^2}} \\
&= \sqrt{bb'}
\end{aligned}
\tag{15.6}
$$

Equation 15.6 indicates that b is not the mere inverse of b' (that is, $b \neq \frac{1}{b'}$), unless the linear relationship between x and y is perfect (i.e., $r = +1$ or -1).

15.4 Statistical Inference

As we have seen, r and b are descriptive statistics that describe different aspects of the linear relationship between two continuous variables, x and y. When $r = 0$ or $b = 0$, there is no linear correlation or mutual interdependence between x and y. When values are obtained that differ from 0, however, we need to ask ourselves whether such a difference is statistically significant; i.e., what is the probability that a difference as large or larger would arise by chance under a null hypothesis of no correlation?

Since r and b are calculated on a sample, we must turn once again to hypothesis testing to provide statistical inferences about the linear relationship between x and y in the target population of which the study subjects are a (hypothetically) random sample. We test the statistical significance of r or b by postulating the null hypothesis that ρ (the population correlation coefficient) or β (the population regression coefficient) is equal to 0.

We can do a t-test on the value of b or r in the study sample, and derive the probability (P value) of obtaining this value of b or r in a random sample from a population in which $\rho=0$ and $\beta=0$. As it turns out, the formula for t is the same for testing either b or r. This makes sense, since the two are mathematically related and since no correlation means no regression (and vice versa).

The formula is as follows:

$$t = r\sqrt{\frac{n-2}{1-r^2}} \tag{15.7}$$

The value of t is then interpreted at $n-2$ degrees of freedom.
For our hemoglobin-creatinine example, $r = -0.779$. Then:

$$t = -0.779\sqrt{\frac{10-2}{1-(-0.779)^2}} = -3.514$$

At $10-2=8$ df, this value of t corresponds to a (two-sided) P value between 0.005 and 0.01. (A one-sided test could be defended here, since the research hypothesis is directional, i.e., increasing renal failure would lead to a *lower* hemoglobin concentration.)

As is evident from Eq. 15.7, the statistical significance of r or b is highly dependent on the sample size. For a given value of r, t rises proportionately with $\sqrt{n}$. Thus, with very large samples, even small degrees of correlation can yield "significant" P values. As in other types of significance tests, the clinical importance of a correlation needs to be considered, as well as its statistical significance. Conversely, even high values of b or r may not achieve statistical significance with very small samples, and the potential for Type II error needs to be kept in mind whenever a decision not to reject H_o is based on small samples.

As discussed previously, the estimation of a confidence interval around an observed measure of association is often more informative than a test of the null hypothesis. For the correlation coefficient, this can be accomplished using Fisher's z-transformation of r:

$$\tfrac{1}{2}\ln\left(\frac{1+r}{1-r}\right) \tag{15.8}$$

which is normally distributed when the sample size is sufficiently large ($n \geq 20$). Then the $100(1-\alpha)\%$ confidence interval for the corresponding population parameter can be computed as follows:

$$\tfrac{1}{2} \ln \left(\frac{1+\rho}{1-\rho}\right) = \tfrac{1}{2} \ln \left(\frac{1+r}{1-r}\right) \pm z_\alpha/\sqrt{n-3} \qquad (15.9)$$

and the equation then solved for ρ.

Let us work through the calculation of a 95% confidence interval for our hemoglobin-creatinine example:

$$\tfrac{1}{2} \ln \left(\frac{1+\rho}{1-\rho}\right) = \tfrac{1}{2} \ln \left(\frac{1-0.779}{1+0.779}\right) \pm 1.96/\sqrt{10-3}$$
$$= \tfrac{1}{2} \ln (0.124) \pm 0.741$$
$$= -1.043 \pm 0.741$$
$$= -1.784 \text{ to } -0.302$$

Hence $\ln \left(\frac{1+\rho}{1-\rho}\right) = -3.568 \text{ to } -0.604$

$\left(\frac{1+\rho}{1-\rho}\right) = 0.028 \text{ to } 0.547$

$1+\rho = (0.028)(1-\rho) \text{ to } (0.547)(1-\rho)$
$\rho = (0.028)(1-\rho) - 1 \text{ to } (0.547)(1-\rho) - 1$
$= -0.028\rho - 0.972 \text{ to } -0.547\rho - 0.453$

Therefore, at the two confidence limits, $1.028\rho = -0.972$ and $1.547\rho = -0.453$

or $\rho = -0.946$ and -0.293

and the 95% confidence interval is -0.293 to -0.946

15.5 Control for Confounding Factors

Just as in the comparison of means or proportions, one or more extraneous variables can confound the linear relationship between two continuous variables. Although matching or stratification can be used to control for such confounding factors, a powerful multivariate statistical technique exists for simultaneous control of any number of confounders: *multiple linear regression.* In addition to this purpose, multiple regression also allows the investigator to assess the separate unconfounded effects of several independent variables on a single dependent variable.

The technique models the dependent variable (y) as a linear function of all the (k) independent variables $(x_i\text{'s})$:

$$\hat{y} = a + b_1x_1 + b_2x_2 + b_3x_3 \ldots b_kx_k$$

The x_i's may be any continuous or dichotomous variables, and the b_i's represent the corresponding regression coefficients. Each b_i is "corrected" simultaneously for the linear relationship between its corresponding x_i and every other x_i, as well as for the linear relationship between the other x_i's and y. An overall r^2 can be calculated for the model and represents the proportion of the total variance of y accounted for by its linear relationship with all the x_i's. Multiple regression is commonly included among the available techniques contained in standard statistical software packages. Further details are available in standard texts [1–3].

As with other measures of exposure-outcome association, including differences in means and proportions, relative risks, and odds ratios, extraneous variables may modify the linear correlation between exposure or outcome without confounding (biasing) the overall correlation. Two variables may be poorly correlated in the overall study sample but highly correlated within one or more subgroups, or the correlation may be "statistically significant" in both but quantitatively much greater in one than the other. In such cases, the magnitudes and significance of the correlation should be reported separately for the different subgroups.

15.6 Rank (Nonparametric) Correlation

The use of r calculated on a study sample to make inferences about the degree of correlation ρ between two continuous variables x and y in the target population is based on the assumption that the joint distribution of x and y is *bivariate normal.* In other words, y should be normally distributed at all values of x and vice versa. Most minor departures from this assumption will not seriously affect the validity of conventional correlation and regression techniques. When the joint distribution shows major departures from normality, however, the investigator has two main choices. Either she can transform (using a logarithmic or other mathematical transformation) x or y or both so that the bivariate normal distributional assumption holds, or she can use a nonparametric form of correlation that does not depend on such an assumption.

Nonparametric correlation is based solely on the ranks of x and y, and thus can be used not only for continuous data that violate the assumption of bivariate normality, but also when x and y are both ordinal variables. It is also useful in examining whether there is a *monotonic* (i.e., consistently in one direction but not necessarily linear) relationship between two continuous or ordinal variables. Moreover, it is far less influenced than r by extreme values of x and y. The usual (Spearman) technique compares the ranks for each of the two variables for each study subject. The closer the ranks, the greater the correlation.

To compute r_s, the *Spearman rank correlation coefficient* (also called *Spearman's rho*), each of the two variables is ranked from lowest (rank = 1) to highest. Subjects with tied values for either of the two variables receive the average of their corresponding ranks (i.e., two subjects tied for the 7th and 8th position would each receive a rank of 7.5). For each subject, we compute the difference d between the ranks of the two variables and then use the following formula:

$$r_s = 1 - \frac{6\Sigma d_i^2}{n^3 - n} \tag{15.10}$$

Table 15.2. Rankings (from Table 15.1) of serum creatinine and hemoglobin concentrations in ten subjects with chronic renal failure

Subject no.	Creatinine (rank)	Hemoglobin (rank)	d_i^a	d_i^2
1	5	5	0	0
2	2	6	−4	16
3	8	2	+6	36
4	1	10	−9	81
5	4	8	−4	16
6	10	1	+9	81
7	7	3	+4	16
8	9	4	+5	25
9	6	7	−1	1
10	3	9	−6	36
				$\Sigma d_i^2 = 308$

[a] d_i = creatinine rank − hemoglobin rank for each subject.

The magnitude of r_s can vary between −1 and +1 and is interpreted in the same way as the Pearson correlation coefficient, r. Its statistical significance can be assessed by consulting tabulated (see Appendix Table A.8) minimum values of r_s required for the usual threshold P values at varying sample sizes (n's). For sample sizes of ten or more, the sampling distribution for the r_s's under the null hypothesis of no correlation is approximated by the standard normal distribution, and a z-test can be used:

$$z = r_s \sqrt{n-1} \tag{15.11}$$

To illustrate the Spearman procedure, the hemoglobin-creatinine data in Table 15.1 have been converted to ranks in Table 15.2. The sum of the squared differences in ranks, Σd_i^2, is 308. Then

$$r_s = 1 - \frac{6\Sigma d_i^2}{n^3 - n} = 1 - \frac{6(308)}{1000 - 10} = -0.867$$

which is not far from the calculated value for r (−0.779). The corresponding P value for this value of r_s can be seen from the Appendix Table A.8 to be <0.01. Or alternatively, using Eq. 15.11:

$$z = r_s \sqrt{n-1} = -0.867 \sqrt{10-1} = -2.60,$$

which corresponds (see Appendix Table A.3) to a two-tailed P value of 0.009.

References

1. Armitage P (1971) Statistical methods in medical research. Blackwell Scientific, Oxford, pp 302–332
2. Snedecor GW, Cochran WG (1980) Statistical methods, 7th edn. Iowa State University Press, Ames, pp 334–364
3. Kleinbaum DG, Kupper LL (1978) Applied regression analysis and other multivariable methods. Duxbury, North Scituate, MA, pp 131–208

Part III

Special Topics

Chapter 16: Diagnostic Tests

16.1 Introduction

Until about 100 years ago, the history and physical examination were the only sources of information available to the clinician confronted with a diagnostic decision. He was thus limited to what he could see, hear, feel, smell, or taste – in other words, to what his own senses could tell him. The development of radiology and bacteriology around the turn of the century enabled him to amplify and extend his sensory input. More recently, with the refinement of sophisticated radiographic, biochemical, and immunologic techniques, the diagnostic test has become an invaluable tool in the detection and definition of disease.

On the other hand, not all tests are equally illuminating, and many are very expensive. Modern clinicians are under increasing attack in many quarters for their indiscriminate use of diagnostic tests. Humane patient care and limited economic resources both demand a more thoughtful, critical approach to testing that examines the relative merits of different tests and their respective costs and benefits.

If we accept the proposition that some tests are better than others for certain disease conditions, and that in certain situations there may be tests that are better left undone, the question is: How do we go about making these comparisons and decisions? This chapter will provide an epidemiologic and statistical framework for evaluating the worth of diagnostic tests.

16.2 Defining "Normal" and "Abnormal" Test Results

Most diagnostic tests have an important requirement in common: the classification of the results of the test as "normal" or "abnormal." Before we consider other requirements of testing, we must first consider how these terms are defined. Many tests consist of the measurement of a continuous variable, such as serum thyroxine or systolic blood pressure. Yet the results of the test are interpreted dichotomously, that is, positive vs negative, abnormal vs normal. This means that so-called normal limits must be established, often arbitrarily. How these limits are defined depends on the statistical model postulated for the distribution of the variable measured.

One of the most commonly used models is a single normal, or Gaussian, distribution. As discussed in Chapter 11, the Gaussian curve was found to describe the distribution of certain measurements, such as height and weight, performed on dif-

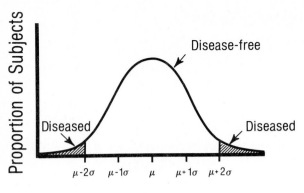

Fig. 16.1. Single Gaussian distribution

ferent subjects, as well as the distribution of results when repeated measurements were performed on a single subject. Gauss and other statisticians of the time used the word "normal" to refer to the bell shape of this distribution. But the word "normal" had already been well established in clinical medicine long before its statistical usage, in reference to a quite different connotation: the distinction between health and disease. These two different meanings of the word "normal," the clinical one and the statistical one, have become blurred over the years, resulting in a number of unfortunate consequences, especially in the interpretation of the results of diagnostic tests.

This statistical model of "abnormality" assumes a single population, with test results falling symmetrically around a mean according to the number of standard deviations from the mean (Fig. 16.1). Approximately 2.5% of the population will lie more than two standard deviations above the mean, and 2.5% will lie more than two standard deviations below the mean. Labeling 2.5% or 5% of the population as diseased (abnormal) merely because of their position in such a postulated distribution makes neither good clinical nor statistical sense, however. For example, use of this model for interpreting the results of serum calcium determinations will automatically establish the prevalence of hypercalcemia and hypocalcemia as 2.5% for each. These prevalences may bear no relation to the proportions of persons with symptoms or with derangements in parathyroid, kidney, or other metabolic functions. Elveback et al. have referred to the frequent use of this inappropriate statistical model of abnormality as the "ghost of Gauss" [1].

The havoc wreaked by Gauss' ghost becomes magnified when multiple diagnostic tests are performed on the same subject. For example, suppose that a "multiphasic screening battery" of 20 serum tests is ordered. If the single Gaussian distribution model is used (as it often is) and the test results are independent of one another, then a subject has a one in 20 chance of having an abnormal value for *each* test. When the 20-test battery is administered, the same subject has a probability of $1 - (0.95)^{20} = 0.64$ of having at least one abnormal result.

Such "statistogenic" disease often results in further testing and occasionally in unnecessary therapy. One wry observer has termed this phenomenon the "Ulysses

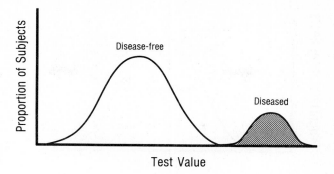

Fig. 16.2. Two nonoverlapping distributions

syndrome" [2]. Ulysses, you will recall, underwent a two-year odyssey between the end of the Trojan War and his return home, during which time he experienced a number of needless, dangerous, but entertaining adventures. *The Odyssey* may make good reading, but foisting such adventures on unsuspecting test subjects makes bad medicine.

The statistical model easiest to deal with is that of two nonoverlapping independent distributions, which may or may not be Gaussian (Fig. 16.2). In this model, there are two distinct populations, a disease-free one and a diseased one, without overlap, so that a given test result will allow a certain decision as to the disease status of the subject tested. Unfortunately, although such a model avoids arbitrary decisions, most diseases do not afford us this luxury. Genetic diseases due to missing or abnormal enzymes may show this pattern. For example, patients with phenylketonuria lack the enzyme tyrosine hydroxylase and are therefore unable to metabolize the amino acid phenylalanine to tyrosine. The distribution of such patients' serum phenylalanine levels is much higher than, and does not overlap with, the distribution of levels in normal subjects.

A more attractive statistical model, and one that seems to pertain to many diseases, is that of a diseased population and a disease-free population with partially overlapping (Gaussian or non-Gaussian) distributions. The overall distribution of test results can take one of two forms, depending on the relative sizes of the two distributions and their degree of overlap: (a) a unimodal distribution skewed toward the direction of abnormality; or (b) a bimodal distribution with recognizable "peaks" corresponding to the modes of the diseased and disease-free populations.

With the unimodal skewed form (Fig. 16.3), it can be exceedingly difficult to distinguish the diseased and disease-free distributions by visual inspection, because they are both "buried" in the overall observed distribution. When the two distributions are both Gaussian, one approach to solving this problem is to plot the overall distribution on cumulative probability graph paper. By "squeezing" the extremely low and high probabilities (*y*-axis) and "stretching out" the middle ones, a Gaussian distribution will be represented by a perfect straight line. A "buried" population with a different Gaussian distribution will appear as a linear deviation from the main line. This procedure is illustrated in Fig. 16.4 with data from a study by Pethybridge et al. of birth weights in southwest England in 1965 [3]. Above about 2500 g, the points fall on a straight line, representing the "normal-birth-weight" ("disease-free") popu-

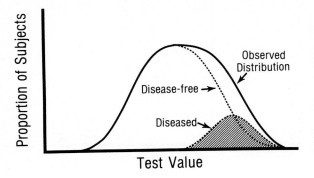

Fig. 16.3. Unimodal skewed distribution

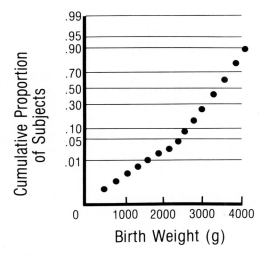

Fig. 16.4. Distribution of birth weights in southwest England, 1965 (plotted on cumulative probability scale)

lation. Below 2000 g, the points also fall on a fairly straight line and indicate a distinct "low-birth-weight" population. Between 2000 and 2500 g, the points appear less linear. This range represents the area of overlap.

When the overall distribution is clearly bimodal (Fig. 16.5), separation of the two populations is somewhat easier. There are some test values that *rule out* or *rule in* the disease. In Fig. 16.5, values below A would lie only within the distribution of the disease-free population, thus ruling out the disease. Conversely, a value above B would lie only within the distribution of the diseased population. The problem remains, however, of how to classify subjects with test values between A and B. Some misclassification is inevitable regardless of what "cutoff" point is used, and the choice will depend largely on the purposes to which the result will be put, as well as on the relative consequences and costs of the two types of misclassification. We will return to this point in Section 16.6.

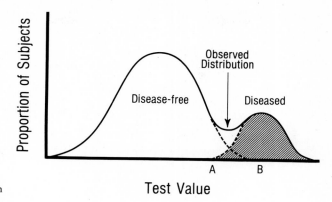

Fig. 16.5. Bimodal distribution

16.3 The Reproducibility and Validity of Diagnostic Tests

As discussed in Chapter 2, the major statistical attributes of any measurement, including the results of diagnostic tests, are reproducibility and validity. The *reproducibility* of a test is its ability to yield the same result on retesting. In general, diagnostic tests that are not reasonably reproducible will have little utility.

The *validity* of a test indicates how close the test result corresponds to some objective diagnostic standard of the disease. Unfortunately, some diseases do not have a readily available "gold standard" by which to assess a test's validity. It is difficult to assess a diagnostic test for pancreatitis, for example, without performing a microscopic examination of a biopsy specimen of the pancreas, and few surgeons are eager to perform a biopsy procedure in patients with suspected pancreatitis. In these types of conditions, the test may have to be validated by its ability to predict prognosis or response to therapy.

When a feasible gold standard does exist, validity can be assessed by comparing the test results with that standard [4]. Validity is usually evaluated *conditionally,* i.e., separately in those subjects with and those without the disease. The proportion of correctly identified diseased persons is called the *sensitivity,* and the proportion of correctly identified disease-free persons is called the *specificity.*

16.3.1 Sensitivity and Specificity

The statistical indices of sensitivity and specificity can be derived from a standard 2×2 table, as illustrated in Table 16.1. Disease presence or absence forms the column headings and test positivity ("abnormal") or negativity ("normal") comprises the rows. *a* is the number of subjects with the disease and a positive test, the so-called *true positives* (TP). Similarly, *b* is the number of *false positives* (FP), *c* the *false negatives* (FN), and *d* the *true negatives* (TN).

Table 16.1. Two-by-two table for evaluating the validity of diagnostic tests

		Disease		
		Present	Absent	
Test	+	a	b	$a+b$
	−	c	d	$c+d$
		$a+c$	$b+d$	N

a, true positives (TP); b, false positives (FP); c, false negatives (FN); d, true negatives (TN).

Sensitivity is defined as the proportion (or percentage)[1] of diseased subjects who have a positive test:

$$\text{sensitivity} = \frac{TP}{TP+FN} = \frac{a}{a+c} \tag{16.1}$$

Specificity is the proportion of disease-free subjects who have a negative test:

$$\text{specificity} = \frac{TN}{TN+FP} = \frac{d}{d+b} \tag{16.2}$$

The perfectly valid diagnostic test would have a sensitivity and specificity both equal to 1. Few if any tests attain these lofty heights, however, and most involve a trade-off between sensitivity and specificity. Usually, the more sensitive a test is (fewer false negatives), the less specific (more false positives) and vice versa. In fact, depending on the setting and purpose of the test (see Section 16.6), the cutoff point for defining positivity or negativity can be changed to increase one or the other of these indexes. These trade-offs will be addressed in greater detail in the following subsection.

16.3.2 The Receiver Operating Characteristics (ROC) Curve

As discussed in Section 16.2, many test results are measured on a continuous scale. The values are then often dichotomized into a normal (negative) or abnormal (positive) result. I have already mentioned the vagaries involved in choosing a cutoff point for defining normal and abnormal. Any single cutoff is by necessity arbitrary,

---

[1] These statistical indexes can be expressed as either proportions or percentages. Equations 16.1 and 16.2 yield proportions; the corresponding percentages are obtained by multiplying by 100.

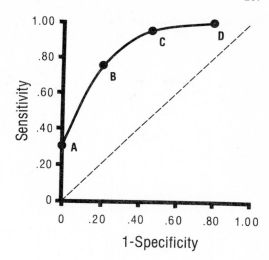

Fig. 16.6. The receiver operating characteristics (ROC) curve

with the consequence that subjects whose test results lie just below or above the cutoff may be misclassified.

In tests for which higher values reflect greater degrees of abnormality, choosing a lower cutoff will result in greater sensitivity, i.e., in missing fewer cases of the disease. Conversely, higher values of the cutoff will result in greater specificity, i.e., less misclassification of people who do not have the disease. This reciprocal relationship between sensitivity and specificity is *always* found when a cutoff point is chosen for the value of a test measured on a continuous scale and can be represented by the test's *receiver operating characteristics curve,* an example of which is shown in Fig. 16.6. Sensitivity is graphed on the *y*-axis and 1 − specificity on the *x*-axis. The greater the sensitivity, the lower the specificity and vice versa.

The term "receiver operating characteristics (ROC) curve" originated in describing performance characteristics of observers using mechanical devices, especially radar detection instruments. Different points on the ROC curve represent different choices of cutoff points, each balanced between maximizing sensitivity and specificity. Point A in Fig. 16.6 represents a point on the curve that results in a specificity of 1 but only .30 sensitivity. At the other extreme, point D represents a point on the curve where sensitivity is 1 but specificity is only .20. Points B and C are intermediate.

It is important to point out that the choice of which of these cutoff points is most appropriate for a diagnostic test may be governed by the purpose for which the test is obtained (see Section 16.6). If sensitivity is important, a point on the curve near C or D is appropriate. When specificity is more important, point A or B would be preferable. It is thus the curve itself, rather than a specific point on the curve, that is characteristic of the test. In other words, the choice of one specific point on this curve does not make the test better or worse. A better test (i.e., one with better overall sensitivity *and* specificity) would have an ROC curve that lies above and to the left of the curve shown in the graph.

In fact, the position of the curve with respect to the diagonal (shown by the dashed line in Fig. 16.6) is an indicator of its informational value. The diagonal rep-

Table 16.2. Die-casting as a "diagnostic test"

		Disease		
		Present	Absent	
	6	10	100	110
Die roll				
	1–5	50	500	550
		60	600	660

$$\text{Sensitivity} = \frac{10}{60} = 0.17$$
$$\text{Specificity} = \frac{500}{600} = 0.83$$
$$\text{Sensitivity} + \text{specificity} = 0.17 + 0.83 = 1$$

resents the line for which sensitivity $= 1 -$ specificity. Rearranging terms, sensitivity $+$ specificity $= 1$. A test for which sensitivity and specificity sum to 1 contributes no more information than pure chance. If our "diagnostic test" consisted of flipping a coin, with heads corresponding to a "positive" (abnormal) test and tails to a "negative" (normal) test, we would expect the test to label half the subjects as diseased and half as disease-free, regardless of whether they do or do not actually have the disease. Thus, the sensitivity and specificity of our "test" would both be 0.5.

Alternatively, if our "test" consisted of casting a die and calling a 6 "positive" and anything below 6 "negative," one out of six subjects would be labeled as diseased and five out of six as disease-free, regardless of their true status. The results of testing 60 diseased and 600 disease-free subjects are shown in Table 16.2. Sensitivity is 0.17, specificity is 0.83, and the total is 1.

The closer a test's ROC curve lies to the diagonal, the less information it provides. The further above and to the left of the diagonal, the more informative it is. (A test whose ROC curve lies below and to the right of the diagonal yields results that are *worse* than those due to chance. In that case, the criteria for "positive" and "negative" should be reversed!)

16.3.3 Spectrum and Bias

The sensitivity and specificity of a diagnostic test are often regarded as "fixed" characteristics of the test. Such is not the case, however. Many tests that appear highly sensitive and specific when first described eventually prove considerably less so after their introduction into the "real world" of clinical practice. Why does such disillusionment occur? The main source of the problem is the design of the studies in which the tests are originally evaluated.

As described in an excellent article by Ransohoff and Feinstein [5], the defects in design of these studies concern *spectrum* and *bias.* Spectrum means: Is the range of patients or subjects tested adequate? A broad spectrum of cases, or persons with the disease, is required to assess adequately the *sensitivity* of a test, while a broad spectrum of controls, or persons without the disease, is necessary for the adequate assessment of its *specificity.* Bias means: Are the diagnosis and test result determined independently of one another? Bias can affect both sensitivity and specificity.

Spectrum includes a number of components. First, we must consider the spectrum of cases studied. An inadequate case spectrum may result in a misleading sensitivity. Here we should examine the *pathologic* spectrum of the disease under study, in other words, its extent, location, and histology. A test for cancer should thus include both patients with local and patients with metastatic disease. The *clinical* spectrum of a disease, that is, its chronicity and severity, are also of obvious importance. If a test is more related to cachexia than to cancer, it may look more sensitive than it really is if only severely cachectic cancer patients are studied. The *co-morbid* spectrum of a disease, that is, the presence of coexisting ailments, can also affect a test's sensitivity. Test results may be different in cancer patients with and without cardiovascular disease, for example.

The spectrum of the controls studied can have profound effects on the specificity of a diagnostic test. An adequate control spectrum should include patients with the same disease process as the cases, but in a different location (for example, patients with breast cancer in a test for colon cancer) and should also include patients with different disease processes in the same location (such as patients with ulcerative colitis in a test for colon cancer). The latter is particularly important, because it is precisely in those patients with similar symptoms (e.g., diarrhea, bloody stools, abdominal pain, and weight loss in the case of colon cancer) that the clinician will want to use the test in practice.

The importance of spectrum in both cases and controls underlines an important principle. The purpose of a diagnostic test, at least in the clinical setting, is to detect a disease that is not otherwise obvious in patients with compatible symptoms. No competent clinician requires a test to distinguish a person with advanced cancer from one who is perfectly healthy. Yet many tests are originally evaluated in a study sample containing just such extreme "cases" and "controls." In attempting to convince their audience of the diseased and disease-free status of their cases and controls, respectively, the original authors may obtain results for both sensitivity and specificity far higher than those to be seen when the test is applied in the real clinical world of patients with less obvious symptoms and early disease.

The second type of design defect in testing a test is bias. Bias can lead to falsely high sensitivity or specificity; it can manifest itself in four ways. In *workup bias,* the result of a test affects the intensity of the subsequent "workup" (i.e., further diagnostic procedures) of the patient, thus increasing the chances for diagnosing the disease. *Nonblind diagnosis* means that the persons making the diagnosis are aware of the test result at the time of diagnosis. This is a potent source of bias when the diagnosis involves a subjective judgment. *Nonblind test interpretation* means that the persons interpreting the test results are aware of the true diagnosis at the time of test interpretation, which is a problem whenever a test is interpreted subjectively. Finally, in *incorporation bias,* the test results are actually incorporated as part of the evidence used to make the diagnosis, i.e., the inferential reasoning is circular.

Ransohoff and Feinstein [5] have shown how problems of spectrum and bias can lead to unjustified enthusiasm for diagnostic tests by examining two prominent examples from the recent past: the CEA test for colonic cancer and the NBT test for bacterial infection. After an optimistic introduction into the medical community, both these tests proved to be disappointing for their originally intended uses. The CEA (carcinoembryonic antigen) test is a blood test that determines (immunologically) the presence or absence of a substance that is normally present only in fetal life. When a cancer of the colon develops, however, the gene for synthesis of this protein is "turned on," and the antigen once again becomes detectable in the blood. When this test was first discovered, it was hoped that it would be a useful marker for the early diagnosis of colonic cancer, thereby enabling early institution of treatment and, hopefully, ultimate cure.

For the CEA test, an adequate spectrum of cases should include patients with both localized and extensive disease. As it turned out, those studies including patients with localized disease reported lower sensitivity than those restricted to patients with extensive and metastatic disease. An adequate spectrum of controls should include patients with other cancers and patients with nonmalignant colonic diseases. Studies including such patients reported low specificity for the CEA test. Since both the CEA test results and the diagnosis of colonic cancer are made fairly objectively, bias did not appear to be a major cause of the decline and fall of this test.

The NBT (nitroblue tetrazolium) test for bacterial infection examines the ability of leukocytes (white blood cells) to reduce the NBT dye to a bluish-black color that is visible on a microscope slide containing these cells. When leukocytes are stimulated during a bacterial infection, the metabolic machinery responsible for dye reduction is "turned on," thus yielding a markedly increased percentage of NBT-positive leukocytes.

For this test, the pathologic spectrum of cases should include patients with infections in different sites, with different bacteria, and with and without bacteremia (bacteria in the blood), while the clinical spectrum should include patients with infections covering a range of severity, and those with and without fever. In most of the studies of the NBT test, the pathologic features were well specified and adequate, but those including a wide clinical spectrum reported lower sensitivity than those studying only febrile patients with severe infections. The control spectrum for the NBT test should include patients with viral and fungal infections and those with other sources of fever, and such a spectrum was investigated in almost all the reported studies. Bias seemed to be a major problem with the studies of NBT. Since the test is interpreted subjectively, it is "at risk" for bias due to nonblinding. Predictably, those studies employing blind test interpretation reported lower sensitivity and specificity of the NBT test.

16.4 The Predictive Value of Diagnostic Tests

As we have seen, the statistical indexes of sensitivity and specificity are extremely useful in assessing the validity and informational value of a diagnostic test. For the clinician, however, these indexes have a major drawback, because the reasoning upon which they are based is the reverse of usual diagnostic reasoning. Sensitivity and specificity start from subjects with and without the disease and determine how often the test is either positive or negative respectively. Unfortunately, a clinician's patients do not usually come to her already bearing labels indicating "diseased" or "disease-free."

Instead, the clinician begins with patients whose disease status is unknown and whose test results must be used to decide whether the disease is present or absent. Clinicians are interested, therefore, in the *predictive value* of a diagnostic test. *Positive predictive value* is defined as the proportion of subjects with a positive test who have the disease. Using the symbols shown in Table 16.1,

$$\text{positive predictive value} = \frac{\text{TP}}{\text{TP} + \text{FP}} = \frac{a}{a+b} \qquad (16.3)$$

Negative predictive value is the proportion of subjects with a negative test who are disease free:

$$\text{negative predictive value} = \frac{\text{TN}}{\text{TN} + \text{FN}} = \frac{d}{d+c} \qquad (16.4)$$

Positive and negative predictive value can thus be considered "horizontal" indexes, since they are defined by row proportions, whereas the "vertical" indexes of sensitivity and specificity are defined by column proportions.

Unlike sensitivity and specificity, positive and negative predictive value are not true indexes of validity, because they depend on the relative proportions of diseased and disease-free persons being tested. Since they are governed by the ratio of true and false positives (positive predictive value) or true and false negatives (negative predictive value), a test with high specificity (few false positives among the disease-free) can have low positive predictive value if the ratio of disease-free to diseased subjects is high. Similarly, a test with high sensitivity (few false negatives among the diseased) can have low negative predictive value if the ratio of disease-free to diseased subjects is low (a very unlikely testing situation).

These relationships are illustrated in Table 16.3. In A, diseased (D) and disease-free ($\overline{D}$) subjects are equally represented, i.e., $D:\overline{D} = 1:1$. Sensitivity, specificity, positive predictive value, and negative predictive value are all high. In B, disease-free subjects predominate ($D:\overline{D} = 1:9$). Sensitivity and specificity remain the same (since they are characteristics of the test in diseased and disease-free persons respectively), but positive predictive value falls, while negative predictive value rises. In fact, in the common clinical situation in which the disease being tested for is rare, $D:\overline{D}$ may be lower than $1:9$, even among patients for whom the clinician is suspicious enough to request the test, with a consequent further reduction in the positive predictive value.

Table 16.3. Sensitivity, specificity, and positive and negative predictive values with three different ratios of diseased (D) and disease-free ($\overline{D}$) subjects

A. D:$\overline{D}$=1:1

Disease

	D	$\overline{D}$	
+	450	100	550
−	50	400	450
	500	500	1000

(Test)

Sensitivity $= \dfrac{450}{500} = 0.90$

Specificity $= \dfrac{400}{500} = 0.80$

Positive predictive value $= \dfrac{450}{550} = 0.82$

Negative predictive value $= \dfrac{400}{450} = 0.89$

B. D:$\overline{D}$=1:9

Disease

	D	$\overline{D}$	
+	90	180	270
−	10	720	730
	100	900	1000

(Test)

Sensitivity $= \dfrac{90}{100} = 0.90$

Specificity $= \dfrac{720}{900} = 0.80$

Positive predictive value $= \dfrac{90}{270} = 0.33$

Negative predictive value $= \dfrac{720}{730} = 0.99$

C. D:$\overline{D}$=9:1

Disease

	D	$\overline{D}$	
+	810	20	830
−	90	80	170
	900	100	1000

(Test)

Sensitivity $= \dfrac{810}{900} = 0.90$

Specificity $= \dfrac{80}{100} = 0.80$

Positive predictive value $= \dfrac{810}{830} = 0.98$

Negative predictive value $= \dfrac{80}{170} = 0.47$

Finally, just to demonstrate the mathematical relationship, C illustrates the rarely encountered situation in which diseased subjects predominate ($D : \overline{D} = 9 : 1$). Positive predictive value becomes very high, while negative predictive value falls.

Many tests are originally evaluated using approximately equal numbers of patients with the disease and disease-free controls, i.e., a disease prevalence of 50% in the evaluation sample. (Even a flip of a coin will have a positive predictive value of 50% in such a sample.) Since most tests intended for clinical diagnosis will be subsequently applied in settings where the disease prevalence is far lower, clinicians are bound to be disappointed by their low positive predictive value. To avoid such disappointment, the test should be evaluated in a setting similar to the one in which it will be applied.

16.5 Bayes' Theorem

The Reverend Thomas Bayes was an eighteenth-century mathematician interested in *conditional probability,* the probability that an event would occur under a given condition. Although neither diagnostic tests nor other aspects of clinical epidemiology were known at the time, *Bayes' theorem* of conditional probabilities has proved useful in these and other domains. In fact, it is the basis of the branch of statistics known as *Bayesian statistics,* which was discussed briefly in Chapter 12.

Before discussing the relevance of Bayes' theorem for diagnostic tests [6], we must explain the notation used to express a conditional probability. Our main interest from the clinical standpoint is the positive predictive value of a diagnostic test. In the language of conditional probability, the positive predictive value of a test is the probability of the disease (D) *given* (i.e., conditional on) a positive test result (T^+). In Bayesian notation, this is written as $P(D|T^+)$, where the vertical line between D and T^+ is read as "given" or "conditional on."

Bayes' theorem applied to diagnostic tests is then expressed as follows:

$$P(D|T^+) = \frac{P(T^+|D) \cdot P(D)}{P(T^+)} \tag{16.5}$$

In other words, Bayes' theorem says that the probability of disease, given a positive test, is the product of the probability of a positive test result given disease, times the probability of disease, divided by the probability of a positive test. That Eq. 16.5 expresses an algebraic truism can be easily seen by converting these probabilities into the familiar symbols of Table 16.1. Thus, $P(D|T^+) = \dfrac{a}{a+b}$, $P(T^+|D) = \dfrac{a}{a+c}$, $P(D) = \dfrac{a+c}{N}$, and $P(T^+) = \dfrac{a+b}{N}$. Hence:

$$\frac{a}{a+b} = \frac{\dfrac{a}{a+c} \cdot \dfrac{a+c}{N}}{\dfrac{a+b}{N}} = \frac{\dfrac{a}{N}}{\dfrac{a+b}{N}} = \frac{a}{a+b}$$

Each of the four components of Eq. 16.5 can be made easily recognizable. As we have already seen, $P(D|T^+)$ is the positive predictive value of the test. Bayesians often refer to it as the *posterior* (or *post-test*) *probability* of disease, because it is known only after (a posteriori) the test result is known. $P(T^+|D)$ is also familiar to us already as sensitivity. Sensitivity is the proportion of diseased subjects with a positive test, which is exactly the same thing as the probability of a positive test given disease.

The third component, $P(D)$, is also called the *prior* (or *pre-test*) *probability* of disease, because it is the probability that the test subject has the disease before (a priori) the test result is known. We use everything we know about the subject prior to the test to arrive at this probability. If we know nothing about the subject other than the population group from which he or she comes, $P(D)$ is the same as the *prevalence* of the disease in that population.

The fourth and last component in Eq. 16.5 is $P(T^+)$, which can be made more easily recognizable by expressing it as the sum of two conditional probabilities. Since any subject must either be diseased (D) or disease-free ($\overline{D}$), the law of total probability states that $P(T^+) = P(T^+|D) \cdot P(D) + P(T^+|\overline{D}) \cdot P(\overline{D})$. As we have seen, $P(T^+|D)$, the probability of a positive test in diseased subjects (i.e., given disease) is already known to us as the sensitivity of the test. $P(T^+|\overline{D})$, the probability of a positive test among the disease-free, is just $1 -$ specificity, since specificity $= P(T^-|\overline{D})$. Thus, Bayes' theorem can be written alternatively as follows:

positive predictive value ($=$ posterior probability of D) $=$

$$\frac{\text{(sensitivity)(prior probability of D)}}{\text{(sensitivity)(prior probability of D)} + (1 - \text{specificity})(\text{prior probability of }\overline{D})} \quad (16.6)$$

where the prior probability of $\overline{D} = 1 -$ prior probability of D. In other words, the positive predictive value of a test depends on its sensitivity and specificity and on the prior probability of the disease (the prevalence of disease among those tested). For a given sensitivity and specificity, positive predictive value will fall as the proportion of diseased subjects falls. This is exactly what we found empirically in Table 16.3.

Bayes' theorem can also be used to calculate the probability that a subject will be disease-free if he has a positive test result:

$$P(\overline{D}|T^+) = \frac{P(T^+|\overline{D}) \cdot P(\overline{D})}{P(T^+)} \quad (16.7)$$

Although $P(\overline{D}|T^+)$ may be of some interest to clinicians in its own right, the reason for introducing Eq. 16.7 here is that it allows the probabilities in which Eq. 16.5 is written to be expressed in terms of odds. An odds, you will recall from Chapter 8, is merely the ratio of a probability to its complement. If we divide Eq. 16.5 by Eq. 16.7, we obtain the following:

$$\frac{P(D|T^+)}{P(\overline{D}|T^+)} = \frac{P(T^+|D)}{P(T^+|\overline{D})} \cdot \frac{P(D)}{P(\overline{D})} \quad (16.8)$$

since the two $P(T^+)$ terms cancel. In other words, Eq. 16.8 says that the *odds* of disease given a positive test (also called the *posterior odds*) is the product of the odds of a positive test under the competing alternatives of disease and nondisease (the so-called *likelihood ratio*) multiplied by the relative proportion of diseased and disease-free subjects tested (the *prior odds*). The Bayesian "translation" of Eq. 16.8 is:

posterior odds = likelihood ratio × prior odds

It can be seen that the likelihood ratio is nothing more than the ratio of sensitivity to $1 -$ specificity.

To illustrate the use of Eq. 16.8, let us work through the calculation of positive predictive accuracy for the test results shown in Table 16.3 B. The sensitivity of the test is 0.90, the specificity is 0.80, and the prior odds of disease is $\frac{100}{900}$. Thus:

$$\text{posterior odds of disease} = \frac{0.90}{(1-0.80)} \cdot \frac{100}{900} = 0.50$$

To convert an odds to a probability, we merely use the formula:

$$\text{probability} = \frac{\text{odds}}{\text{odds}+1}$$

(4:1 odds *against* a horse is the same as a 1/5 probability that the horse will win). Hence:

$$\text{positive predictive value} = \text{posterior probability of disease} = \frac{0.50}{0.50+1} = 0.33,$$

which is the same result we obtained from the 2×2 table.

Formulating Bayes' theorem in terms of odds (Eq. 16.8) provides an instant index of the informational value of a positive test result, since of the two terms on the right side of the equation, the test contributes only to the first (the likelihood ratio). If the test adds no information (likelihood ratio = 1), the posterior odds and the prior odds are the same. In other words, the test result does not change the probability that the subject has the disease. If the likelihood ratio = 1, then sensitivity = $1 -$ specificity, and sensitivity + specificity = 1. This is exactly the same situation as that represented by the diagonal line in the ROC curve (Fig. 16.6). As we saw in Section 16.3.2, a test whose sensitivity and specificity sum to 1 provides no information.

The overall usefulness of a diagnostic test depends on both its informational content and the prior odds of disease. The informational content is determined by the likelihood ratio (LR). Although we have focused on the LR associated with a positive test result (LR$^+$), Eq. 16.8 could be recast using a negative test result. Then:

$$\text{LR}^- = \frac{P(\text{T}^-|\text{D})}{P(\text{T}^-|\overline{\text{D}})} = \frac{1\text{-sensitivity}}{\text{specificity}}$$

The lower (i.e., the closer to 0) the LR$^-$, the greater the informational value of a negative test. The total information content of a diagnostic test can therefore be defined by either its LR$^+$ or its LR$^-$.

When combined with the prior odds, LR^+ and LR^- provide an instant index to the impact of a positive or negative test result. If the prior odds is low (e.g., testing an asymptomatic, healthy "volunteer") and the test is highly discriminatory (high LR^+ and low LR^-), a positive test result will yield a large increase in the posterior odds (relative to the prior odds), but a negative test result will succeed only in making a remote possibility even more remote. Conversely, if the prior odds is very high (e.g., a patient with "classic" signs and symptoms), a positive test will result in very little change in the posterior odds, although a negative test will substantially reduce it.

The overall clinical utility of a test is therefore greatest when the prior odds is near 1, i.e., when the clinician is most uncertain (a virtual "toss-up" between disease presence or absence) prior to the test. A positive test then makes the disease likely, and a negative test makes it unlikely. This is consistent with common sense: the less certain we are, the more we are swayed by new information.

Another advantage of the Bayesian approach to the interpretation of diagnostic tests is that it is not necessarily tied to the dichotomous ("positive" vs "negative," "abnormal vs normal") characterization of the results (see Section 16.2). For diagnostic tests whose results are expressed on a continuous scale, no cutoff point is necessarily required. Instead, the actual result can be evaluated in terms of its differential diagnostic value, i.e., its consistency with disease vs nondisease. The likelihood merely needs to be expressed as the probability of obtaining the observed test result T_i under the competing hypotheses of disease and nondisease:

$$LR = \frac{P(T_i|D)}{P(T_i|\overline{D})}$$

with the probabilities estimated from the underlying distribution of values for the diseased and disease-free populations.

In addition to its use in evaluating diagnostic tests, Bayes' theorem has applications to other aspects of clinical decision-making and to causality inference. These will be considered in Chapters 17 and 19 respectively.

16.6 The Uses of Diagnostic Tests

As outlined by Sackett and Holland [7], diagnostic tests can be used for clinical diagnosis, case-finding, screening, or epidemiologic study. Each of these different settings has its own characteristics and requirements, and the criteria used for evaluating a test will depend not only on the setting but also on the nature of the disease and its treatment.

The main use of diagnostic tests in clinical practice is in *clinical diagnosis,* i.e., to identify the disease responsible for causing a specific complaint. A patient with a persistent cough, for example, may consult a physician. In addition to taking a careful medical history and performing a physical examination, the physician may obtain a chest roentgenogram. It is this use of diagnostic tests that has been the focus of our discussion thus far.

Case-finding is the testing of patients for diseases unrelated to their specific complaint. A woman who consults her physician because of pain and stiffness in her knees may have her blood pressure taken, not because the physician suspects hypertension as the cause of her symptoms, but because hypertension that is undetected and untreated carries a significant risk of subsequent morbidity and mortality.

The major purpose of case-finding is early (presymptomatic) detection. Obviously, the disease tested for should have a treatment that does more good than harm to those who are afflicted by it; there is no advantage to early detection of an untreatable disease. A treatment that improves survival, reduces morbidity, or improves physical or social functioning (performance) should therefore exist *before* case-finding is undertaken. Merely advancing the time of diagnosis without delaying death, morbidity, or functional impairment (the so-called *zero-time shift* or *lead-time bias*) does not constitute an improvement in outcome. In fact, early detection by itself may do more harm than good if it results in adverse psychological effects due to "labeling."

The zero-time shift is illustrated in Fig. 16.7. The top diagram represents the natural history of a disease without effective treatment. The time axis runs from left to right, and the usual sequence is seen of onset of disease, followed by onset of symptoms. The symptoms lead to a visit to a clinician who then establishes the diagnosis. Death or morbidity occurs at some later time. The lower diagram shows what happens when a test leads only to early detection. Note that onset of disease, onset of symptoms, and death or morbidity occur at exactly the same points along the time axis. The sole change has been an earlier time of diagnosis. If survival time (or morbidity-free time) is measured from the time of diagnosis, the patient whose disease was detected early will *appear* to go longer before experiencing death or morbidity. We must be on the lookout for this artifact of early detection; such a change does not qualify as a beneficial change in outcome.

Screening is the testing of asymptomatic subjects from the general population for the purpose of early detection of a particular disease. Although it is similar to case-finding in its aim to detect disease in asymptomatic subjects, it is different in several important respects. In case-finding, the patient seeks health care, and the clinician's

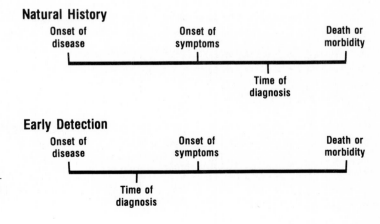

Fig. 16.7. The zero-time shift (lead-time bias)

main responsibility relates to the symptom or other problem that prompted the patient's visit. Early detection of an unrelated disease may be useful to the patient but is clearly secondary to the main "contract" [7].

In screening, on the other hand, early detection of asymptomatic disease is the main goal. False-negative test results are far less acceptable with screening, since failure to detect the disease screened for vitiates the principal objective. Consequently, the sensitivity of a screening test must be very high [8].

As with case-finding, screening requires the *prior* existence of a treatment with an overall favorable effect on mortality, morbidity, or performance. Early detection of an untreatable disease not only is of no benefit, but may even prolong the suffering caused by a patient's awareness of his diagnosis. Once again, the zero-time shift artifact should be considered in evaluating any screening test to ensure that outcome is truly improved.

One major difference from case-finding, however, is that even if a potentially beneficial treatment exists, true improvement in outcome requires referral of the diseased subject to an appropriate clinician, a decision by the clinician to prescribe the treatment, and adequate compliance by the patient. In case-finding, no referral is required, the clinician can decide a priori to treat patients in whom she detects the disease, and she may be selective in testing only those patients for whom her prior experience indicates a high probability of treatment compliance. Although the distinction between case-finding and screening can sometimes be blurred, e.g., in the case of the periodic health examination ("annual checkup"), their differences should be kept in mind.

Diagnostic tests can also be used to measure disease incidence or prevalence as part of an *epidemiologic study.* Whenever a given disease represents the study outcome, the results of a diagnostic test can be used to classify study subjects as diseased or disease-free. Descriptive surveys in representative samples of defined population groups can be used to provide incidence and prevalence rates for particular diseases. This may be important for public health purposes, such as in allocating resources, providing baseline data prior to some planned intervention, or supporting (or refuting) claims of a perceived epidemic in communities exposed to a suspected toxic agent. In analytic cohort studies and clinical trials, diagnostic tests can be used to standardize surveillance and provide an unbiased outcome assessment in different exposure groups. The main interest here is the *rate* of disease in the study groups rather than the presence or absence of disease in any individual. Thus, reproducibility, sensitivity, and specificity are less important than in other settings. If these indexes are too low, however, the resulting misclassification may lead to erroneous rates and inferences.

For all of the above test settings, the advantages and disadvantages of each test should be carefully weighed before deciding whether or not to perform the test. In addition to the probabilities of disease given the possible test results, which are determined by the prevalence of the disease and the test's sensitivity and specificity, the clinician or public health policy maker must also consider the *consequences* of correct and incorrect disease classification, the values that individual patients and society as a whole attach to these consequences, and the monetary costs involved. Issues such as the *acceptability* (risk of serious adverse consequences, pain, convenience, embarrassment) and *complexity* (logistic and mechanical difficulties, required expertise of personnel) of the test will weigh heavily in these evaluations [7, 8]. The technique for balancing the benefits and risks of available management options is called *decision analysis* and forms the basis of the following chapter.

References

1. Elveback LR, Guillier CL, Keating FR (1970) Health, normality, and the ghost of Gauss. JAMA 211: 69–75
2. Rang M (1972) The Ulysses syndrome. Can Med Assoc J 106: 122–123
3. Pethybridge RJ, Ashford JR, Fryer JG (1974) Some features of the distribution of birth weight of human infants. Br J Prev Soc Med 28: 10–18
4. Feinstein AR (1975) Clinical biostatistics. XXXI. On the sensitivity, specificity, and discrimination of diagnostic tests. Clin Pharmacol Ther 17: 104–116
5. Ransohoff DF, Feinstein AR (1978) Problems of spectrum and bias in evaluating the efficacy of diagnostic tests. N Engl J Med 199: 926–930
6. Sox HC (1986) Probability theory in use of diagnostic tests. Ann Intern Med 104: 60–66
7. Sackett DL, Holland WW (1975) Controversy in the detection of disease. Lancet 2: 170–172
8. Sackett DL (1975) Laboratory screening: a critique. Fed Proc 34: 2157–2161

Chapter 17: **Decision Analysis**

17.1 Strategies for Decision-Making

Mrs. Smith is a 75-year-old widow with mitral stenosis (narrowing of the left atrio-ventricular heart valve) complicated by left ventricular dysfunction (markedly reduced ejection fraction), which has been leading to progressive heart failure for the past 2 years. She is being treated by her cardiologist with standard medical therapy (digitalis and diuretics), but she is finding it increasingly difficult to climb the stairs to her apartment and often wakes up at night short of breath. A cardiovascular surgeon has seen Mrs. Smith in consultation. He believes that a successful commissurotomy (a surgical operation to widen the valvular opening) would relieve her symptoms and prolong her survival but is worried that her age and unstable cardiovascular status would substantially increase the risk of operative death. What should her physicians do, continue medical therapy or operate?

A variety of strategies could be used for making this decision. Several of the most common are discussed in the following subsections (D. A. Lane, 1983, The Foundations of Decision Analysis, unpublished manuscript).

17.1.1 Distilled "Clinical Judgment": Global Introspection

The decision strategy most commonly used by practitioners is based on global "clinical judgment," by which the knowledge base and previous experience of a seasoned clinician are somehow carefully weighed and considered to yield the proper course of action. The factors considered by Mrs. Smith's cardiologist and surgeon would probably include knowledge of her previous medical history, the extent of her current suffering, estimates of her probable survival with continued medical therapy, the expertise and experience of the surgeon, Mrs. Smith's chances of surviving the operation, and published studies in which the two treatments are compared. The physicians would discuss the case between them, perhaps consulting the views of other colleagues at a joint medical-surgical conference, and eventually reach a decision. The various considerations are mixed up together in the cauldron of the clinicians' brains, and the end product is a brew that hopefully represents the best decision for Mrs. Smith.

17.1.2 Avoid Disaster: The Conservative Approach

Another approach seeks to minimize the risk of the worst possible outcome. In statistical parlance, this strategy is called *minimax;* it chooses the decision with the minimum probability of the maximum loss. In Mrs. Smith's case, the decision would be to continue medical therapy. Although her condition is slowly deteriorating, her risk of dying in the next few weeks or months is low with her current treatment. Since she might not survive an operation, her risk of early death is much higher with surgery. Even if a successful operation prolongs her life, avoidance of early death mandates a decision for medical therapy.

17.1.3 "Go for Broke": The Gambling Approach

The opposite to the conservative (or minimax) decision strategy is the approach of the gambler: "go for broke." The gambler chooses the decision that maximizes the probability of the most favorable outcome. This approach is often frowned upon by clinicians, who are understandably reluctant to recommend risk-taking by their patients, even in the face of substantial potential gains. Nonetheless, Mrs. Smith, along with her cardiologist and surgeon, might decide that her expected course under medical therapy is so inexorably downhill that the potential gain in survival with surgery is worth the risk of operative death.

17.1.4 Is $P < 0.05$? The "Significance" Approach

A more "scientific" strategy would assemble evidence from the published literature, preferably from randomized clinical trials comparing surgical and medical therapy for mitral stenosis. If the evidence suggests that the outcome is different with one therapy vs another, and sampling variation can be safely ruled out as an explanation for the difference (i.e., $P < 0.05$), then this strategy would select the treatment associated with the better outcome. But what about Mrs. Smith's case? Does the published literature pertain to 75-year-old women with Mrs. Smith's poor left ventricular function and current symptoms? If (as is likely) medical treatment is significantly better for short-term survival, while surgery is better for long-term survival, which is better overall for Mrs. Smith? And how are her current suffering and impaired functioning to be weighed against the chances of either short- or long-term survival? Unfortunately, the significance strategy does not provide answers to these questions.

17.1.5 Decision Analysis: Maximize Expected Utility

Decision analysis (or *risk-benefit analysis*) is a systematic strategy by which the ramifications of each possible decision are compared for all relevant outcomes [1–4]. After estimating the *probability* of these outcomes for each decision and assigning a *utility* to each outcome, the decision is chosen that maximizes expected utility. For Mrs. Smith, decision analysis would consider not only the short-term risks of surgery, the probabilities of long-term survival, the persistence of relief of symptoms, and her ability to care for herself, but also the relative value (i.e., utility) that she and her physicians attach to these outcomes.

Of all the decision strategies considered thus far, decision analysis is the only one that guarantees logical consistency in balancing benefits and risks. Another way of saying this is that use of any other strategy will, on average, yield a lower utility. Global introspection may result in maximum utility, but since all relevant outcomes (along with their probabilities and utilities) are not necessarily considered, there is no guarantee that it will do so. The significance approach will maximize utility only if the difference in the outcome chosen as a basis for comparison outweighs the probabilities and utilities of all other outcomes. Avoiding disaster will often result in suboptimal average utility, because the utilities of outcomes other than the disastrous one are not considered. The gambling approach yields suboptimal results for the opposite reason; i.e., it does not take account of outcomes other than the favored one.

As we have seen, the basic building blocks of decision analysis consist of probabilities and utilities. Before these building blocks can be assembled, the decision analyst requires a "blueprint" indicating how and where they are to be used. This blueprint is called a *decision tree,* and its construction is the subject of the following section.

17.2 Constructing a Decision Tree

A decision tree is a visual representation of the logical and temporal consequences of each decision being considered. It reads from left to right, with smaller branches representing consequences of the larger branch from which they originate. The first (left-most) branch point represents the decision being analyzed. This point is called the *decision node* and is usually represented by a square. The number of choices available to the decision maker is the number of initial "branches" emanating from the decision node. In our example, Mrs. Smith's physicians have two choices: medical therapy or surgery, as shown schematically in Fig. 17.1.

The next step in constructing the tree is to list the possible consequences of each decision. These are shown as branches emanating to the right from a *chance node* along each main branch defined by the decision node. Chance nodes are designated as such because the events taking place beyond them (i.e., to the right of them in the tree) are determined by chance or are otherwise beyond the control of the decision-maker. Chance nodes are conventionally represented by a circle or point. Each immediate consequence may give rise to further consequences, and these are represented by chance nodes lying along the corresponding branches. Further branching is accomplished by adding subsequent chance nodes until the *terminal branches* represent the final clinical outcomes of interest.

The end result is a tree with smaller branches lying to the right of larger ones. The event represented by each branch is conditional upon the branch that precedes (i.e., gives rise to) it. Both the logical and temporal sequences proceed from left to

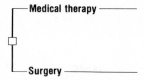

Fig. 17.1. The decision node: medical therapy vs surgery for Mrs. Smith

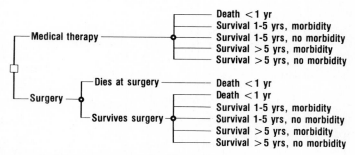

Fig. 17.2. Full decision tree: medical therapy vs surgery for Mrs. Smith

right, from the largest branches representing the decisions to the smallest terminal branches representing the final outcomes.

In our example, we shall simplify the decision tree by considering five final outcomes: death before 1 year, survival for 1–5 years with morbidity, survival for 1–5 years without (significant) morbidity, survival for more than 5 years with morbidity, and survival for more than 5 years without morbidity. Operative death will be included in the "death before 1 year" category. The full decision tree incorporating these outcomes is shown in Fig. 17.2.

Two of the branches shown in Fig. 17.2 are superfluous. Although we have not yet discussed how we estimate the probabilities associated with each branch of the tree, it is apparent that morbidity-free survival with medical therapy is virtually impossible (i.e., probability = 0), since Mrs. Smith has severe symptoms now with medical treatment. Consequently, the branches corresponding to morbidity-free survival for 1–5 years and > 5 years with medical therapy can be "pruned." The final decision tree obtained after pruning these branches is shown in Fig. 17.3.

The decision tree we have constructed has been simplified for heuristic purposes. Outcomes have been limited to five categories, and neither the morbid sequelae of surgery nor the side effects of medication have been considered. If the probabilities and utilities of other outcomes might affect the decision, including them would be important. The resulting tree would then be "bushier" (i.e., have more branches) and hence more comprehensive.

It is also important to point out that decisions may involve diagnostic, as well as therapeutic, choices, such as the decision to order a certain diagnostic test. Four outcomes arise from each decision mode involving a diagnostic test, corresponding to the true and false positives and true and false negatives discussed in Chapter 16.

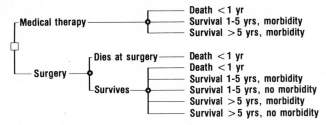

Fig. 17.3. Pruned decision tree: medical therapy vs surgery for Mrs. Smith

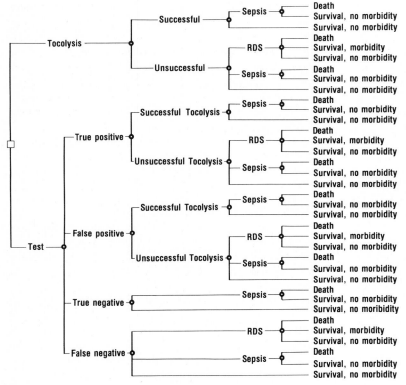

Fig. 17.4. Decision tree for L:S ratio test vs immediate tocolysis in women with spontaneous rupture of membranes and preterm labor

Consider the following example, the decision tree for which is shown in Fig. 17.4. Pregnant women who present with spontaneous rupture of fetal membranes (i.e., the amniotic sac) and premature labor represent a difficult dilemma for the obstetrician. If she lets nature take its course, many of these women will deliver a premature infant, with a high risk of respiratory distress syndrome (RDS), a condition caused by lung immaturity and associated with significant morbidity and mortality. If the obstetrician administers tocolytic (labor-inhibiting) drugs, she may succeed in delaying delivery until the lungs have matured and thus avoid RDS. But prolonged membrane rupture increases the risk of neonatal sepsis (systemic bacterial infection), which has an even higher mortality than RDS. (We will assume for simplicity that a neonate who survives a bout of sepsis will have no residual morbidity, and that the coincidence of RDS and sepsis is sufficiently unlikely to ignore.)

An alternative to immediate tocolysis is a diagnostic test of fetal lung maturity. The amniotic fluid is tested for the ratio of lecithin to sphingomyelin (called the L:S ratio). An L:S ratio $\leq 2:1$ (a positive test) indicates immature fetal lungs and a high risk of RDS. But, like other diagnostic tests, the L:S ratio is neither perfectly sensitive nor specific for RDS. In particular, many infants with a positive test will not develop RDS (i.e., the positive predictive value of the test is not high). If the test is positive (whether true positive or false positive), the obstetrician will institute tocolytic therapy, which may or may not be successful in delaying delivery until the lungs have matured. In the case of the false positives, successful tocolytic therapy will have unnecessarily increased the risk of sepsis. If the test is negative (true negative or false negative), the obstetrician will attempt to deliver the baby as soon as possible, using oxytocin augmentation if necessary, to minimize the risk of sepsis. In the case of false negatives, however, this will result in the birth of some infants with RDS.

The decision tree for this analysis is obviously more complicated than the one we constructed for our first example involving Mrs. Smith. Even the tree shown in Fig. 17.4 is an oversimplification, however, since it does not consider such issues as amniocentesis prior to tocolytic therapy, the use of betamethasone (a corticosteroid) to promote lung maturation, the differential morbidity and mortality of preterm and full-term infants, or the range of possible morbidities. In fact, many clinical decisions would look almost impossibly complex if displayed in their full arboreal splendor.

What this means, though, is that the decisions themselves are complex. The decision tree merely displays the complexities; it does not create them. Decisions can be (and usually are) made without decision trees. But all decisions weigh probabilities and utilities, although most do so only implicitly. Even if the tree is not used to carry out the full analysis, however, its construction can be helpful to the clinician by forcing her to consider all relevant consequences of her decision choices. Finally, many complex trees can be made more manageable by careful pruning of nonessential branches.

17.3 Probabilities and Utilities

Once the decision tree has been constructed, the next step in decision analysis is to estimate the probabilities of its branches and assign utilities to the possible final outcomes. These will be discussed in the following two subsections.

17.3.1 Probabilities

A variety of sources exist for estimating the probabilities of events occurring as consequences of the decisions being analyzed. Published clinical trials, observational studies, and descriptive case series can all be used, with priority given to data representing the best combination of methodologic rigor and clinical relevance to the case or cases being analyzed. In Mrs. Smith's case, for example, our preference would be for a randomized trial in which surgery and medical therapy were compared for short-term and long-term mortality, relief of symptoms, and functional performance, preferably in women around 75 years of age with similar past history, current symptomatology, and associated left ventricular dysfunction.

The chance of finding such a trial, of course, is slim. Instead, a variety of published literature must often be searched to provide the best probability estimates. In the absence of reliable published data, it may be necessary to solicit the opinion of an expert or panel of experts. Although such a process might appear dangerously similar to the global introspection approach discussed earlier, there are important differences. For one thing, the introspection is far less global. The expert is being asked for an opinion concerning a specific probability, not a recommendation for an overall decision. By breaking down a global task into a series of small ones, each becomes more manageable (i.e., the branch probability assessment is more reproducible and valid). Second, the expert is consulted only in the area of his or her expertise. No one person is being asked to know and properly weigh all the relevant facts.

Although such procedures for estimating probabilities may appear "sloppy" after the epidemiologic and statistical principles outlined earlier in this text, there is no readily available alternative. After all, some decision has to be made. Decision analysis provides a logical framework for weighing the available information, even if that information is fuzzy. To be sure, the better the probability estimates, the more reliance we can place on the results of the analysis. As we shall see later on, however, *ranges* of feasible probability estimates can be assessed to see if the preferred decision changes with different estimates.

Regardless of how the individual probability estimates are derived, their combination must conform to the rules of probability theory. Since the branches emanating from a given chance node represent mutually exclusive events, the probability of *either* of two such events occurring is the sum of their individual probabilities. If the two events are represented by A and B, then using the probability notation introduced in Chapter 16:

$$P(\text{A or B}) = P(\text{A}) + P(\text{B}) \tag{17.1}$$

Furthermore, since a chance node gives rise to a branch for each possible consequent event, and one of the events *must* occur, the sum of the probabilities of all the branches emanating from a chance node must sum to 1. If there are n such branches.

$$P(\text{A or B or C} \ldots \text{or } n) = P(\text{A}) + P(\text{B}) + P(\text{C}) \ldots + P(n) = 1 \tag{17.2}$$

Returning to our example, let us estimate the probabilities for the branches at each of the three chance nodes shown in the Fig. 17.3 decision tree. Let us say that, based

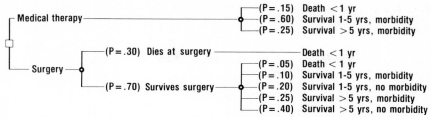

Fig. 17.5. Figure 17.3 decision tree containing branch probabilities

on our review of the literature and consultation with experts, the probabilities of death before 1 year, survival for 1–5 years (with morbidity), and survival for more than 5 years are 0.15, 0.60, and 0.25, respectively, for medical therapy. Note that these three probabilities sum to 1. For surgery, the first chance node concerns the probability of surviving surgery. The literature and expert opinion indicate that a 75-year-old woman in Mrs. Smith's current condition would have only a 70% (i.e., $P = 0.70$) chance of surviving a mitral valve commissurotomy. By the law of additivity (Eq. 17.2), the probability of operative death must be 0.30.

If she survives surgery, Mrs. Smith may experience any of the five possible outcomes. Let us say that our estimates of the probabilities of these outcomes, conditional on her surviving the operation, are 0.05 for death before 1 year, 0.10 for surviving 1–5 years with morbidity, 0.20 for surviving 1–5 years without morbidity, 0.25 for surviving more than 5 years with morbidity, and 0.40 for surviving more than 5 years without morbidity. Note once again that these probabilities sum to 1. The branch probabilities are often written into the decision tree just after the branch point (chance nodes), as shown in Fig. 17.5.

The second rule for combining probabilites concerns events that occur subsequent to, and possibly conditional upon, prior events. This rule will tell us how to calculate overall probabilities for the final outcomes representing the terminal branches of the decision tree. If B is an event that can occur in a person who has already experienced event A, then the probability that both A and B will occur is the product of the probability of A and the conditional probability of B (given A). In the notation of conditional probability,

$$P(\text{A and B}) = P(\text{A}) \times P(\text{B}|\text{A}) \tag{17.3}$$

The probability of each branch of the tree is conditional on the probabilities of the preceding larger branches, i. e., the branches lying to its left on the tree, all the way back to the first chance node. Thus, the number of probabilities multiplied together for each terminal branch is the same as the number of chance nodes occurring between the decision node and the terminal branch.

In our example, the terminal branches representing the possible final outcomes for surgery are conditional on surviving the operation. The overall probabilities associated with these terminal branches are calculated by multiplying the probability of surviving surgery ($P = 0.70$) by the conditional probability of each outcome. Thus, for death before 1 year the overall probability is $(0.70)(0.05) = 0.035$. The

Table 17.1. Overall probabilities of terminal branches in decision tree shown in Fig. 17.5

Terminal branch	Probability
Medical therapy	
Death <1 year	0.15
Survival 1–5 years, morbidity	0.60
Survival >5 years, morbidity	0.25
Surgery	
Dies at surgery (death <1 year)	0.30
Survives surgery	
Death <1 year	0.035
Survival 1–5 years, morbidity	0.070
Survival 1–5 years, no morbidity	0.140
Survival >5 years, morbidity	0.175
Survival >5 years, no morbidity	0.280

probabilities of each of the nine terminal branches of the decision tree in Fig. 17.5 are listed in Table 17.1. Note that, consistent with the additivity rule, the sum of the overall probabilities for the five terminal branches for operative survival is 0.70, the probability of operative survival itself.

17.3.2 Utilities

The other major constituents required for decision analysis are utilities. When only a single dichotomous outcome is involved, utility assessment is straightforward. One need only decide which of the two outcome categories is preferred, and the decision that yields the highest average probability of that outcome category is favored. In the case of Mrs. Smith, if 5-year survival (yes or no) were the single outcome of interest, we would need "only" find out whether medical therapy or surgery is associated with a higher 5-year survival rate in women like Mrs. Smith, and then act accordingly.

As we have seen, however, other outcomes *are* important. Mrs. Smith is already 75 years old and may care far more about 1-year survival than 5-year survival. Since she is a widow who lives alone, she is also likely to prefer a treatment that reduces her breathlessness and enables her to go out, walk up the stairs to her apartment, and care for herself without assistance. Decision analysis requires that all outcomes be rated on a single utility scale. How can this be achieved? In other words, how can we consider all these outcomes simultaneously, and how do we go about weighting their relative utilities?

The best way of answering these questions is to consult the persons who will be directly affected by the decision under analysis. Whereas clinicians, researchers, and other experts are required for estimating probabilities, patients and the "general public" are often best able to assign utilities to various outcomes. In the case of Mrs. Smith, the best decision for *her* will depend on the relative weight *she* places on 1-year survival, 5-year survival, symptoms, and functional independence. Similarly, if the decision is a public health intervention, it might be wise to poll a representative sample of the community in which the intervention will take place.

Assignment of utilities according to a single utility scale is usually facilitated by first ranking the outcomes in order of preference. Although any scale can be used, a frequent strategy is to "anchor" the utility scale by assigning a utility of zero ($u=0$) to the least desirable outcome and $u=1$ to the most desirable outcome. People usually have no trouble deciding the outcomes they find least and most desirable, so this "anchoring" is easily accomplished.

Assigning utility weights for intermediate outcomes is a bit trickier. Nonmathematically inclined persons may find it difficult to assign numerical values to the possible outcomes, and clinicians often feel awkward asking them to do so. Translating each outcome into a lottery provides an operational definition of utility: given the "anchoring" outcomes assigned utilities of 0 and 1, the utility of any intermediate outcome is equivalent to the probability of winning the most favored outcome (i.e., the one with $u=1$) over the least favored one ($u=0$) in a lottery in which the respondent would be indifferent between trying the lottery and being guaranteed the outcome of unknown utility. For example, if the patient is indifferent between a 0.7 chance of winning the lottery and a promise of the outcome of unknown utility, the latter outcome has a utility of 0.7.

In fact, if this "indifference point" accurately reflects the patient's values, the assignment of any utility other than 0.7 would lead to incoherence. If the utility scale were in dollars, and the patient were willing to pay any price other than 70 cents for the outcome in question, another party could make a "dutch book" against him (i.e., would be guaranteed to make money off him) if the lottery were repeated many times. The other party would choose the lottery (with a probability of 0.7 of winning a dollar) whenever the patient's price dropped below 70 cents and would choose the outcome in question whenever the price rose above 70 cents.

Returning to the decision tree for Mrs. Smith, her physicians would need to elicit her utilities for each of the five possible final outcomes: (1) death before 1 year; (2) survival for 1–5 years with continued morbidity (symptoms and functional impairment); (3) survival for 1–5 years without significant morbidity; (4) survival for >5 years with morbidity; and (5) survival for >5 years without morbidity. Mrs. Smith would have no trouble ranking (1) as the least desirable and (5) as the most desirable, so these would be assigned utilities of 0 and 1 respectively.

She might then be asked how many years with morbidity she would trade (i.e., be indifferent to exchanging) for 1 year without symptoms or functional impairment. Suppose she said two, indicating that morbidity-free survival was worth twice as much to her as survival with morbidity. Then outcome 2 should have a utility half that of outcome 3, and outcome 4 should have a utility half that of outcome 5.

The only problem remaining is asking her to indicate and quantitate her preference for outcome 3 vs outcome 4. Would she prefer 1–5 years without morbidity or >5 years with morbidity, and by how much? If we assume that the average length of survival in patients in outcome group 4 (>5 years) is double that in group 3 (1–5 years), then consistency dictates that their respective utilities should be equivalent.

So the entire utility scale problem is now solved. According to Mrs. Smith's preference, the five outcomes should have utilities of 0, 0.25, 0.50, 0.50, and 1 (see

Table 17.2. Assigned utilities (u_i's) of five possible final outcomes for Mrs. Smith

Outcome	u_i
1. Death <1 year	0
2. Survival 1–5 years, morbidity	0.25
3. Survival 1–5 years, no morbidity	0.50
4. Survival >5 years, morbidity	0.50
5. Survival >5 years, no morbidity	1

Table 17.2). The combination of morbidity and mortality into a single utility scale is analogous to a concept known as *quality-adjusted life years*. Instead of using a utility scale from 0 to 1, we might have "translated" each outcome into an equivalent number of quality-adjusted life years and used the latter itself as the scale. The advantage of the 0-to-1 u-scale, however, is the equivalence to the "indifference" lottery probabilities discussed earlier.

17.4 Completing the Analysis

17.4.1 Maximizing Expected Utility

To complete the decision analysis, we simply calculate the *expected utility* U_{E_k} for each of the k decision branches of the tree by multiplying the probability P_{i_k} of each terminal branch by its corresponding utility u_{i_k} and then summing over all terminal branches leading to that decision:

$$U_{E_k} = \Sigma(P_{i_k} \times u_{i_k}) \tag{17.4}$$

Table 17.3 shows the calculation of expected utilities for our example. For medical therapy, $U_{E_m} = 0 + 0.150 + 0.125 = 0.275$. For surgery, $U_{E_s} = 0 + 0 + 0.0175 + 0.070 + 0.0875 + 0.280 = 0.455$.

The final step is to choose the decision that maximizes average utility. Since 0.455 is higher than 0.275, surgery is chosen over medical therapy for Mrs. Smith.

17.4.2 Sensitivity and Threshold Analyses

The "correctness" of a decision based on maximizing expected utility depends on the probability and utility assessments used in the analysis. Both types of assessments are fraught with uncertainty. The subjective nature of utility assessments is readily apparent, but even probabilities often require either expert opinion or subjective adjustment of frequency data reported in epidemiologic studies that contain methodologic imperfections and whose pertinence to the particular type of patient under analysis may be questionable. Faced with such uncertainty, it is important to consider the impact that different probability or utility assessments could have on

Table 17.3. Expected utilities (U_{E_i}'s) for decision tree shown in Fig. 17.5

Terminal branch	$P_i \times u_i$
Medical therapy	
Death <1 year	$0.15 \times 0 = 0$
Survival 1–5 years, morbidity	$0.60 \times 0.25 = 0.150$
Survival >5 years, morbidity	$0.25 \times 0.50 = 0.125$
	$U_{E_m} = \Sigma(P_{i_m} \times u_{i_m}) = 0.275$
Surgery	
Dies at surgery	$0.30 \times 0 = 0$
Survives surgery	
Death <1 year	$0.035 \times 0 = 0$
Survival 1–5 years, morbidity	$0.070 \times 0.25 = 0.0175$
Survival 1–5 years, no morbidity	$0.140 \times 0.50 = 0.070$
Survival >5 years, morbidity	$0.175 \times 0.50 = 0.0875$
Survival >5 years, no morbidity	$0.280 \times 1 = 0.280$
	$U_{E_s} = \Sigma(P_{i_s} \times u_{i_s}) = 0.455$

the analysis, especially when the expected utility of the preferred decision is only slightly higher than the others. The process of varying the probabilities and utilities is called *sensitivity analysis.*

Sensitivity analysis assesses whether the decision choice would change with (i.e., is sensitive to) feasible changes in the component probabilities or utilities. It is somewhat analogous to using confidence intervals around means, proportions, or relative risks. We may be able to provide reasonable ranges for probabilities and utilities that incorporate our uncertainties, and we may be far more comfortable with the range than we are with any single point estimate. If the decision associated with the maximum expected utility remains unchanged, we can then be more confident that that decision is the correct one.

Returning to our example, if the probability of dying at surgery were 0.50 instead of 0.30, would surgery still be preferred over medical therapy? The expected utility for the surgical decision branch now becomes five sevenths (i.e., 0.50/0.70) of 0.455 (the value obtained with a probability estimate of surviving surgery of 0.70), or 0.325. Since 0.325 is still higher than 0.275, surgery would still be preferred over medical therapy for Mrs. Smith. In other words, the decision favoring surgery is not sensitive to an operative mortality of 50%. If operative mortality were as high as 70%, however, the average utility of surgery would be only (0.30/0.70) of 0.455 = 0.195, and medical therapy would be preferred.

We can also test the sensitivity of the decision to changes in utilities. In Mrs. Smith's case, we need only consider a reduction in the utility of morbidity-free survival (since any increase in that utility would further favor surgery) and an increase in the relative "disutility" of death in less than 1 year. If, for example, survival for at least 1 year were of paramount importance to Mrs. Smith, and subsequent survival with morbidity were only slightly less valuable to her than survival without symptoms, the utilities of the five outcomes listed in Table 17.2 might be 0, 0.60, 0.70, 0.90, and 1, instead of 0, 0.25, 0.50, 0.50, and 1. If the probabilities remained unchanged from those shown in Fig. 17.5, the expected utility for medical therapy would be $(0.15)(0) + (0.60)(0.60) + (0.25)(0.90) = 0.585$, and that for surgery $(0.30)(0) + (0.70)(0.05)(0) + (0.70)(0.10)(0.60) + (0.70)(0.20)(0.70) + (0.70)(0.25)(0.90) + (0.70)(0.40)(1) = 0.5775$. In other words, the two decisions would have approximately equal expected utilities, with medical therapy very slightly preferred.

Finally, probabilities and utilities can be varied simultaneously. Although changes in individual probability or utility assessments may not alter the final decision, the effect of combined changes in several utilities and probabilities can create a "worst-case" scenario that maximally stresses the sensitivity of the analysis. If the "worst-case" combination does not result in a change in decision, the analyst can be quite confident that the decision chosen is the correct one.

Usually, however, sensitivity analysis will indicate that the decision *would* change under different probability or utility assessments. This does not signal defeat for the analyst. Rather, it helps focus the attention of the decision-maker on the crucial factors upon which the decision hinges. If changes in one key probability estimate would lead to a different decision, for example, attempts should be made to obtain a more confident estimate (i.e., better information), perhaps by carrying out further research. If utility values are the key, more careful questioning of the patient or the target population may yield more valid utility assessments. Even when better assessments are not achievable, however, it is often helpful for the decision-maker to recognize the sources of uncertainty leading to the chosen decision.

Once it is apparent that some change can affect a decision, it is often useful to determine the *threshold* probability or utility at which two decisions will have equal expected utilities, i.e., the point at which the decision-maker would be indifferent between the two. This aspect of sensitivity testing is known as *threshold analysis* and is achieved by assigning an unknown value to the probability or utility in question, expressing the expected utility for each decision algebraically, setting the algebraic terms for the two decisions as equal, and solving for the unknown (threshold) value.

For our example, suppose we wanted to know the operative survival rate at which Mrs. Smith's physicians should be indifferent between surgery and medical therapy. We assume that all other probabilities and utilities remain unchanged. The expected utility for medical therapy would still be 0.275, of course. If we let x be the probability of surviving surgery, then the expected utility of surgery would be:

$$(1 - x)(0) + (x)(0.05)(0) + (x)(0.10)(0.25) + (x)(0.20)(0.50) + (x)(0.25)(0.50) + (x)(0.40)(1) = 0.65x$$

We then set the two expected utilities as equal:

$$0.65x = 0.275$$

Solving for x, $x = \dfrac{0.275}{0.65} = 0.423$

Thus, at a surgical survival rate of 42.3%, the two decisions result in equal expected utilities. This is useful information. It indicates that, assuming the other probabilities and utilities are valid, any surgical survival rate above 42.3% should favor surgery. If the surgeon is sure that Mrs. Smith's chance of surviving the operation is higher than this figure, he should operate; if it is lower, he should not.

17.5 Cost-Benefit Analysis

Comparing the average utility of two or more decisions is not the only type of analysis required by the decision-maker. Even if a decision analysis indicates which decision among two or more is to be preferred, it does not indicate the financial costs of carrying out the decision or whether the expected health benefits of the decision will be worth those costs.

Cost-benefit analysis is a method of computing the net costs or benefits of a given clinical decision or health practice [5–7]. These costs and benefits can be considered from the vantage point of the individual patient or of society at large (depending on who is paying and who is benefiting), although the societal perspective is far more frequent. Like decision analysis, it makes use of expected utilities. Since costs and benefits must be compared directly, however, it requires that all utilities, including years of life, morbidity, and functional performance, be valued *monetarily*. This may be fairly straightforward for such benefits as savings in hospitalization and other medical costs associated with a given favorable outcome, but how does one go about assigning monetary values to increased life span or freedom from pain or disability?

Putting price tags on human life, death, and suffering is exceedingly difficult at best. Many clinicians or patients may consider it distasteful or even unethical. Nonetheless, financial resources for health care are not unlimited and must be balanced against other needs of individuals and societies. Just because a given practice produces health benefits does not necessarily justify paying for it. No one would spend his or her life savings to get rid of a hangnail. Similarly, some cost threshold must exist above which the expected benefit of a decision or practice is not worth its price. Furthermore, even if the price of a certain benefit is reasonable, a society may not be able to afford all such benefits. Priority may have to be given to those with the highest ratio of benefits to costs.

Cost-benefit analysis can facilitate these types of decisions by making costs and benefits explicit [5–7]. *Health benefits* (the differences in expected utility achieved when the health service or practice is provided vs when it is not) are expressed in monetary terms. They include savings in medical care costs realized by the health service or practice under analysis. Prolonged survival and decreased morbidity are often valued by considering the anticipated corresponding increase in productivity, i.e., earning power. (Unfortunately, relief of pain, anxiety, and functional dependence then count for nothing unless productivity is affected.)

On the cost side of the "ledger" are included such items as equipment, personnel, and indirect costs (e.g., paying for rent, utilities, and other overhead at the site at which the practice or service will be carried out). Choices have to be made between using average costs or marginal costs (the costs of paying for one additional unit of the service) for these items, and expenditures must be adjusted for future inflation and discounted over the duration of the service to compensate for the lost future earning power of the money expended. Sensitivity analysis can be carried out to assess the extent to which the service becomes more or less cost beneficial with changes in the underlying assumptions about expected benefits, costs, and discount rates.

As an example, consider the example of annual mammography (breast roentgenography) screening for breast cancer. The anticipated benefits associated with early diagnosis and treatment of breast cancer include lower mortality and less need for subsequent hospitalization, surgery, radiation therapy, and chemotherapy. The lower mortality must be valued in monetary terms by estimating the average increase in earnings, plus the savings of costs that would have been incurred in paying someone else to carry out usual domestic tasks, associated with the number of women-years gained by screening. The costs are all the direct and indirect costs incurred by the population-wide screening program. If the monetary value of the total anticipated benefits exceeds the costs (after adjustment for inflation and the discount rate), the screening is declared to be cost-beneficial.

Cost-benefit analyses are best accomplished by collaboration among clinicians, economists, and medical or public health administrators. Politicians are often particularly interested in such analyses, because it is they who have to determine budgets and thus make choices about how much to spend on medical care in general and specific services in particular. The major problem with cost-benefit analysis, however, arises in considering the value of human life and physical and psychological suffering. The analyst must either give them a price tag or ignore them completely. Neither of these solutions is entirely satisfactory, either ethically or scientifically.

17.6 Cost-Effectiveness Analysis

Cost-effectiveness analysis is a hybrid between cost-benefit analysis and decision analysis [7–9]. As in cost-benefit analysis (with which it is often confused), utility is expressed in terms of expected health *benefit*, i.e., the difference in expected utility obtained when a service is provided and when it is not, and expected health benefits are balanced against expected costs. It is also similar to cost-benefit analysis in that costs and benefits are usually considered from a societal vantage point (although either technique can be based on the perspective of the individual patient if he or she will be paying the bill out of pocket). Like decision analysis, cost-effectiveness analysis compares two or more health services or policies. Also like decision analysis, but unlike cost-benefit analysis, health benefits are valued on a nonmonetary utility scale. The service or practice associated with the lowest monetary cost per unit of benefit achieved is judged to be most cost-effective.

As an example, consider the decision of a public health official in a developing country who wishes to reduce the infant mortality rate (IMR) in his country. He has only a limited budget and wants to know whether he would be better off providing caloric supplementation or tetanus immunization to pregnant women. His country cannot afford both, so he wants to provide the service with the greatest impact for a given monetary input. Caloric supplementation would increase intrauterine growth;

since infant mortality is inversely proportional to birth weight, the IMR would be correspondingly reduced. Tetanus immunization would not affect birth weight, but birth weight-specific IMR should be reduced by eliminating the neonatal tetanus that can occur after deliveries in unsanitary settings (often at home in developing countries).

To carry out the analysis, each service must be assessed in terms of the target benefit and the associated costs. It is often convenient to base the calculations on an arbitrary number of persons served. For a population of 10 000, the benefit of each service would be the number of infants who would die without the service but live with it. The cost of each service would be calculated as in cost-benefit analysis and would include personnel, equipment, and indirect costs and would take both inflation and the discount rate into account. The service associated with the lower cost per unit benefit is then declared more cost-effective. For our example, the public health official would choose between caloric supplementation and tetanus immunization by comparing the cost of saving one infant life with one service vs the other. Sensitivity analyses could then be carried out by varying estimates both of the costs and the reduced IMR achieved for each service and observing the effect on the overall result.

As with decision analysis, morbidity, pain, suffering, and functional impairment can be combined with mortality on a single health utility scale. The benefits can be expressed in terms of quality-adjusted life years, for example, with the target population polled to derive the formula for quantitative adjustment. The fact that such outcomes do not have to be valued in monetary terms makes cost-effectiveness analysis more palatable than cost-benefit analysis to many clinicians and lay persons. Since procedures for estimating costs are identical to those used in cost-benefit analysis, consultation with a health economist is often essential to arrive at valid estimates.

References

1. Weinstein MC, Fineberg HV (1980) Clinical decision analysis. Saunders, Philadelphia
2. Lindley DV (1985) Making decisions, 2nd edn. Wiley, London
3. Pauker SG, Kassirer JP (1987) Decision analysis. N Engl J Med 316: 250–258
4. Lane DA (1987) Utility, decision, and quality of life. J Chronic Dis 40: 585–591
5. Dunlop DW (1975) Benefit-cost analysis: a review of its applicability in policy analysis for delivering health services. Soc Sci Med 9: 133–139
6. Pliskin N, Taylor AK (1977) General principles: cost-benefit and decision analysis. In: Bunker JP, Barnes BA, Mosteller F (eds) Costs, risks, and benefits of surgery. Oxford University Press, New York, pp 5–27
7. Drummond MF, Stoddart GL, Torrance GW (1986) Methods for economic evaluation of health care programmes. Oxford University Press, Oxford
8. Weinstein MC, Stason WB (1977) Foundations of cost-effectiveness analysis of health and medical practices. N Engl J Med 296: 716–721
9. Shepard DS, Thompson MS (1979) First principles of cost-effectiveness analysis in health. Public Health Rep 94: 535–543

Chapter 18: **Life-Table (Survival) Analysis**

18.1 Introduction

In Chapter 6 we considered a variety of ways of analyzing the results of a cohort study. When the outcome variable is continuous and the exposure is dichotomous, the main comparison is the mean outcome in the two groups defined by exposure status. We later devoted nearly an entire chapter (Chapter 13) to inferential statistical techniques used in testing an observed difference in means.

When the exposure is dichotomous and the outcome variable is categorical, the main analysis is a comparison of rates in the two exposure groups. In the common situation of a dichotomous outcome, the ratio of the two rates becomes a relative risk, the statistical significance of which can be tested using a χ^2 or Fisher exact test or by constructing an appropriate confidence interval (see Chapter 14).

In this chapter, we shall once again focus on cohort studies with dichotomous outcomes. But the kind of cohort study we are considering here is a special, albeit quite common, type in which the duration of follow-up varies among individuals in the cohort. Rarity of "exposure" may require that enrollment of the study cohort be spread over a considerable period of time, such as in studying survival among patients with a rare disease or the risks and benefits of a complex or costly treatment. If the outcome requires many months or years to develop, study subjects will have been followed for varying lengths of time. The first subject enrolled will have the longest *potential* duration of follow-up (i.e., if he does not develop the outcome and does not withdraw from the study), and the most recently enrolled subject will have the shortest. Since the investigator must close the study at some date, she cannot know if the subjects who have not yet developed the outcome at study termination *would have* done so had they been followed up longer.

Life-table analysis (also called *survival analysis*) is a statistical technique that allows the investigator to calculate a probability of developing a given outcome that takes into account the duration of follow-up. It makes maximum use of all data on a cohort, including those members who withdraw from the study or are lost to follow-up for other reasons. Although the technique owes its origin and name to vital status as the study outcome (death vs survival, hence the terms *life*-table and *survival* analysis), it can be used to examine the distribution of time to occurrence of any dichotomous outcome. It can be used for either descriptive (single exposure group) or analytic (two or more exposure groups) cohort studies and applies equally well to observational and experimental (clinical trial) designs.

Before discussing the anatomy and physiology of life tables, I shall begin with a clinical example and then examine the various ways in which the data could be analyzed. After a review of the limitations of each of the alternative strategies, the rationale for life-table analysis should be evident.

18.2 Alternative Methods of Analysis: an Example

Consider a descriptive study of survival in a cohort of 15 adolescents with osteogenic sarcoma (a rare bone cancer) of the femur treated with a combination of leg amputation and a new chemotherapy regimen at a single tertiary care referral center. The first patient to receive the regimen began treatment on October 9, 1979. As shown in Fig. 18.1, 14 additional patients received a similar treatment, with the most recent enrolled on January 18, 1985. The study was terminated on October 9, 1985, exactly 6 years after its inception.

How could the survival experience of this cohort best be summarized? Several commonly used approaches are listed below, along with a brief discussion of their strengths and limitations.

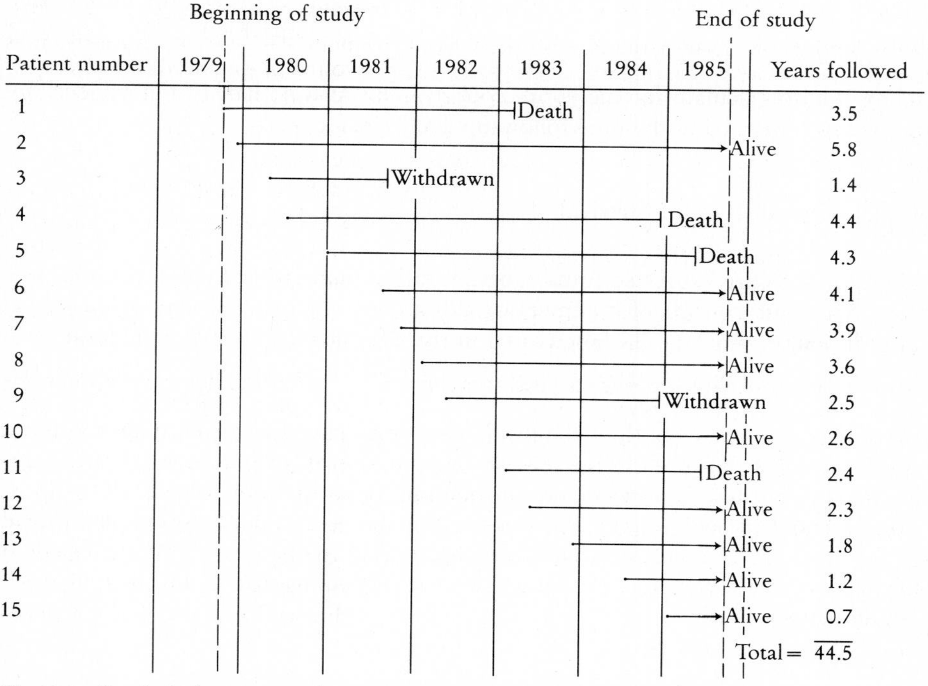

Fig. 18.1. Survival of 15 osteogenic sarcoma patients receiving new treatment regimen

18.2.1 Mean (Average) Duration of Survival

Mean survival is probably the least desirable alternative. The main problem is what to do about the two patients who moved away and the nine who are still alive at the end of the study. Should they be used in calculating the mean? Their duration of survival is, of course, unknown. If the duration of their follow-up is used instead, the overall mean will be underestimated, since all of the lost or still-living patients would have lived at least slightly longer than they were actually followed up. If, on the other hand, these patients are omitted, the mean will be based only on the four patients who were known to have died during the 6 years of follow-up. This mean would be unrepresentative of the entire cohort and would be biased toward short survivals, since it was based on those patients who were known to have died soonest.

The other problem with using the mean is the effect of outliers. Patients with very short or very long survival will have an undue impact on the mean for the cohort. The four deaths in our example occurred at 2.4, 3.5, 4.3, and 4.4 years after the start of treatment, for an overall mean of 3.7 years. If the first patient had died at 0.2 years instead of 2.4 years, the mean would have been only 3.1 years. Mean survival time is probably the least desirable method of analysis.

18.2.2 Median Duration of Survival

Although use of the median instead of the mean eliminates the potent effect of outliers (if the first death had occurred at 0.2 years instead of 2.4 years, the median survival among the four patients who died would remain $\frac{3.5+4.3}{2} = 3.9$ years), it is impossible to calculate for the entire cohort unless at least half of the subjects are known to have died at the time follow-up is terminated.

18.2.3 Overall Rate of Survival

Here the data are expressed in categorical, rather than continuous, form, i.e., as a rate. But a rate consists of a numerator and a denominator, and here again we get into difficulty. Who should be counted in the denominator? If we include the two patients lost to follow-up, the survival rate will be $\frac{11}{15}$, or 73%. This may be too optimistic, because one or both of the lost patients may have subsequently died without our knowing it. But even in the absence of study losses, overall survival rate is unsatisfactory because it contains no information about the *duration* of follow-up. If our patients had been followed up for a maximum of 2 years, for example, instead of 5.8 years, all (i.e., 100%) would have been classified as survivors. Conversely, if all had been followed for 100 years, survival (including that of the investigator!) would have been 0%.

18.2.4 *n*-Year Survival Rate

The most commonly used approach is to calculate a rate of survival for a given length of time (less, of course, than the duration of the study). For our example, we could calculate a 1-year, 2-year, or 5-year survival rate. This approach overcomes the major objection to the overall survival rate, because it includes duration of follow-up in its definition. It does not resolve the "denominator problem," however, of how we deal with patients who are lost to follow-up before *n* years elapse or with those patients who are still alive at study termination but who have been followed for fewer than *n* years.

For example, only one of the osteosarcoma patients in our example was known to survive 5 years or more. Four more were known to have died in less than 5 years, while the remaining ten either were lost (two) or were still alive at the end of the study (eight). If the latter ten are included in the denominator, the 5-year survival rate is only $\frac{1}{15}$, or 6.7%. This is overly pessimistic, since one or more of the ten lost or remaining patients might well have lived $\geqq 5$ years. Conversely, the 5-year mortality of $\frac{4}{15}$, or 27%, is overly optimistic, since it assumes that the ten incompletely followed patients would all have survived at least 5 years. If the ten patients are excluded from the denominator, the 5-year survival rate becomes $\frac{1}{5}$, or 20%. This is also too low, however, because it does not take into account the known years of survival among the exclusions. The same result would have been obtained if all ten had been lost immediately after enrollment and had had no observed survival.

18.2.5 Person-Years Approach

Another approach (discussed in Chapter 6) uses the length of follow-up for each subject, sums this value for each member of the cohort to obtain a total number of person-years of follow-up, and then uses this figure as the denominator. Subjects lost to follow-up or remaining alive at study termination thus contribute to the denominator and appropriately reduce the mortality rate. Consequently, this method is generally superior to the four discussed previously. In our example, the total number of person-years is 44.5, and the mortality would thus be $\frac{4}{44.5}$, or 0.090 deaths per person-year.

The major limitation of the person-years approach arises in situations where the risk of death (or other study outcome) is not constant over time. Since the same 100 person-years can accumulate from two subjects followed for 50 years or 50 subjects followed for 2 years, a mortality expressed in terms of person-years can be misleading. In our example, eight of the 15 patients contributed <3 years to total follow-up time for the cohort. If relapses and death are expected to occur mostly after 3 years, the calculated mortality of 0.090 per person-year may be too optimistic.

This type of problem is particularly likely to occur for exposures with long latent periods. If most radiation-induced cancers occur 20 years or longer after exposure, for example, a cohort study with a sample size of 1000 but only a 15-year average, and a 20-year maximum, follow-up might detect few or no excess cases of cancer per 15 000 person-years. A cohort of 500 followed for an average of 30 years, however, would detect a much higher number of excess cases for the same 15 000 person-years.

18.2.6 Life-Table Analysis

Life-table analysis has many of the same attractive features as the person-years approach. It utilizes information available on all study subjects, including those withdrawn from the study, regardless of duration of follow-up. But it has one additional advantage: it does not require a constant risk over time. All person-years are not treated as equivalent; those occurring soon after exposure are counted differently from those occurring later in the course of follow-up. It is thus the analysis of choice whenever there are unequal duration of follow-up and study withdrawals and when constancy of risk over time cannot be assumed.

There are two principal techniques for carrying out a life-table analysis: the *actuarial method* [1, 2] and the *Kaplan-Meier* (or *product-limit*) *method* [2–4]. These will be described in turn in the following two sections.

18.3 The Actuarial Method

18.3.1 Requirements and Assumptions

The first requirement for any life-table analysis is a clear indication of the starting point. This is often called the *zero time* and usually corresponds to the time of first exposure. When the exposure is a treatment and the study is a randomized clinical trial, the time of randomization is usually preferred.

When the exposure is a disease, ascertainment of zero time becomes problematic. Should it be the onset of symptoms? Time of diagnosis? First presentation for treatment? Since patients often differ as to when symptoms are first noticed (or retrospectively recalled) in the course of their disease, onset of symptoms is usually a poor choice for zero time. Similarly, time of diagnosis will vary with the intensity of medical surveillance, the diagnostic acumen of the patient's clinician, and the use of laboratory tests capable of early detection (i.e., screening or case-finding). Date of first treatment for the disease is often used as zero time, because it is usually easy to determine objectively and because treatment is often (although not always) begun at a similar point in the disease's natural history.

The second requirement is a well-defined study outcome. Not only must it be dichotomous; it must also not be subject to multiple episodes. Thus, death and chronic diseases are outcomes ideally suited to analysis by life tables. Diseases subject to multiple remissions and relapses can be studied using this technique, providing the outcome is defined as the occurrence or nonoccurrence of a *first* relapse. Examples of other outcomes for which life-table analysis is appropriate include first metastasis, first hospitalization, and first physician visit. When several dichotomous outcomes are involved, each must be analyzed separately or the outcome must be defined in such a way as to incorporate a specific combination of interest, e.g., death *or* first relapse.

Regardless of what outcome event is chosen, a decision must be made about whether all such events will be counted, only those from specific causes (e.g., death from myocardial infarction), or only those "attributable" to exposure. Suppose, for example, that one of the osteosarcoma patients in our example had died in an automobile accident. If the investigator is convinced that this death was totally unrelated to the underlying disease, then it should probably be counted as a loss to follow-up (withdrawal). Suppose further, however, that the patient was depressed because his disease was progressing and that he deliberately crashed the family car into a telephone pole. Counting the death as a study withdrawal would lead to an overly optimistic estimate of survival for the cohort. In other words, the suicide was actually caused by the osteosarcoma.

This leads us more generally to the third requirement for the life-table analysis: losses to follow-up should be independent of the study outcome. If subjects who drop out are those doing particularly well or particularly poorly, then their loss will bias the results in the overall cohort. If our osteosarcoma patients had been transferred to a hospice facility as soon as their disease became unresponsive to treatment, all four deaths would have been counted as withdrawals, and survival would have been calculated as 100%! Thus, life-table analysis assumes that lost subjects have an identical prognosis to those remaining in the cohort at that time. Actually, this assumption is also shared by other cohort analytic approaches (i.e., mean or median survival, overall or *n*-year survival rates, and person-years) whenever losses to follow-up occur.

The fourth requirement is that the risk of the outcome is independent of calendar time. In other words, the prognosis of subjects entering the study early should be no different from that of those enrolled toward the end. Although life tables do not assume that risk remains constant for any given subject over time, they do assume no major secular changes in prognosis for the overall cohort. If advances in supportive care or in treatment of adverse reactions to therapy resulted in a better prognosis among our osteosarcoma patients enrolled since 1982, for example, the overall survival of the cohort would largely reflect deaths occurring among patients treated earlier and thus would be overly pessimistic.

The fifth and final requirement is that the risk of the study outcome remain constant *within* intervals used in constructing the life table (see following subsection). Risk need not be constant from one interval to the next, but it must remain so within each interval. This is not a major restriction, since intervals of any length can be constructed and can vary within a given life table. Consequently, if the investigator suspects a possible variation in risk within one or more intervals, these intervals should be subdivided into smaller ones with constant risk, so that the constant risk requirement is satisfied.

With these five requirements and assumptions in mind, we are now ready to construct the life table.

18.3.2 Constructing the Actuarial Life Table

The first step in constructing the life table is to refer the timing of all "events" (including time to outcome, loss to follow-up, or end of study) to the zero time, rather than to calendar time. Figure 18.2 makes this conversion for the 15 patients of the osteosarcoma cohort. The corresponding life table is shown in Table 18.1; each column of the table will be discussed in turn.

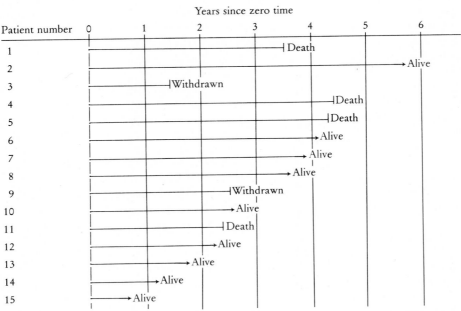

Fig. 18.2. Survival of 15 osteogenic sarcoma patients with respect to time of initiating treatment (zero time)

Table 18.1. Life table for 15 patients with osteogenic sarcoma (actuarial method)

(1) x Interval (years)	(2) l_x Subjects living at start of interval	(3) w_x Subjects withdrawn during interval	(4) $r_x = l_x - \dfrac{w_x}{2}$ Subjects at risk during interval	(5) d_x Deaths during interval	(6) $q_x = \dfrac{d_x}{r_x}$ Death rate during interval	(7) $p_x = 1 - q_x$ Survival rate during interval	(8) $S_{x_i} = (p_{x_i})$ $(p_{x_2}) \ldots (p_{x_i})$ Cumulative survival rate to end of interval
0–1	15	1	14.5	0	0	1	1
1–2	14	3	12.5	0	0	1	1
2–3	11	3	9.5	1	0.105	0.895	0.895
3–4	7	2	6	1	0.167	0.833	0.746
4–5	4	1	3.5	2	0.571	0.429	0.320
5–6	1	1	0.5	0	0	1	0.320

Column (1): Interval (x)

This is the interval since zero time. As discussed in Section 18.2, the intervals need not be of equal length, but they should be short enough so that the risk of outcome is constant throughout (requirement 5). The intervals should be established a priori, i.e., before examination of the data. Otherwise, the investigator could influence the calculated survivals just by changing the interval boundaries. For our osteosarcoma example we have chosen yearly intervals.

Column (2): Subjects Living at Start of Interval (l_x)

For the first interval, this is the number of total subjects enrolled in the study. For succeeding intervals,

$$l_x = l_{x-1} - (w_{x-1} + d_{x-1}) \qquad (18.1)$$

i.e., the number of subjects entering the previous interval minus the number withdrawn (w) or developing the outcome (d) in the previous interval.

Column (3): Subjects Withdrawn During Interval (w_x)

Withdrawn subjects include not only those who drop out or are lost to follow-up during the interval but also those still free of the outcome who were in that interval when the study ended. Withdrawn subjects are also referred to as *censored* subjects in much of the life-table literature.

Column (4): Subjects at Risk During Interval (r_x)

Under the assumption that the risk remains constant within intervals (requirement 5), subjects who withdraw during an interval will be at risk, on average, for half the interval. Thus, the effective number at risk will be the number who enter the interval (l_x) minus half the number who withdraw $\left(\dfrac{w_x}{2}\right)$.

Column (5): Deaths During Interval (d_x)

This is simply the number of subjects developing the outcome (e.g., death) during the interval.

Column (6): Death Rate During Interval (q_x)

This is also called the *hazard* and is equivalent to the probability of a subject's developing the study outcome (death or other) during the given interval, conditional on his or her being free of the outcome (e.g., alive) at the start of the interval (i.e., $q_x = \dfrac{d_x}{r_x}$).

Column (7): Survival Rate During Interval (p_x)

Since the outcome is dichotomous, the probability of *not* developing the outcome (e.g., of surviving) during the interval is simply $1 - q_x$. It, too, can be thought of as a conditional probability, since it depends on a subject being free of the outcome at the start of the interval.

Column (8): Cumulative Survival Rate to End of Interval (S_x)

Because the p_x's (column 7) represent successive conditional probabilities of remaining outcome-free (e.g., of survival), the cumulative probability can be calculated using Eq. 17.3, the multiplicative rule for combining conditional probabilities:

$$S_{x_i} = (p_{x_1})\,(p_{x_2})\,(p_{x_3}) \cdots (p_{x_i}) \tag{18.2}$$

The S_x's are the main quantities of interest in life-table analysis. They represent the rates (or probabilities) of survival through the end of each interval in the table. Thus, for our osteosarcoma cohort, the 1-year life-table survival rate is 100%, the 3-year rate is 89.5%, and the 5-year rate is 32.0%. Note that the latter rates are substantially different from (in this case, better than) those calculated without using the life table. For example, the ordinary (i.e., non-life-table) 5-year survival rate, even excluding the ten subjects not observed for ≥ 5 years, was 20% (see Section 18.2). The difference arises because outcome-free duration is included for subjects lost to follow-up and for those followed for < 5 years at the end of the study.

Life tables can be used to calculate cumulative rates of survival up to and including the longest duration of follow-up. We were able to calculate an overall 5-year survival for the entire cohort even though only one patient was followed for 5 or more years. Therein lies the great advantage of life-table analysis. The paucity of observations at long durations, however, will lead to a loss in reproducibility of the sample estimate, i.e., a wide confidence interval (see Section 18.5). Life tables cannot, of course, be used to estimate survival beyond the longest duration of follow-up.

The S_x's are often depicted graphically, as shown for our example in Fig. 18.3. The graph is also sometimes called a "life table" but usually goes under the name of *survival curve*.

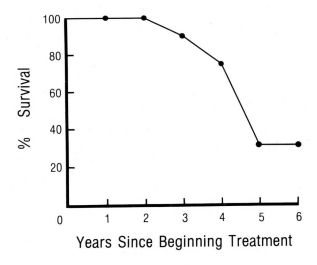

Fig. 18.3. Survival curve for 15 patients with osteogenic sarcoma (actuarial method)

18.4 The Kaplan-Meier (Product-Limit) Method

The *Kaplan-Meier* (or *product-limit*) *method* [2–4] of life-table analysis is very similar to the actuarial method. There are two main differences:

1. The Kaplan-Meier method does not group the times in which outcome events occur into intervals. Each row in the life table is defined by the time at which the next subject (or subjects) experiences the study outcome. Obviously, the exact time the outcome occurs must be known for each subject. (With the actuarial method, we need know only in which pre-established interval to place each subject experiencing the outcome.) This feature, of course, obviates the assumption of constant risk within intervals (requirement 5).
2. Withdrawn subjects (once again, including those lost to follow-up and those still free of the outcome at the end of the study) are assumed to be at risk for the outcome up to and including the time they are withdrawn. Since the rows in the table are determined by the next occurring outcome event(s), subjects who are withdrawn between the times corresponding to two successive rows are used to calculate the outcome rate for the first of the two rows, but not the second. In other words, only those subjects known to be at risk at the time each outcome event occurs are used to calculate the rate at that time.

The data from Figs. 18.1 and 18.2, depicting survival times in 15 osteosarcoma patients, have been analyzed using the Kaplan-Meier approach in Table 18.2. Patients who are known to have died during the period of follow-up are ranked in ascending order of the time of death. The columns are then calculated as follows:

Column (1): Time of the Next Occurring Death (t)
The shortest time after beginning treatment at which death was known to occur was 2.4 years. The other three deaths observed during follow-up occurred at 3.5, 4.3, and 4.4 years after the start of treatment.

Column (2): Number at Risk for Death at Time t (r_t)
This includes all patients known to be alive just prior to time t and is thus equal to the number known to be alive at t plus the number of deaths at t.

Table 18.2. Kaplan-Meier life-table analysis of survival in 15 osteogenic sarcoma patients

(1) t Time (years)	(2) r_t Number at risk	(3) d_t Deaths	(4) $q_t = \dfrac{d_t}{r_t}$ Death rate	(5) $p_t = 1 - q_t$ Survival rate	(6) $S_{t_i} = (p_{t_1})(p_{t_2}) \ldots (p_{t_i})$ Cumulative survival rate
2.4	10	1	0.100	0.900	0.900
3.5	7	1	0.143	0.857	0.771
4.3	3	1	0.333	0.667	0.514
4.4	2	1	0.500	0.500	0.257

Column (3): Number of Deaths at Time t (d_x)
For our example, no two patients died at exactly the same time after beginning treatment, and thus all the entries in this column are 1's.

Column (4): Death Rate at Time t (q_t)
This is analogous to the interval death rate or hazard (q_x) calculated using the actuarial method. It can be interpreted as the *instantaneous hazard* at time t and is the probability of dying at time t conditional on having survived until t.

Column (5): Survival Rate at Time t (p_t)
The instantaneous survival rate p_t is analogous to the actuarial (interval) survival rate p_x and is calculated as $1 - q_t$.

Column (6): Cumulative Survival Rate up to and Including Time t (S_t)
As with the actuarial method, the cumulative survival is obtained by multiplying p_t by the survival rates at all previous times.

Because the S_t's are computed for exact times, rather than for time intervals, survival curves based on the Kaplan-Meier method show abrupt drops ("steps") in percent survival corresponding to the times at which deaths actually occurred in the cohort under analysis. These steps become progressively larger as the number of subjects still at risk diminishes, i.e., toward the right side of the curve. Figure 18.4 shows the survival curve drawn from Table 18.2, along with the curve derived using the actuarial method (Fig. 18.3) for comparison. As can be seen, the two methods yield fairly similar curves.

As with the actuarial method, Kaplan-Meier life-table analysis can be used for dichotomous outcomes other than death. When exact times for outcome events are known, the Kaplan-Meier method obviates the need for arbitrary intervals. It may

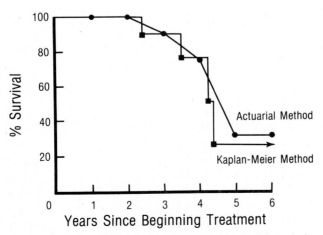

Fig. 18.4. Comparison of Kaplan-Meier and actuarial survival curves for 15 osteogenic sarcoma patients

also result in improved statistical efficiency (analogous to analyzing continuous data in their native continuous form vs after they have been categorized), but this gain is counterbalanced by the fact that follow-up that ends between times when outcome events occur is ignored. In general, however, the Kaplan-Meier and actuarial methods give comparable results.

18.5 Statistical Inference

The techniques used for statistical inference are identical for the actuarial and Kaplan-Meier methods of life-table analysis, and they will thus be presented together. Interpretation of the results will differ somewhat for the two methods, however, corresponding to their basis on either time intervals (x's) or exact time points (t) respectively.

18.5.1 Parametric Estimation

Peto et al. [4] provide an easily calculated approximation for the standard error (SE) of S_x or S_t:

$$SE(S_x) = S_x \sqrt{\frac{1 - S_x}{r_x}}$$

$$SE(S_t) = S_t \sqrt{\frac{1 - S_t}{r_t}}$$

(18.3)

Thus, the SE for the 3-year survival in Table 18.1 can be computed as follows:

$$SE(S_3) = 0.895 \sqrt{\frac{1 - 0.895}{9.5}} = 0.094$$

That for the 5-year survival is

$$SE(S_5) = 0.320 \sqrt{\frac{1 - 0.320}{3.5}} = 0.141$$

As is often the case with longer durations of follow-up and correspondingly fewer observations, the standard error is larger for the 5-year survival.

Once the standard error has been calculated, the standard normal (z-) distribution can be used to estimate a confidence interval around the S_x or S_t observed in the study sample. (This assumes a normally distributed sampling distribution of S_x's or S_t's.) The $100(1 - \alpha)\%$ confidence interval will include the "true" (target population) S_x or S_t with a probability of $1 - \alpha$, where α is 0.05, 0.01, or some other chosen value. The 95% confidence intervals for the 3- and 5-year actuarially derived survivals from our example are:

$S_3 = 0.895 \pm 1.96(0.094) = 0.895 \pm 0.184 = 0.711$ to 1.000
    (since the survival rate cannot exceed 100%)
$S_5 = 0.320 \pm 1.96(0.141) = 0.320 \pm 0.276 = 0.044$ to 0.596

18.5.2 Differences Between Two Survival Curves: z-Test

Life tables can also be used to calculate the difference in survival (or other outcome) between two exposure or treatment groups. To illustrate, we shall introduce a new example of a randomized trial comparing first-relapse rates (defined as need for hospitalization) in chronic schizophrenics in remission treated with antipsychotic drugs alone ($n = 18$) vs those treated with drugs plus individual psychotherapy ($n = 22$). The trial was terminated 48 months after inception, and the remission durations (times of first relapse) in months were as follows, with withdrawals (patients lost to follow-up or still in remission at the end of the trial) indicated with an asterisk:

Drug therapy alone: 1*, 3, 6*, 7, 7*, 7*, 11, 14*, 15, 18, 24, 27*, 30, 32, 35*, 40, 42, 45*
Drug plus psychotherapy: 3*, 4, 7*, 9, 9*, 10*, 11*, 12*, 17, 19*, 20*, 22, 25*, 30*, 34, 38, 38*, 39*, 41*, 42, 42, 44*

The actuarial life tables and survival curves for the two groups are shown in Table 18.3 and Fig. 18.5. Patients relapsing or withdrawing at the common boundaries between intervals (e.g., 6 months) are assumed to have been in remission at that time but to have relapsed or withdrawn sometime in the succeeding month. They are thus "credited" to the next succeeding interval.

Judging from Fig. 18.5 or from the last column of Table 18.3, the combination treatment (drug plus psychotherapy) appears superior. How likely is it that the observed difference is due to chance? In other words, what is the probability of obtaining a difference at least as large as the one observed, under the null hypothesis that the treatment groups represent random samples from target populations having the same probability of survival?

There are two main approaches to testing two S_x's or S_t's for a statistically significant difference, i.e., to calculating the probability that sampling variation can explain the observed difference under the null hypothesis of no difference. The first assumes a normally distributed sampling distribution of S_x's or S_t's and involves a z-test of the difference between two S_{x_i}'s or S_{t_i}'s at any given x_i or t_i:

$$z = \frac{S_{x_{i1}} - S_{x_{i2}}}{\sqrt{[SE(S_{x_{i1}})]^2 + [SE(S_{x_{i2}})]^2}}$$

$$z = \frac{S_{t_{i1}} - S_{t_{i2}}}{\sqrt{[SE(S_{t_{i1}})]^2 + [SE(S_{t_{i2}})]^2}}$$

(18.4)

where $S_{x_{i1}}$ and $S_{x_{i2}}$ (or $S_{t_{i1}}$ and $S_{t_{i2}}$) are the S_x's (or S_t's) in the two groups being compared.

Table 18.3. Actuarial life tables for randomized clinical trial comparing drug therapy alone with drug plus psychotherapy in 40 chronic schizophrenics

	(1) x Interval (months)	(2) l_x Number entering interval	(3) w_x Number with- drawn	(4) r_x Number at risk	(5) d_x Relapses during interval	(6) q_x Relapse rate	(7) p_x Contin- ued remis- sion rate	(8) S_x Cumula- tive continued remission rate
1. Drug	0– 6	18	1	17.5	1	0.057	0.943	0.943
therapy	6–12	16	3	14.5	2	0.138	0.862	0.813
alone	12–18	11	1	10.5	1	0.095	0.905	0.736
	18–24	9	0	9	1	0.111	0.889	0.654
	24–30	8	1	7.5	1	0.133	0.867	0.567
	30–36	6	1	5.5	2	0.364	0.636	0.361
	36–42	3	0	3	1	0.333	0.667	0.241
	42–48	2	1	1.5	1	0.667	0.333	0.080
2. Drug plus	0– 6	22	1	21.5	1	0.047	0.953	0.953
psychotherapy	6–12	20	4	18	1	0.056	0.944	0.900
	12–18	15	1	14.5	1	0.069	0.931	0.838
	18–24	13	2	12	1	0.083	0.917	0.768
	24–30	10	1	9.5	0	0	1	0.768
	30–36	9	1	8.5	1	0.118	0.882	0.677
	36–42	7	3	5.5	1	0.182	0.818	0.554
	42–48	3	1	2.5	2	0.800	0.200	0.111

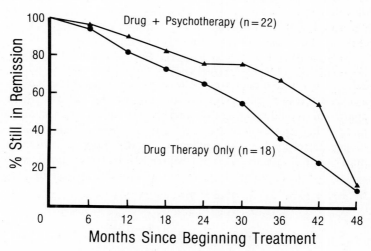

Fig. 18.5. Survival curves for RCT comparing drug therapy alone with drug plus psychotherapy in 40 chronic schizophrenics (actuarial method)

For the actuarial continued remission rate at 24 months in our example:

$$S_{24_1} = 0.654 \text{ and } SE(S_{24_1}) = 0.654 \sqrt{\frac{1-0.654}{9}} = 0.128$$

$$S_{24_2} = 0.768 \text{ and } SE(S_{24_2}) = 0.768 \sqrt{\frac{1-0.768}{12}} = 0.107$$

$$z = \frac{0.654 - 0.768}{\sqrt{(0.128)^2 + (0.107)^2}} = -0.683$$

The corresponding two-tailed P value is 0.495, and thus the difference is not statistically significant. In other words, we cannot reject the null hypothesis. A one-tailed test could be justified here, since there is no reason to think that drug therapy alone would be *more* efficacious than drug plus psychotherapy. The one-tailed P value would remain nonsignificant at $P=0.247$. A relative risk can also be calculated for the outcome through the end of any interval x or at any time t:

$$RR_x = \frac{1-S_{x_1}}{1-S_{x_2}}$$

$$RR_t = \frac{1-S_{t_1}}{1-S_{t_2}}$$

(18.5)

For our example, the actuarial relative risk for relapse through 24 months is

$$RR_{24} = \frac{1-0.654}{1-0.768} = 1.49$$

Of course, the time at which the curves are to be tested should be established a priori, i.e., before the data are collected. Otherwise, the temptation would be great to examine the two curves visually and choose the interval where they are farthest apart. This would maximize the opportunity for finding a statistically significant difference, but the P value resulting from such post hoc significance testing would no longer correspond to the probability of obtaining the observed result by chance under the null hypothesis (see Chapter 12). If, for example, we had tested the two schizophrenic treatment regimens at 36 months, instead of 24 months, we would have obtained the following result:

$$S_{36_1} = 0.361 \text{ and } SE(S_{36_1}) = 0.361 \sqrt{\frac{1-0.361}{5.5}} = 0.123$$

$$S_{36_2} = 0.677 \text{ and } SE(S_{36_2}) = 0.677 \sqrt{\frac{1-0.677}{8.5}} = 0.132$$

$$z = \frac{0.361 - 0.677}{\sqrt{(0.123)^2 + (0.132)^2}} = -1.751$$

$$RR_{36} = \frac{1-0.361}{1-0.677} = 1.98$$

The corresponding two-tailed P value $= 0.080$, and the one-tailed P value $= 0.040$. We thus might have (unfairly) rejected the null hypothesis.

The other approach to significance testing is called the *log-rank test* [2, 4]. Despite its being a nonparametric test, the log-rank test is more efficient than the z-test, because it compares the entire survival curve, rather than just a single point on the curve (such as 24 months). It is also, therefore, less arbitrary. For each interval or time in the table, the observed (O) number of relapses (or deaths, or other outcome) in each group is compared with the number expected (E) based on the total number of relapses observed and the number of subjects at risk in each group:

$$E_{x_i} = \left[\frac{r_{x_i}}{r_{x_1} + r_{x_2}} \right] (O_1 + O_2)$$

$$E_{t_i} = \left[\frac{r_{t_i}}{r_{t_1} + r_{t_2}} \right] (O_1 + O_2) \tag{18.6}$$

Thus, if there are an equal number of subjects at risk for a given interval, half of the observed relapses would be expected to occur in each group. The observed (O) and expected (E) relapses for each group are then summed over all intervals in the table and an overall χ^2 is calculated as follows:

$$\chi^2 = \frac{(\Sigma O_1 - \Sigma E_1)^2}{\Sigma E_1} + \frac{(\Sigma O_2 - \Sigma E_2)^2}{\Sigma E_2} \tag{18.7}$$

Finally, the calculated value of χ^2 is compared with tabulated critical values at one degree of freedom to obtain the corresponding P value.

The log-rank test will be illustrated using our same example. The calculations using the actuarial life table (Table 18.3) are shown in Table 18.4. Despite the improved efficiency of the log-rank test, the calculated value of χ^2 is only 1.573 and does not achieve statistical significance, even with a one-tailed test. Similar results are obtained using the Kaplan-Meier life table.

An overall relative risk can also be calculated using the log-rank approach:

$$RR_{\text{overall}} = \frac{\Sigma O_1 / \Sigma E_1}{\Sigma O_2 / \Sigma E_2} \tag{18.8}$$

For Table 18.4, $RR_{\text{overall}} = \dfrac{10/7.383}{8/10.617} = 1.80$

This relative risk is probably clinically important. It indicates an 80% higher risk of relapse with drug therapy alone as compared with drug plus psychotherapy. The fact that this difference between the two treatments is not statistically significant, however, should make us concerned about inferring that the two treatments are equivalent. Although P is not low enough to warrant rejection of the null hypothesis, the small sample size (low statistical power) has enabled a clinically important difference to "escape" statistical significance. In other words, the risk of a Type II error is high (see Chapter 12).

Table 18.4. Calculation of log-rank test for RCT comparing drug therapy alone (group 1) with drug plus psychotherapy (group 2) in 40 chronic schizophrenics (actuarial method)

Interval (months)	Number at risk			Observed relapses			Expected relapses $= \left[\dfrac{r_{x_i}}{r_{x_1} + r_{x_2}} \right](O_1 + O_2)$		
x	r_{x_1}	r_{x_2}	Total $(r_{x_1} + r_{x_2})$	O_1	O_2	Total $(O_1 + O_2)$	E_1	E_2	Total $(E_1 + E_2)$
0–6	17.5	21.5	39	1	1	2	0.897	1.103	2
6–12	14.5	18	32.5	2	1	3	1.338	1.662	3
12–18	10.5	14.5	25	1	1	2	0.840	1.160	2
18–24	9	12	21	1	1	2	0.857	1.143	2
24–30	7.5	9.5	17	1	0	1	0.441	0.559	1
30–36	5.5	8.5	14	2	1	3	1.179	1.821	3
36–42	3	5.5	8.5	1	1	2	0.706	1.294	2
42–48	1.5	2.5	4	1	2	3	1.125	1.875	3
				$\Sigma = 10$	$\Sigma = 8$	$\Sigma = 18$	$\Sigma = 7.383$	$\Sigma = 10.617$	$\Sigma = 18$

$$\chi^2 = \frac{(\Sigma O_1 - \Sigma E_1)^2}{\Sigma E_1} + \frac{(\Sigma O_2 - \Sigma E_2)^2}{\Sigma E_2} = \frac{(10 - 7.383)^2}{7.383} + \frac{(8 - 10.617)^2}{10.617} = 1.573; \text{ at 1 } df, P > 0.10$$

$$RR = \frac{\Sigma O_1 / \Sigma E_1}{\Sigma O_2 / \Sigma E_2} = \frac{10/7.383}{8/10.617} = 1.80$$

18.5.3 Control for Confounding Factors

Just as in the case of comparing two means or two proportions, a comparison of two survival curves may be biased by one or more confounding factors associated with both exposure and (independently of exposure) outcome. There are two main methods used for controlling for such confounding effects.

The first method is stratification [4]. A separate life table is constructed for each stratum defined by the confounder or combination of confounders. (Obviously, continuous confounders must first be categorized.) Equation 18.6 is used to calculate stratum-specific expected values for each interval or time in the life table. The stratum-specific observed and expected totals are then added together for all strata to get an overall total of observed and expected for each exposure group. These totals can be used in Eq. 18.7 to calculate an overall χ^2, which is referred to critical values of χ^2 at one degree of freedom to derive the corresponding P value. This technique is analogous to the Mantel-Haenszel procedure (see Sections 6.3 and 14.2.8). Finally, the overall relative risk can be estimated by applying the observed and expected totals to Eq. 18.8.

The second method of controlling for confounding is a multivariate statistical technique based on the *proportional hazards model*. As we have seen, life-table analysis does not require that the risk (hazard) of the outcome remain constant throughout the period of follow-up. Use of the actuarial method does assume a constant risk *within* intervals defining the life table, but not necessarily *between* intervals. That is why the slope of the actuarial survival curve changes from one interval to another, as seen in Figs. 18.3 and 18.5.

In comparing two survival curves, however, it is reasonable to assume that RR, the relative risk of developing the outcome, does remain constant over time. In other words, even if the slope *(instantaneous hazard)* of a given curve changes over time, the ratio of two slopes (the *proportional hazard*) corresponding to the survival of two exposure groups should remain fairly constant. Cox has formulated a regression procedure somewhat analogous to multiple logistic regression analysis (see Section 14.2.8) that models the proportional hazard (relative risk) as a function of exposure and any number of continuous and categorical confounders. The details of the Cox regression procedure are beyond the scope of this text, and the interested reader is referred to more specialized references [5, 6].

References

1. Cutler SJ, Ederer F (1958) Maximum utilization of the life-table method in analyzing survival. J Chronic Dis 8: 699–712
2. Coldman AJ, Elwood JM (1979) Examining survival data. Can Med Assoc J 121: 1065–1071
3. Kaplan EL, Meier P (1958) Nonparametric estimation from incomplete observations. JASA 53: 457–481
4. Peto R, Pike MC, Armitage P, Breslow NE, Cox DR, Howard SV, Mantel N, McPherson K, Peto J, Smith PG (1977) Design and analysis of randomized clinical trials requiring prolonged observation of each patient. II. Analysis and examples. Br J Cancer 35: 1–39
5. Cox DR (1972) Regression models and life tables. JR Stat Soc (Series B) 34: 187–202
6. Anderson A, Auquier A, Hauck WW, Oakes D, Vandaele W, Weisberg HI (1980) Statistical methods for comparative studies: techniques for bias reduction. Wiley, New York, pp 214–230

Chapter 19: Causality

19.1 What is a "Cause"?

Most of this text has concerned the design and analysis of epidemiologic studies of a possible relationship between exposure to an agent, maneuver, or treatment and the development of a particular health outcome. Usually the hypothesis of interest is whether exposure is *causally* related to the outcome, which we can indicate by the following symbols:

$$E \longrightarrow O$$

It is important to realize that the terms "exposure" and "outcome" do not denote distinct types of events or states. A variable considered an exposure in one situation can serve as the putative outcome in another. For example, in a study of cigarette smoking as a cause of lung cancer, the exposure variable is obviously cigarette smoking. In a study of some health education intervention intended to reduce smoking, however, smoking is the outcome. Thus, deciding which variable is the exposure and which is the outcome involves a choice by the clinician or investigator. The only a priori constraint on this choice is *temporality:* exposure must be known to precede outcome.

Given this understanding of the terms "exposure" and "outcome," the following definition of cause can then be offered:

> Exposure is a cause of outcome if exposure at a given level results in a different outcome (or level of outcome) than *would have* occurred without that (level of) exposure.

We can summarize this definition as follows:

$$E_1 \longrightarrow O_1 \text{ if and only if } E_2 \longrightarrow O_2$$

where $E_1 \neq E_2$ and $O_1 \neq O_2$.

Although the definition seems unobjectionable, it is different from some conventional notions of cause in that it insists on an alternative. No exposure-outcome relationship can be thought about in isolation. Before making a causal inference about whether a given exposure is the cause of an outcome, one must ask: "Compared with what?" For example, smoking one pack of cigarettes per day is a cause of lung cancer compared with not smoking, but not compared with smoking two packs a day.

At first glance, the definition may appear truly operational, because it indicates the steps that should be taken before making a causal inference. Change the exposure (E_1 to E_2) and observe the outcome; if the outcome changes (O_1 to O_2), then causality can be inferred. The definition has intuitive appeal, because it is based on an experimental paradigm. The experimenter changes one factor and observes the effect on another.

But things are not as straightforward as they appear. The definition is based on what would have occurred if the *same* exposed individuals had instead experienced the comparative exposure. But this is obviously not possible, at least not at the same period of time; the same individuals cannot experience two mutually exclusive exposures simultaneously. Even a crossover experiment in which the same individuals *successively* experience different exposures cannot exclude the possibility that something else changed either in the individuals or in the environment to explain an observed change in outcome. It was just this impossibility, in fact, that led the philosopher Hume to argue for the empirical nonverifiability of cause and effect [1].

It is evident that the choice of the comparative exposure requires a choice by the clinician or investigator. How should the comparative exposure differ from the observed one? Should the difference be qualitative (e.g., a different agent) or quantitative (a different dose of the same agent)? If quantitative, should the level be higher or lower? By how much? Should it be total nonexposure? There are no right or wrong answers to these questions. The choice of comparative exposure is necessarily subjective and fraught with uncertainty. But it is also unavoidable.

The choice of comparative exposure can and should be guided by prior notions about what changes in exposure are feasible in the "real" world. After all, why is causal inference important in the first place?

Two principal justifications can be offered. First, an understanding of cause is essential for *change*. In fact, we even defined the causal relationship between exposure and outcome in terms of the change in the latter that occurs when the former is altered. A deliberate intervention (change in exposure) will be successful in altering outcome only to the extent that the exposure is a true cause of that outcome.

We need to understand cause in order to act in the best interest of individual patients and of society at large. Engineers refer to this as "control" to distinguish it from "prediction." Exposure can be an excellent marker, or predictor, of outcome without necessarily being a true cause. But prediction does not necessarily imply control. (This is another way of relating the familiar epidemiologic maxim that association does not prove causation, and I shall have more to say about this issue later in discussing how causality assessments are actually made.)

So, either as clinicians intervening to improve the health of individual patients or as a society implementing a policy to improve the public health, causal inference is essential. This orientation toward change dictates which comparative exposures should be contemplated. It is pointless to compare outcome between two exposures unless both of those exposures can be feasibly implemented. For example, in addressing the question of whether a serum cholesterol level of 350 mg/dl is a cause of coronary artery disease, it makes little sense to compare individuals with a serum cholesterol of 0 mg/dl, since there is no real possibility of reducing serum cholesterol to that level.

The second justification for studying cause is to learn about *mechanism.* For exposures that are not manipulable by man, change occurs, but it is nature's doing, not ours. When nature is doing the controlling, causal inference should involve a comparison of outcomes between two exposures that occur naturally. Thus, in inferring whether the presence of a valine residue at position 6 of the beta chain of hemoglobin is the cause of sickle cell anemia, the appropriate comparison involves otherwise identical individuals with a glutamic acid residue in position 6, since it is glutamic acid (and not some other amino acid) that is usually found in this position.

Understanding fundamental biological processes is important not only to satisfy human curiosity about what makes nature "tick," but also to enable us to adapt ourselves better to its requirements. Moreover, the history of science in general and of medical science in particular has amply demonstrated that knowledge of underlying causal mechanisms often serves as a basis for generating new hypotheses for interventions. For example, elucidation of the biochemical pathways of intermediary metabolism has led to specific nutritional and pharmacologic interventions to correct, at least partially, a variety of inborn metabolic errors. Consequently, this second justification for understanding cause "feeds back" to the first. Epidemiologic research and clinical practice have always benefited, and should continue to benefit, from a knowledge of basic biologic mechanisms and the resulting improvement in the ability of the human species to adapt to and change the world around us.

19.2 Necessary, Sufficient, and Multiple Causes

In the definition offered in Section 19.1, the *locus* of cause was considered to be a group of individuals. This is the conventional framework for causal inference in epidemiology. But as discussed in Chapter 1, clinicians are primarily concerned with individual patients and thus often make causality assessments about individuals. An exposure that is known to cause a given outcome in groups can be necessary, sufficient, both, or neither as a cause of that outcome in a given individual.

A given exposure is considered a *necessary cause* of an outcome if the outcome does not occur in its absence. It is a *sufficient cause* if it always (i.e., in all individuals) leads to the outcome without requiring the presence or absence of any other factors.

Exposure to the tubercle bacillus is a necessary cause of tuberculosis in any individual, but it is usually not sufficient. Otherwise, all family members and health providers who came in contact with the organism would develop the disease, which fortunately is not the case. Nutrition, living conditions, and immune status all play a role in determining whether an exposed person becomes infected. As discussed in Section 6.4, such factors are called *effect modifiers,* because they modify the effect of exposure among the individuals within a group [2]. Using our usual notation:

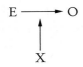

In biologic terms, we refer to such a relationship as *synergism*. Statistically, the relationship is identified by demonstrating an *interaction* between the two factors. (In a multivariate statistical model, inclusion of the *product* of the two variables would explain a significantly greater proportion of the total variance in outcome than a model containing only the two variables by themselves.)

Intrauterine rubella infection at a critical time during the first trimester of pregnancy is sufficient to cause intrauterine growth retardation (IUGR) in all fetuses of nonimmune women. No other factor is required; the infected mother may not be short or undernourished and may not smoke or engage in other harmful practices during pregnancy. Since these other factors, alone or in combination, can themselves suffice to cause IUGR, however, intrauterine rubella infection cannot be considered a necessary cause of IUGR.

For exposure to be both necessary and sufficient as a cause, its relationship with outcome must be perfectly specific, i.e., one-to-one. In other words, an individual can never be exposed without developing the outcome, and the outcome can never occur in a person who has not been exposed. We can then in fact consider the exposure to be *the* cause of the outcome. This kind of exposure-outcome specificity is extremely rare. The relationship between microorganisms and specific infectious diseases was originally thought to be a one-to-one correspondence and formed the basis of the famous Koch postulates. But as we have seen, even the organism that Koch discovered (the tubercle bacillus) does not automatically result in infection in persons who are exposed to it. Certain (but not all) genetic mutations causing so-called inborn errors of metabolism, however, probably fit the bill; the inability to synthesize a particular enzyme results in a metabolic derangement that is highly specific for the missing enzyme.

For many health outcomes, causality is *multifactorial;* causes are neither necessary nor sufficient for any given individual. Such is the case for many chronic diseases. For example, cigarette smoking, high blood pressure, a diet high in saturated fat, insufficient exercise, high serum cholesterol, stress, and genetic predisposition may all contribute to coronary artery disease. Coronary artery disease can occur in the absence of any one of these factors, and none by itself may suffice. Each factor may independently contribute to augment the risk, however, and thus each can be considered a true cause. As we have seen, IUGR is another outcome with a complex, multifactorial "web of causation."

The multifactorial model can be represented as follows:

$$
\left.
\begin{array}{l}
E_1 \longrightarrow \\
E_2 \longrightarrow \\
E_3 \longrightarrow \\
E_4 \longrightarrow \\
\quad\vdots \\
E_n \longrightarrow
\end{array}
\right\} \quad O
$$

As in the case of single exposure factors, the multifactorial model can be complicated by interactions (effect modification) among the various factors, as well as between one or more of them and other variables.

19.3 Patterns of Cause

19.3.1 Causal Paths

Exposure may cause a certain outcome by first affecting an intermediate factor (also called a *mediating* variable) that in turn leads to the outcome:

$$E \longrightarrow X \longrightarrow O$$

A series of causally linked variables is called a *causal path* or *causal chain*. Causal paths can be contemplated either in terms of the individual or in terms of the group.

Very young maternal age, for example, appears to affect birth weight through its impact on several mediating variables. Pregnant adolescents who have just recently passed their menarche have not completed their physical growth and tend, therefore, to be shorter and thinner than older women. Their caloric intake may also be less. Short stature, low weight-for-height, and low caloric intake then subsequently lead to impaired intrauterine growth. In other words, young teenage mothers are likely to have lighter babies *because* they are short and thin and consume an insufficient diet [3].

Socioeconomic status (SES) is a typical example of an exposure variable that tends to lie somewhat removed from ("distal" to) the outcome in most causal paths. For many health outcomes, persons of low SES fare worse than those of higher SES. It is difficult to imagine a biologic mechanism, however, whereby low educational attainment, income, or social standing has a direct influence on health. Rather, it appears that low-SES persons have more crowded living conditions, consume poorer diets, have less access to medical care, and experience more psychological stress, and that these latter factors are the mediators (more "proximal" causes) of the SES effects.

Many authors refer to exposures whose effect on an outcome is not known to be mediated by other factors as *direct causes* [4]. Exposures lying more distal on the causal path, i.e., those whose causal effects involve recognized mediating variables, are called *indirect causes* [4]. In fact, however, if one continues to probe at a more basic scientific level, most of the factors we consider "directly" causal are mediated by physiologic or biochemical processes. In this narrower sense, only the last molecular event preceding an outcome can be called a direct cause, and even then such an inference must remain tentative, pending possible discovery of further intermediate steps in the final molecular pathway. Thus, the distinction between direct and indirect causes is somewhat artificial. It depends on both the "level" of factor (environmental agent, personal characteristic, biochemical reaction) and the state of knowledge at the time of inference. But within a given level (e.g., two environmental factors such as SES and nutrition), such a distinction can be useful in constructing causal paths and, hence, in understanding biologic mechanisms and contemplating possible interventions.

Some exposures may operate through more than one causal path:

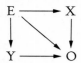

In this diagram, exposure causes outcome through three different paths: one mediated by X, a second mediated by Y, and a third "direct" (i.e., without any identified mediating variable). To return to our birth weight example, maternal cigarette smoking is believed to reduce intrauterine growth (as reflected in birth weight) by several mechanisms, including carbon monoxide-mediated fetal hypoxia, nicotine-induced uterine vasoconstriction, and appetite suppression (the latter also in part due to nicotine). A statistical technique known as *path analysis* is sometimes useful for testing postulated causal paths. It is based on multiple linear regression, and interested readers are referred to several standard references [5, 6].

19.3.2 Causal Networks

A description of all the known causal paths and effect modifiers leading to a given outcome (in groups of individuals) is called a *causal network* or *causal web*. The causal network for an outcome for which a given exposure constitutes a necessary cause will consist of a single causal path (accompanied by relevant effect modifiers). For multifactorial outcomes, causal networks may be represented by several exposure variables, linked through numerous causal paths and interacting with a variety of effect modifiers.

A multifactorial causal network can also include one or more exposures that are sufficient to cause the outcome. As we have seen, intrauterine growth retardation (IUGR) can be caused by a variety of factors. First-trimester rubella infection is a sufficient cause (assuming the mother is nonimmune), and thus the causal path to IUGR is a single line without effect modifiers. Since rubella infection is not a necessary cause, however, the causal network for IUGR also contains numerous other causal paths involving other exposures and their effect modifiers, such as maternal short stature, low prepregnancy weight, insufficient caloric intake during pregnancy, primiparity, and cigarette smoking [3].

19.4 Probability and Uncertainty

Most persons tend to think about causality in dichotomous terms: either an exposure causes an outcome or it does not. Clinicians in particular tend to think this way, because many of the events they observe and the decisions they make are yes-or-no dichotomies. A patient either lives or dies, a surgeon decides either to operate or not. In nature, of course, an exposure is either a cause or not, and an omniscient being would know which. Unfortunately, we mortals can never be certain beyond all doubt. If I throw a stone into a window and it breaks, I am reasonably certain that my missile caused the window to break. For all practical purposes, I can assign a probability *(P)* of 1 to such a statement. It is possible (although exceedingly improbable), however, that the window would have broken on its own at that very moment, perhaps from some inherent structural defect, or that, unbeknownst to me, someone else simultaneously fired a bullet at the same window.

Absolute proof of causality is thus elusive, and assessment of causality inevitably involves a statement of probability, i.e., uncertainty, rather than certainty. The fact that causality is more continuous than dichotomous, however, need not result in nihilism or paralysis. The probability need not be 1 to justify action. Clinicians may institute treatment to combat a cause that seems reasonably likely, such as beginning antibiotic treatment for suspected bacterial meningitis before the diagnosis is confirmed by bacteriologic culture results one or two days later. Similarly, an industrial plant may reduce potentially hazardous vapor or dust levels based on a preliminary epidemiologic study demonstrating adverse health effects. In these situations and many others like it, the probability of causality needs to be weighed in a decision analysis (risk-benefit analysis) along with the efficacy and side effects of available treatments, as well as the consequences of withholding treatment.

Deciding that exposure causes outcome, therefore, usually requires a probability assessment. Even for genetic diseases where a given mutation appears to be both necessary and sufficient, the laboratory evidence may not be completely unequivocal. The probability assessment is most useful when it is made quantitative, in the sense of assigning a probability P between 0 and 1. Such a quantitative assessment expresses the degree of belief in causality. It usually involves a subjective component, but pretending that causality is either yes ($P=1$) or no ($P=0$) is usually neither helpful for understanding nor necessary for action. Dichotomous causality thinking can in fact be harmful, because it is likely to lead to errors in clinical or public health decisions and consequent disillusionment with the clinician or scientific community supplying the "evidence."

The probability of causality can be assessed in terms of three different questions relating exposure to outcome [7, 8]:

1. *Can it?* (*potential* causality assessment): What is the probability that exposure can, at least in certain persons under certain circumstances, cause the outcome?
2. *Will it?* (*predictive* causality assessment): What is the probability that the next person exposed will develop the outcome because of the exposure? In more general terms, is the exposure a quantitatively *important* cause of the outcome?
3. *Did it?* (*retrodictive* causality assessment): What is the probability that a given person who has already developed the outcome did so because of exposure?

Each of these three types of causality assessment may be important, depending on the setting and the intended purpose (e.g., decision). All three depend, at least in part, on evidence gathered from epidemiologic studies. As we shall see, even the *Did it?* assessment, which appears to bridge the gap between epidemiologic and clinical reasoning (see Chapter 1), makes use of such evidence. The three assessments, *Can it?*, *Will it?*, and *Did it?* will be discussed in turn in the following sections.

19.5 Can Exposure Cause Outcome?

Because the *Can it?* question is not posed with respect to any individual in particular, its response usually requires assessment of groups or populations of sufficient size and diversity to enhance the likelihood of propitious effect modifiers. The data bearing on these population-based assessments are often obtained in epidemiologic studies. If reduction or elimination of exposure alone leads to a lower risk (when dichotomous) or to a lesser degree (if continuous) of the outcome in a given population, the exposure *can* cause the outcome in that population. Since the "if" part of this statement can never be known with absolute certainty, however, some probability must be assigned to it. The statement is cast in a way that suggests two important and interrelated features of *Can it?* probability. First, an experimental design (clinical trial) provides the strongest evidence for or against causality. Second, it leads to a prediction: intervening on exposure should lead to a change in outcome.

Epidemiologic studies traditionally focus on the *Can it?* question, and the elements relevant to weighing the evidence from such studies have been discussed by many authors, most notably Sir Austin Bradford-Hill [9]. Although Hill did not conceptualize causality in probabilistic terms, the stronger the epidemiologic evidence favoring causality, the higher the *Can it?* probability. These relevant elements are summarized below.

19.5.1 Analytic Bias

Analytic bias exists in four types (see Chapter 5): information bias, sample distortion bias, confounding bias, and reverse causality ("cart-vs-horse") bias. Given an association between exposure and outcome, the evidence that the association is causal will be strengthened to the extent that each of these sources of bias is eliminated or reduced. Measurements of exposure and outcome should be reproducible and valid, and neither measurement should be influenced by the other. Sloppy (imprecise) measurements may obscure true causal relationships; systematically biased measurements may either create or obscure associations, depending on the direction of the bias. Sample distortion bias can arise in assembling the study sample or from differential loss to follow-up.

Confounding bias is an ever-present danger in observational studies, and its control requires adequate design and statistical analytic techniques. Confounding results in an exposure-outcome association because exposure and outcome are both caused by a third factor X:

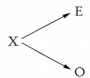

For example, anemia and iron deficiency have frequently been reported to be associated with low birth weight (birth weight < 2500 g). The evidence suggests, however, that iron deficiency is a result of generally poor nutritional status, and that insufficient caloric intake is often accompanied by low iron intake. The deficient diet causes both iron deficiency and low birth weight, but the iron deficiency itself has no causal role [3]. Iron deficiency or anemia may thus be an *indicator* or *marker* of risk for low birth weight, but it is not a *cause*. The distinction is important, because iron supplementation will correct the iron deficiency and anemia but have no effect on birth weight.

Confounding also occurs whenever the exposure factor is tightly linked to a third factor that, although unrecognized, is the true cause of the outcome. This is merely a special case of the general concept of confounding that can be indicated as follows:

$$
\begin{array}{l}
X \longrightarrow O \\
| \\
E
\end{array}
$$

This type of confounding can occur, for example, when an adverse reaction attributed to the active pharmacologic ingredient of a drug is actually caused by a preservative or other component contained in the preparation administered. As another illustration, consider the relationship between alcohol consumption and lung cancer. Because heavy drinkers are likely to be cigarette smokers, failure to consider the confounding effect of smoking might lead to the erroneous inference that heavy drinking causes lung cancer. High alcohol consumption may be a marker of risk, but it is not a true causal factor.

Randomized clinical trials (RCTs) provide the best protection against confounding bias. When combined with double blinding, standardized detection methods (to protect against information bias), and vigorous follow-up (to reduce sample distortion occurring after randomization), RCTs provide the most convincing epidemiologic evidence of *Can it?* causality.

A given exposure can cause an outcome only if it precedes it. Sorting out which is the cart and which is the horse is occasionally quite difficult, especially in cross-sectional studies. Unless the exposure factor is known to have been present since birth (e. g., sex, blood type, or racial origin), uncertainty as to whether exposure preceded outcome or vice versa will result in a lower probability estimate for *Can it?* Case-control studies can protect themselves against reverse causality bias, at least to some extent, by using newly occurring (incident) outcomes and specifically inquiring about *prior* exposure. Such exposure histories, however, depend on adequate records or valid subject recall. Cohort studies can avoid this problem if the study sample is known to be free of the outcome at the time exposure begins. Once again, clinical trials provide the best evidence, since exposure is assigned by the investigator.

19.5.2 Strength of Association

The strength of association between exposure and outcome relates to the size of the effect on outcome produced by a given amount of exposure. For dichotomous exposures and outcomes, this refers to the relative risk. For dichotomous exposures and continuous outcomes, the mean difference in outcome is the corresponding indicator. All else (i.e., other elements for weighing the epidemiologic evidence) being equal, the larger the effect size, the greater the likelihood that exposure can cause the outcome. Small relative risks or mean differences always raise the question as to whether some hidden or incompletely controlled source of bias might explain the results. Large effects are less likely to be entirely explained away by such factors.

19.5.3 Biologic Gradient

When exposure is ordinal (ranked) or continuous, the probability of *Can it?* causality is often increased by demonstrating a graded effect on outcome with different degrees of exposure, i.e., a dose-response relationship. When the outcome is dichotomous, the relative risk should increase with higher categories of exposure. When both exposure and outcome are continuous, the slope (regression coefficient) indicates the amount of change in outcome resulting from a given increase or decrease in exposure. It should be emphasized, however, that threshold, ceiling, optimum (inverted "U"), and nonlinear graded effects are possible. Consequently, steady increases in relative risk or a constant slope are not necessary to demonstrate a biologic gradient. Furthermore, even the total absence of any dose-response relationship may not weigh heavily against the *Can it?* probability if the underlying biologic mechanism is independent of the dose of exposure, such as with anaphylactic or idiosyncratic adverse drug reactions.

19.5.4 Statistical Significance

When exposure-outcome associations are found, causality is obviously strengthened by demonstrating a low probability of obtaining an association at least as large as the one observed merely by chance. The lower the *P* value obtained in a test of statistical significance, the less likely the association is to be a chance occurrence if the null hypothesis is in fact true, i.e., the less likely the risk of a type I error. The absence of statistical significance, however, is not proof that an association does not exist. A clinically important effect may not achieve statistical significance if the sample size is small or (for continuous variables) the variance is high. Any claim that exposure and outcome are not associated, and hence not causally related, should therefore be backed up by demonstrating an appropriately low risk of type II error, and the relative likelihoods of the null (no effect) and alternative (clinically important effect) hypotheses should be kept in mind before accepting the null.

19.5.5 Consistency

No matter how unbiased, strong, graded, and statistically significant a given exposure-outcome association appears to be from a single epidemiologic study, *Can it?* causality is strengthened by replication. If several investigators in different settings and (preferably) using different methods all find a significant association, the probability that exposure can cause outcome is increased. In Bayesian terms, positive results of each previous study increase the prior odds favoring the alternative hypothesis (H_A), and new data favoring H_A continue to raise its posterior odds. Replication is particularly helpful in excluding chance as an explanation. Repeated failure to control for sources of bias, however, can lead to consistent findings that are invalid. Many studies from developing countries, for example, have reported an association between maternal anemia and low birth weight. None that reported such an association, however, controlled for the confounding effect of poor prepregnant and gestational nutrition. Consistency alone, therefore, is an insufficient criterion of causality.

19.5.6 Biologic Plausibility and Coherence

The exposure-outcome association should be plausible and coherent with current knowledge about the biology of the exposure and outcome. The physiologic or molecular mechanism need not be known, but the *Can it?* probability should be reduced whenever an association contradicts established biologic facts or principles, at least until the alleged association has been confirmed. John Snow provided convincing evidence that cholera was transmitted by contaminated water long before microbiologic demonstration of the infecting organism. Similarly, aspirin was used by countless arthritis victims generations before prostaglandins were discovered. On the other hand, given the known proliferative effects of estrogen on the endometrium, a single study showing that postmenopausal estrogens *protect* against subsequent endometrial cancer should be considered dubious, even in the absence of obvious bias or other explanation.

19.5.7 Similarity to "Known" Cause

This is a corollary to the previous criterion and concerns the biologic similarity of the exposure factor under assessment to another factor whose causal effect on the outcome is well established. Suppose, for example, that an association is demonstrated between a newly marketed drug and neutropenia (a low concentration of neutrophilic white blood cells). Knowledge that the new agent has a chemical structure very similar to that of one or more long-standing drugs with recognized neutropenic effects will increase the probability that the association with the new drug is indeed causal.

19.6 Is Exposure an Important Cause of Outcome?

The quantitative importance of a given exposure as a cause of outcome obviously depends on the answer to the *Can it?* question (Section 19.5). If the probability is very low that E *can* cause O, then it follows that the probability is also very low that it is an important cause. If the *Can it?* probability is sufficiently high, then its importance also merits consideration.

It is the magnitude of the causal effect that will enter into risk-benefit calculations in making decisions about preventing an undesirable outcome or promoting a desirable one (see Chapter 17). If a particular treatment or preventive maneuver is dangerous, painful, or expensive, for example, the benefits will not be worth the risks or costs if only a marginal change in outcome can be expected.

How do we go about assessing the importance, i.e., measuring the magnitude, of a causal effect? Actually, this issue has already been discussed, to some degree, in Chapters 6–9. The answer depends on whether the outcome under consideration is categorical (usually dichotomous) or continuous, and these will be discussed separately.

For dichotomous outcomes, the importance of a cause can be gauged by assessing the probability that the next exposed person will develop the outcome because of the exposure (or, equivalently, the number of persons out of the next 100 exposed who will develop the outcome because of the exposure). In other words, *Will it?*

The *Will it?* probability is the difference in the probability of the outcome occurring in an exposed person, i.e., the probability of outcome given exposure $[P(O|E)]$, and the probability of it occurring without exposure $[P(O|\overline{E})]$: $P(O|E) - P(O|\overline{E})$. It can thus be estimated by the attributable risk, i.e., the difference in incidence of the outcome in otherwise similar exposed and nonexposed persons, which depends on both the relative risk of exposure and the incidence of the disease in the unexposed population. In Table 6.3, we examined data on lung cancer and cardiovascular disease mortality among smoking and nonsmoking male British physicians. Despite a very high relative risk (32.43) for lung cancer death among smokers, the attributable risk was only 2.20 per 1000 per year. In other words, smoking can be expected to *add* 2.2 lung cancer deaths per year for each 1000 smoking male British physicians. The cardiovascular death attributable risk is higher at 2.61 per 1000 per year, despite a much lower relative risk (1.36), because cardiovascular deaths occur far more frequently than lung cancer deaths (7.32 vs 0.07 per 1000 per year among nonsmokers).

For continuous variables, the importance of exposure as a cause of outcome can be formulated by the question *How much will it?* and is determined by the difference in outcome due to exposure. Although the expected difference in outcome actually represents an entire probability distribution of expected differences in outcome between exposed and nonexposed persons, we usually base our estimate on the mean difference. Thus, if the mean difference in birth weight between infants of smoking and those of nonsmoking mothers that is attributable to smoking (i.e., unconfounded by other factors) is 150 g, the estimate of the expected smoking effect will be − 150 g.

19.7 Did Exposure Cause Outcome in a Specific Case?

In essence, this is the setting of clinical diagnosis, in which the clinician attempts to determine the cause of a given complaint. The *Did it?* causality assessment is necessarily individualized, since it refers to a specific case in which the outcome is already known to have occurred. Despite this focus on individuals, evidence from epidemiologic studies can be very useful in carrying out a *Did it?* probability assessment. In fact, Bayes' theorem enables the merging of individual case information with epidemiologic data in assessing the *Did it?* causality question.

Suppose that a given individual has developed the outcome. Without knowing whether that individual was exposed, what is the probability that the exposure was the cause? Although this question is posed in terms of the individual, the *Did it?* probability can be estimated by measuring the proportion of persons developing the outcome who do so because of exposure. This proportion is called the *etiologic fraction* (EF) or *population attributable risk;* it is already familiar to us from Chapter 6 and can be calculated as follows, using Eq. 6.4:

$$EF = \frac{P_E(RR-1)}{P_E(RR-1)+1}$$

where RR is the relative risk of the outcome in otherwise similar exposed vs nonexposed individuals and P_E is the probability (i.e., prevalence) of exposure in the population of interest [10].

For a fixed relative risk, EF increases as the probability of exposure increases, reaching a theoretical maximum of 1. Consequently, even an exposure with a high relative risk may not have a high EF if the exposure is rare. First-trimester intrauterine rubella infection is associated with a very high relative risk of intrauterine growth retardation (IUGR), but because such infection is rare, the corresponding EF is quite low. Conversely, maternal cigarette smoking may only double or triple the risk of IUGR, but it is so common that a large proportion of IUGR may be caused by it in populations where many women smoke during pregnancy [3].

When outcome and exposure are both known to have occurred in an individual, an improved (over the EF) estimate of the probability that exposure caused outcome in that individual can be derived using the *etiologic fraction among the exposed* (EF$_E$) obtained from epidemiologic data [11]. EF$_E$ represents the proportion of all exposed persons in a population developing the outcome who do so because of exposure. It can be calculated as follows:

$$EF_E = \frac{RR-1}{RR} \tag{19.1}$$

Thus, in the absence of any other information about a specific individual from that population who developed the outcome other than the fact that he or she was exposed, EF$_E$ provides an estimate of the probability that the exposure caused the outcome. If the relative risk of lung cancer is 10 in smokers vs nonsmokers, for example, the probability that a smoker who develops lung cancer did so *because* of smoking would be $\frac{10-1}{10} = 0.90$.

Often, however, we know much more relevant information about a specific case of an outcome than merely whether or not exposure occurred. We also probably know something about the dose of exposure (if not purely dichotomous) and its timing, in addition to background factors concerning the subject's age, sex, socioeconomic status, and past medical history. How can these be used to refine our *Did it?* probability assessment?

Various informal and formal methods have been used in this regard. In fact, clinicians usually take into account some, if not all, of the above factors in making a causality assessment. But a clinician's "global introspection" tends to become less reliable as the problem gets more complex. It is difficult or impossible for most clinicians to simultaneously consider and properly weigh all the relevant facts, let alone possess those facts.

The construction of algorithms (branched logic trees) can be helpful in improving the reproducibility and validity of diagnostic judgments. One particular area that has received considerable attention in this regard is that of adverse drug reactions (ADRs). A variety of algorithms or equivalent checklists have been developed to help clinicians, drug manufacturers, and regulatory agencies judge whether a given drug caused an observed adverse event in specific cases [12]. Although these schemes appear to yield more reproducible causality assessments than global introspection (even that of clinical pharmacology experts), their assessment procedures are somewhat arbitrary and often lead to different results from one method to another.

A potentially more rewarding approach is to use Bayesian techniques for manipulating conditional probabilities (see Chapter 16). The posterior odds that an outcome was caused by exposure can be decomposed into a prior odds and a likelihood ratio (see Eq. 16.8). The knowledge that a specific case was exposed can be incorporated into the prior odds, i.e., the odds that exposure caused the outcome given only the background information (B):

$$\text{prior odds} = \frac{P(E{\rightarrow}O|B)}{P(E{\nrightarrow}O|B)}$$

where $E{\rightarrow}O$ and $E{\nrightarrow}O$ denote the opposing propositions that exposure did and did not, respectively, cause the outcome. As with the etiologic fraction in the exposed (EF_E), the prior odds is usually based on epidemiologic data derived from otherwise similar exposed individuals. In fact, $P(E{\rightarrow}O|B) = EF_E$ and $P(E{\nrightarrow}O|B) = 1 - P(E{\rightarrow}O|B) = 1 - EF_E$.

The specific case information (C) concerning dose, timing, background, and other relevant factors can then be included in computing the likelihood ratio (LR):

$$LR = \frac{P(C|E{\rightarrow}O)}{P(C|E{\nrightarrow}O)}$$

The posterior odds then incorporates both the background and case information:

$$\frac{P(E{\rightarrow}O|B,C)}{P(E{\nrightarrow}O|B,C)} = \frac{P(E{\rightarrow}O|B)}{P(E{\nrightarrow}O|B)} \times \frac{P(C|E{\rightarrow}O)}{P(C|E{\nrightarrow}O)} \tag{19.2}$$

For ADRs, for example, the likelihood term would include information about the age, sex, and medical history of the patient; the dosage and timing of drug administration; and the results of dechallenge (stopping the drug) and rechallenge (restarting it).

For continuous outcomes, *Did it?* usually means *How much did it?* If a smoking mother delivers an infant whose birth weight is 2800 g, what is our best estimate of what the weight would have been had the mother not smoked during pregnancy? Once again, we should use all the relevant factors at our disposal to make this estimate. Based on the mean difference in birth weight in infants of smoking vs nonsmoking mothers, or far better, the decrease in birth weight per cigarette smoked per day for the precise time during pregnancy that the mother smoked, an average expected effect of her pregnancy smoking history can be estimated. This estimate can be further refined by knowledge about any factors known to modify the effect of exposure (effect modifiers).

Did it? causality assessments are assuming increasing prominence for a variety of scientific and nonscientific reasons. One major reason is that clinicians are seeking to improve on global introspection as a diagnostic method. Another reason is related to liability. Harmful exposures or treatments can be caused by industry, government, or individuals. Even if it is known ($P=1$) that a given exposure *can* cause an outcome, exposed persons who develop the outcome will naturally wish to know whether their exposure was the cause. They may even wish to sue the party they believe to be responsible for exposing them. A patient developing a serious adverse reaction to a drug, for example, may bring suit against the treating physician, the drug's manufacturer, and perhaps even the government agency regulating its availability on the market. Although the courts do not easily deal with concepts such as numerical probabilities or average expected differences, *Did it?* causality assessment will probably become more important in the future for legal, as well as scientific, reasons.

In this regard, one major difference between *Did it?* and either *Can it?* or *Will it?* is that the *Did it?* assessment cannot be used for prediction and therefore cannot be tested. Sensitivity testing or distributional assumptions can be used to estimate a range of *Did it?* probabilities (analogous to a confidence interval). The figures can even be revised in the light of new epidemiologic evidence. But the probability estimate remains a hypothesis; it can never be confirmed or refuted.

A final comment about *Did it?* causality assessment will bring us back full circle to the introductory remarks made in Chapter 1. The discussion there focused on the clinical vs the epidemiologic approaches to problem solving. Clinical reasoning is fundamentally individualized and attempts to answer a question based on the facts of a single case. Epidemiologic reasoning is probabilistic; it is founded on relationships in groups between exposure and outcome. In deciding whether a given exposure caused an observed outcome in a specific case, the Bayesian approach brings epidemiologic reasoning to the clinical "bedside," the individual subject. The best estimate of the prior odds of causality is usually based on the best epidemiologic, probabilistic data available. But the facts of the individual case are then used to alter the prior odds (through the likelihood ratio) to arrive at a final assessment of the posterior odds of causation for that case.

Did it? causality assessment represents an excellent example of the essential compatibility of the clinical and epidemiologic approaches. The marriage is quite recent, and the two parties have much to learn from one another, but the prospects for fertility appear excellent.

References

1. Hume D (1946) A treatise of human nature. Selby-Bigge CA (ed) Claredon Press, Oxford
2. Miettinen OS (1974) Confounding and effect modification. Am J Epidemiol 100: 350–353
3. Kramer MS (1987) Determinants of low birth weight: methodological assessment and meta-analysis. Bull WHO 65: 663–737
4. Susser M (1973) Causal thinking in the health sciences. Oxford University Press, New York
5. Turner ME, Stevens CD (1959) The regression analysis of causal paths. Biometrics 15: 236–238
6. Duncan OD (1986) Path analysis: sociological examples. Am J Sociol 72: 1–16
7. Kramer MS, Hutchinson TA (1984) The Yale algorithm. Drug Inf J 18: 283–291
8. Lane DA (1984) A probabilist's view of causality assessment. Drug Inf J 18: 323–330
9. Hill AB (1977) A short textbook of medical statistics. Hodder and Stoughton, London, pp 285–296
10. Levin ML (1953) The occurrence of lung cancer in man. Acta Unio Int Contra Cancrum 9: 531–541
11. Miettinen OS (1974) Proportion of disease caused or prevented by given exposure trait or intervention. Am J Epidemiol 99: 325–332
12. Venulet J, Berneker G-C, Ciucci AG (1982) Assessing causes of adverse drug reactions with special references to standardized methods. Academic, London

Appendix Tables

Table A.1. Random numbers arranged in groups of 5 digits

85967	73152	14511	85285	36009	95892	36962	67835	63314	50162
07483	51453	11649	86348	76431	81594	95848	36738	25014	15460
96283	01898	61414	83525	04231	13604	75339	11730	85423	60698
49174	12074	98551	37895	93547	24769	09404	76548	05393	96770
97366	39941	21225	93629	19574	71565	33413	56087	40875	13351
90474	41469	16812	81542	81652	45554	27931	93994	22375	00953
28599	64109	09497	76235	41383	31555	12639	00619	22909	29563
25254	16210	89717	65997	82667	74624	36348	44018	64732	93589
28785	02760	24359	99410	77319	73408	58993	61098	04393	48245
84725	86576	86944	93296	10081	82454	76810	52975	10324	15457
41059	66456	47679	66810	15941	84602	14493	65515	19251	41642
67434	41045	82830	47617	36932	46728	71183	36345	41404	81110
72766	68816	37643	19959	57550	49620	98480	25640	67257	18671
92079	46784	66125	94932	64451	29275	57669	66658	30818	58353
29187	40350	62533	73603	34075	16451	42885	03448	37390	96328
74220	17612	65522	80607	19184	64164	66962	82310	18163	63495
03786	02407	06098	92917	40434	60602	82175	04470	78754	90775
75085	55558	15520	27038	25471	76107	90832	10819	56797	33751
09161	33015	19155	11715	00551	24909	31894	37774	37953	78837
75707	48992	64998	87080	39333	00767	45637	12538	67439	94914
21333	48660	31288	00086	79889	75532	28704	62844	92337	99695
65626	50061	42539	14812	48895	11196	34335	60492	70650	51108
84380	07389	87891	76255	89604	41372	10837	66992	93183	56920
46479	32072	80083	63868	70930	89654	05359	47196	12452	38234
59847	97197	55147	76639	76971	55928	36441	95141	42333	67483
31416	11231	27904	57383	31852	69137	96667	14315	01007	31929
82066	83436	67914	21465	99605	83114	97885	74440	99622	87912
01850	42782	39202	18582	46214	99228	79541	78298	75404	63648
32315	89276	89582	87138	16165	15984	21466	63830	30475	74729
59338	42703	55198	80380	67067	97155	34160	85019	03527	78140
58089	27632	50987	91373	07736	20436	96130	73483	85332	24384
61705	57285	30392	23660	75841	21931	04295	00875	09114	32101
18914	98982	60199	99275	41967	35208	30357	76772	92656	62318
11965	94089	34803	48941	69709	16784	44642	89761	66864	62803
85251	48111	80936	81781	93248	67877	16498	31924	51315	79921
66121	96986	84844	93873	46352	92183	51152	85878	30490	15974
53972	96642	24199	58080	35450	03482	66953	49251	63719	57615
14509	16594	78883	43222	23093	58645	60257	89250	63266	90858
37700	07688	65533	72126	23611	93993	01848	03910	38552	17472
85466	59392	72722	15473	73295	49759	56157	60477	83284	56367

Source: Daniel WW (1974) Biostatistics: a foundation for analysis in the health sciences. John Wiley
& Sons, New York, p 417.

Table A.2. Areas in one tail ($\geq +z$ or $\leq -z$) of the standard normal distribution

z	0.00	0.01	0.02	0.03	0.04	0.05	0.06	0.07	0.08	0.09
0.0	0.500	0.496	0.492	0.488	0.484	0.480	0.476	0.472	0.468	0.464
0.1	0.460	0.456	0.452	0.448	0.444	0.440	0.436	0.433	0.429	0.425
0.2	0.421	0.417	0.413	0.409	0.405	0.401	0.397	0.394	0.390	0.386
0.3	0.382	0.378	0.374	0.371	0.367	0.363	0.359	0.356	0.352	0.348
0.4	0.345	0.341	0.337	0.334	0.330	0.326	0.323	0.319	0.316	0.312
0.5	0.309	0.305	0.302	0.298	0.295	0.291	0.288	0.284	0.281	0.278
0.6	0.274	0.271	0.268	0.264	0.261	0.258	0.255	0.251	0.248	0.245
0.7	0.242	0.239	0.236	0.233	0.230	0.227	0.224	0.221	0.218	0.215
0.8	0.212	0.209	0.206	0.203	0.200	0.198	0.195	0.192	0.189	0.187
0.9	0.184	0.181	0.179	0.176	0.174	0.171	0.169	0.166	0.164	0.161
1.0	0.159	0.156	0.154	0.152	0.149	0.147	0.145	0.142	0.140	0.138
1.1	0.136	0.133	0.131	0.129	0.127	0.125	0.123	0.121	0.119	0.117
1.2	0.115	0.113	0.111	0.109	0.107	0.106	0.104	0.102	0.100	0.099
1.3	0.097	0.095	0.093	0.092	0.090	0.089	0.087	0.085	0.084	0.082
1.4	0.081	0.079	0.078	0.076	0.075	0.074	0.072	0.071	0.069	0.068
1.5	0.067	0.066	0.064	0.063	0.062	0.061	0.059	0.058	0.057	0.056
1.6	0.055	0.054	0.053	0.052	0.051	0.049	0.048	0.048	0.046	0.046
1.7	0.045	0.044	0.043	0.042	0.041	0.040	0.039	0.038	0.038	0.037
1.8	0.036	0.035	0.034	0.034	0.033	0.032	0.031	0.031	0.030	0.029
1.9	0.029	0.028	0.027	0.027	0.026	0.026	0.025	0.024	0.024	0.023
2.0	0.023	0.022	0.022	0.021	0.021	0.020	0.020	0.019	0.019	0.018
2.1	0.018	0.017	0.017	0.017	0.016	0.016	0.015	0.015	0.015	0.014
2.2	0.014	0.014	0.013	0.013	0.013	0.012	0.012	0.012	0.011	0.011
2.3	0.011	0.010	0.010	0.010	0.010	0.009	0.009	0.009	0.009	0.008
2.4	0.008	0.008	0.008	0.008	0.007	0.007	0.007	0.007	0.007	0.006
2.5	0.006	0.006	0.006	0.006	0.006	0.005	0.005	0.005	0.005	0.005
2.6	0.005	0.005	0.004	0.004	0.004	0.004	0.004	0.004	0.004	0.004
2.7	0.003	0.003	0.003	0.003	0.003	0.003	0.003	0.003	0.003	0.003
2.8	0.003	0.002	0.002	0.002	0.002	0.002	0.002	0.002	0.002	0.002
2.9	0.002	0.002	0.002	0.002	0.002	0.002	0.002	0.001	0.001	0.001
3.0	0.001									

Source: Colton T (1974) Statistics in medicine. Little, Brown, Boston, p 345.

Table A.3. Areas in two tails ($\geq +z$ plus $\leq -z$) of the standard normal distribution

z	0.00	0.01	0.02	0.03	0.04	0.05	0.06	0.07	0.08	0.09
0.0	1.000	0.992	0.984	0.976	0.968	0.960	0.952	0.944	0.936	0.928
0.1	0.920	0.912	0.904	0.897	0.889	0.881	0.873	0.865	0.857	0.849
0.2	0.841	0.834	0.826	0.818	0.810	0.803	0.795	0.787	0.779	0.772
0.3	0.764	0.757	0.749	0.741	0.734	0.726	0.719	0.711	0.704	0.697
0.4	0.689	0.682	0.674	0.667	0.660	0.653	0.646	0.638	0.631	0.624
0.5	0.617	0.610	0.603	0.596	0.589	0.582	0.575	0.569	0.562	0.555
0.6	0.549	0.542	0.535	0.529	0.522	0.516	0.509	0.503	0.497	0.490
0.7	0.484	0.478	0.472	0.465	0.459	0.453	0.447	0.441	0.435	0.430
0.8	0.424	0.418	0.412	0.407	0.401	0.395	0.390	0.384	0.379	0.373
0.9	0.368	0.363	0.358	0.352	0.347	0.342	0.337	0.332	0.327	0.322
1.0	0.317	0.312	0.308	0.303	0.298	0.294	0.289	0.285	0.280	0.276
1.1	0.271	0.267	0.263	0.258	0.254	0.250	0.246	0.242	0.238	0.234
1.2	0.230	0.226	0.222	0.219	0.215	0.211	0.208	0.204	0.201	0.197
1.3	0.194	0.190	0.187	0.184	0.180	0.177	0.174	0.171	0.168	0.165
1.4	0.162	0.159	0.156	0.153	0.150	0.147	0.144	0.142	0.139	0.136
1.5	0.134	0.131	0.129	0.126	0.124	0.121	0.119	0.116	0.114	0.112
1.6	0.110	0.107	0.105	0.103	0.101	0.099	0.097	0.095	0.093	0.091
1.7	0.089	0.087	0.085	0.084	0.082	0.080	0.078	0.077	0.075	0.073
1.8	0.072	0.070	0.069	0.067	0.066	0.064	0.063	0.061	0.060	0.059
1.9	0.057	0.056	0.055	0.054	0.052	0.051	0.050	0.049	0.048	0.047
2.0	0.046	0.044	0.043	0.042	0.041	0.040	0.039	0.038	0.038	0.037
2.1	0.036	0.035	0.034	0.033	0.032	0.032	0.031	0.030	0.029	0.029
2.2	0.028	0.027	0.026	0.026	0.025	0.024	0.024	0.023	0.023	0.022
2.3	0.021	0.021	0.020	0.020	0.019	0.019	0.018	0.018	0.017	0.017
2.4	0.016	0.016	0.016	0.015	0.015	0.014	0.014	0.014	0.013	0.013
2.5	0.012	0.012	0.012	0.011	0.011	0.011	0.010	0.010	0.010	0.010
2.6	0.009	0.009	0.009	0.009	0.008	0.008	0.008	0.008	0.007	0.007
2.7	0.007	0.007	0.007	0.006	0.006	0.006	0.006	0.006	0.005	0.005
2.8	0.005	0.005	0.005	0.005	0.005	0.004	0.004	0.004	0.004	0.004
2.9	0.004	0.004	0.004	0.003	0.003	0.003	0.003	0.003	0.003	0.003
3.0	0.003									

Source: Colton T (1974) Statistics in medicine. Little, Brown, Boston, p 346.

Table A.4. Critical values of t required for certain P values, according to number of degrees of freedom (df)

df	P value One-tailed	0.25	0.1	0.05	0.025	0.01	0.005	0.0025	0.001	0.0005
	Two-tailed	0.5	0.2	0.1	0.05	0.02	0.01	0.005	0.002	0.001
1		1.000	3.078	6.314	12.706	31.821	63.657	127.32	318.31	636.62
2		0.816	1.886	2.920	4.303	6.965	9.925	14.089	22.327	31.598
3		0.765	1.638	2.353	3.182	4.541	5.841	7.453	10.214	12.924
4		0.741	1.533	2.132	2.776	3.747	4.604	5.598	7.173	8.610
5		0.727	1.476	2.015	2.571	3.365	4.032	4.773	5.893	6.869
6		0.718	1.440	1.943	2.447	3.143	3.707	4.317	5.208	5.959
7		0.711	1.415	1.895	2.365	2.998	3.499	4.029	4.785	5.408
8		0.706	1.397	1.860	2.306	2.896	3.355	3.833	4.501	5.041
9		0.703	1.383	1.833	2.262	2.821	3.250	3.690	4.297	4.781
10		0.700	1.372	1.812	2.228	2.764	3.169	3.581	4.144	4.587
11		0.697	1.363	1.796	2.201	2.718	3.106	3.497	4.025	4.437
12		0.695	1.356	1.782	2.179	2.681	3.055	3.428	3.930	4.318
13		0.694	1.350	1.771	2.160	2.650	3.012	3.372	3.852	4.221
14		0.692	1.345	1.761	2.145	2.624	2.977	3.326	3.787	4.140
15		0.691	1.341	1.753	2.131	2.602	2.947	3.286	3.733	4.073
16		0.690	1.337	1.746	2.120	2.583	2.921	3.252	3.686	4.015
17		0.689	1.333	1.740	2.110	2.567	2.898	3.222	3.646	3.965
18		0.688	1.330	1.734	2.101	2.552	2.878	3.197	3.610	3.922
19		0.688	1.328	1.729	2.093	2.539	2.861	3.174	3.579	3.883
20		0.687	1.325	1.725	2.086	2.528	2.845	3.153	3.552	3.850
21		0.686	1.323	1.721	2.080	2.518	2.831	3.135	3.527	3.819
22		0.686	1.321	1.717	2.074	2.508	2.819	3.119	3.505	3.792
23		0.685	1.319	1.714	2.069	2.500	2.807	3.104	3.485	3.767
24		0.685	1.318	1.711	2.064	2.492	2.797	3.091	3.467	3.745
25		0.684	1.316	1.708	2.060	2.485	2.787	3.078	3.450	3.725
26		0.684	1.315	1.706	2.056	2.479	2.779	3.067	3.435	3.707
27		0.684	1.314	1.703	2.052	2.473	2.771	3.057	3.421	3.690
28		0.683	1.313	1.701	2.048	2.467	2.763	3.047	3.408	3.674
29		0.683	1.311	1.699	2.045	2.462	2.756	3.038	3.396	3.659
30		0.683	1.310	1.697	2.042	2.457	2.750	3.030	3.385	3.646
40		0.681	1.303	1.684	2.021	2.423	2.704	2.971	3.307	3.551
60		0.679	1.296	1.671	2.000	2.390	2.660	2.915	3.232	3.460
120		0.677	1.289	1.658	1.980	2.358	2.617	2.860	3.160	3.373
∞		0.674	1.282	1.645	1.960	2.326	2.576	2.807	3.090	3.291

Source: Pearson ES, Hartley HO (eds) (1976) Biometrika tables for statisticians, vol. 1. Biometrika Trust, London, p 146.

Table A.5. Critical values of U for certain P values, according to sample sizes (n_1 and n_2) of two compared groups (for Mann-Whitney U-test)

A. $P = 0.05$ (one-tailed) or 0.10 (two-tailed)

n_2	3	4	5	6	7	8	9	10	11	12	13	14	15	16	17	18	19	20
n_1																		
2		0	0	0	0	1	1	1	1	2	2	2	3	3	3	4	4	4
3	0	0	1	2	2	3	3	4	5	5	6	7	7	8	9	9	10	11
4		1	2	3	4	5	6	7	8	9	10	11	12	14	15	16	17	18
5			3	5	6	8	9	11	12	13	15	16	18	19	20	22	23	25
6				7	8	10	12	14	16	17	19	21	23	25	26	28	30	32
7					11	13	15	17	19	21	24	26	28	30	33	35	37	39
8						15	18	20	23	26	28	31	33	36	39	41	44	47
9							21	24	27	30	33	36	39	42	45	48	51	54
10								27	31	34	37	41	44	48	51	55	58	62
11									34	38	42	46	50	54	57	61	65	69
12										42	47	51	55	60	64	68	72	77
13											51	56	61	65	70	75	80	84
14												61	66	71	77	82	87	92
15													72	77	83	88	94	100
16														83	89	95	101	107
17															96	102	109	115
18																109	116	123
19																	123	130
20																		138

B. $P = 0.025$ (one-tailed) or 0.05 (two-tailed)

n_2	3	4	5	6	7	8	9	10	11	12	13	14	15	16	17	18	19	20
n_1																		
2						0	0	0	0	1	1	1	1	1	1	2	2	2
3			0	1	1	2	2	3	3	4	4	5	5	6	6	7	7	8
4		0	1	2	3	4	4	5	6	7	8	9	10	11	11	12	13	13
5			2	3	5	6	7	8	9	11	12	13	14	15	17	18	19	20
6				5	6	8	10	11	13	14	16	17	19	21	22	24	25	27
7					8	10	12	14	16	18	20	22	24	26	28	30	32	34
8						13	15	17	19	22	24	26	29	31	34	36	38	41
9							17	20	23	26	28	31	34	37	39	42	45	48
10								23	26	29	33	36	39	42	45	48	52	55
11									30	33	37	40	44	47	51	55	58	62
12										37	41	45	49	53	57	61	65	69
13											45	50	54	59	63	67	72	76
14												55	59	64	67	74	78	83
15													64	70	75	80	85	90
16														75	81	86	92	98
17															87	93	99	105
18																99	106	112
19																	113	119
20																		127

Table A.5. (continued)
C. $P = 0.01$ (one-tailed) or 0.02 (two-tailed)

n_2	3	4	5	6	7	8	9	10	11	12	13	14	15	16	17	18	19	20
n_1																		
2											0	0	0	0	0	0	1	1
3					0	0	1	1	1	2	2	2	3	3	4	4	4	5
4			0	0	1	2	3	3	4	5	5	6	7	7	8	9	9	10
5			1	2	3	4	5	6	7	8	9	10	11	12	13	14	15	16
6				3	4	6	7	8	9	11	12	13	15	16	18	19	20	22
7					6	8	9	11	12	14	16	17	19	21	23	24	26	28
8						10	11	13	15	17	20	22	24	26	28	30	32	34
9							14	16	18	21	23	26	28	31	33	36	38	40
10								19	22	24	27	30	33	36	38	41	44	47
11									25	28	31	34	37	41	44	47	50	53
12										31	35	38	42	46	49	53	56	60
13											39	43	47	51	55	59	63	67
14												47	51	56	60	65	69	73
15													56	61	66	70	75	80
16														66	71	76	82	87
17															77	82	88	93
18																88	94	100
19																	101	107
20																		114

Source: Smart JV (1963) Elements of medical statistics. Charles C. Thomas, Springfield, MA, pp 125–127.

Table A.6. Critical values of sums of ranks for certain P values, according to sample size (n) in each of two pair-matched groups (for Wilcoxon signed rank test). Entry before comma represents maximum value for lower sum; entry after comma is minimum value for higher sum

n (number of pairs)	P value	One-tailed Two-tailed	0.025 0.05	0.01 0.02	0.005 0.01
6			0, 21	– –	– –
7			2, 26	0, 28	– –
8			3, 33	1, 35	0, 36
9			5, 40	3, 42	1, 44
10			8, 47	5, 50	3, 52
11			10, 56	7, 59	5, 61
12			13, 65	9, 69	7, 71
13			17, 74	12, 79	9, 82
14			21, 84	15, 90	12, 93
15			25, 95	19, 101	15, 105
16			29, 107	23, 113	19, 117
17			34, 119	28, 125	23, 130
18			40, 131	32, 139	27, 144
19			46, 144	37, 153	32, 158
20			52, 158	43, 167	37, 173
21			58, 173	49, 182	42, 189
22			66, 187	55, 198	48, 205
23			73, 203	62, 214	54, 222
24			81, 219	69, 231	61, 239
25			89, 236	76, 249	68, 257

Source: Colton T (1974) Statistics in medicine. Little, Brown, Boston, p 350.

Table A.7. Critical values of χ^2 required for certain P values (two-tailed only), according to number of degrees of freedom *(df)*

df	Two-tailed P value			
	0.10	0.05	0.01	0.001
1	2.71	3.84	6.63	10.83
2	4.61	5.99	9.21	13.82
3	6.25	7.81	11.34	16.27
4	7.78	9.49	13.28	18.47
5	9.24	11.07	15.09	20.52
6	10.64	12.59	16.81	22.46
7	12.02	14.07	18.48	24.32
8	13.36	15.51	20.09	26.13
9	14.68	16.92	21.67	27.88
10	15.99	18.31	23.21	29.59
11	17.28	19.68	24.73	31.26
12	18.55	21.03	26.22	32.91
13	19.81	22.36	27.69	34.53
14	21.06	23.68	29.14	36.12
15	22.31	25.00	30.58	37.70
16	23.54	26.30	32.00	39.25
17	24.77	27.59	33.41	40.79
18	25.99	28.87	34.81	42.31
19	27.20	30.14	36.19	43.82
20	28.41	31.41	37.57	45.32
21	29.62	32.67	38.93	46.80
22	30.81	33.92	40.29	48.27
23	32.01	35.17	41.64	49.73
24	33.20	36.42	42.98	51.18
25	34.38	37.65	44.31	52.62

Source: Colton T (1974) Statistics in medicine. Little, Brown, Boston, p 348.

Table A.8. Critical values of Spearman rank correlation coefficient (r_s) for certain P values, according to sample size (n)

n (number of pairs)	P value	One-tailed	0.025	0.005
		Two-tailed	0.05	0.01
6			0.886	1.000
7			0.786	0.929
8			0.738	0.881
9			0.683	0.833
10			0.648	0.794
11			0.623	0.818
12			0.591	0.780
13			0.566	0.745
14			0.545	0.716
15			0.525	0.689
16			0.507	0.666
17			0.490	0.645
18			0.476	0.625
19			0.462	0.608
20			0.450	0.591
21			0.438	0.576
22			0.428	0.562
23			0.418	0.549
24			0.409	0.537
25			0.400	0.526
26			0.392	0.515
27			0.385	0.505
28			0.377	0.496
29			0.370	0.487
30			0.364	0.478

Sources: Colton T (1974) Statistics in medicine. Little, Brown, Boston, p 353.
Snedecor GW, Cochran WG (1980) Statistical methods, 7th edn. Iowa State University Press, Ames, p 478.

Subject Index